Quick Guide to the Management of Keratoconus

Mazen M. Sinjab

Quick Guide to the Management of Keratoconus

A Systematic Step-by-Step Approach

Springer

Author
Mazen M. Sinjab, M.D., M.S., CABOphth, Ph.D.
Assistant Professor
Al Zahra Eye Center
Mysat Square
Al Tal 167 Damascus
Behind Quiti Mosque
Syrian Arab Republic
mazen.sinjab@yahoo.com

ISBN 978-3-642-21839-2 e-ISBN 978-3-642-21840-8
DOI 10.1007/978-3-642-21840-8
Springer Heidelberg Dordrecht London New York

Library of Congress Control Number: 2011941189

Printed on acid-free paper

Springer is part of Springer Science+Business Media (www.springer.com)

Preface

Keratoconus is a common disease, and its prevalence increases day by day due to the huge development in diagnostic and screening tools. Management of keratoconus has also developed; new approaches have raised either to halt the progression of the disease or to rehabilitate the cornea or to achieve both.

It is easy to diagnose the disease, but it is not that easy to classify and grade it. Nevertheless, each treatment modality has its own indications, conditions, contraindications, and complications. All of that put the doctor in many cases on crossroads and make a challenge in choosing the modality(s) that may give the patient the desired optimal result.

There are – of course – general guidelines, but tricky things are so many, hence the aim of this book: that is to clarify and specify those guidelines and to build up a mesh among specific criteria that the doctor should look for.

The way that this book deals with this topic is systematic and academic. First, it mentions the disease and its diagnostic tools with the related clinical interpretation. Second, it goes through treatment modalities in a classified and listed manner rather than an elaborating one. Third, it builds up a mesh in a flow chart manner and suggests a checklist together with a three-step approach. The checklist and the three-step approach are finally applied on nine cases taken as examples and studied following the systematic approach.

The strategy in compiling this book is combining excellence in pictorial quality with a concise but ordered text.

I have aimed the book at all those who need some initial assistance in approaching keratoconus. There are sure to be some errors; as the ophthalmology editor, I take full responsibility for these and look forward to being further educated.

Damascus, Syrian Arab. Rep. Mazen M. Sinjab

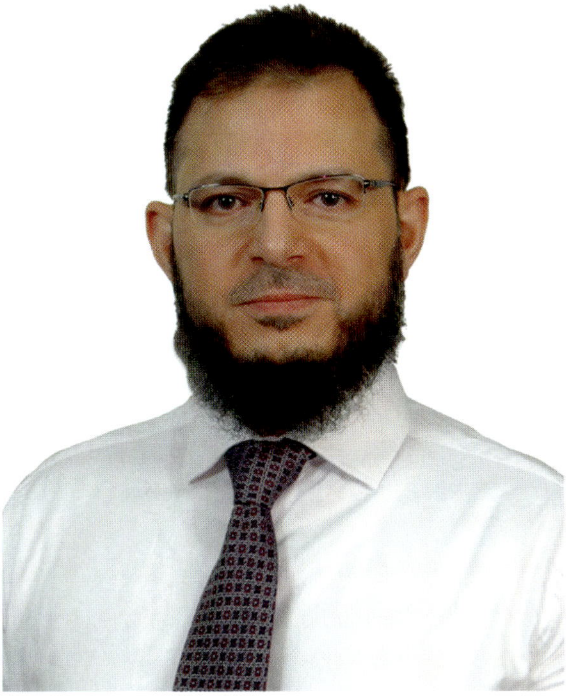

Mazen M. Sinjab M.D., M.S., CABOphth, Ph.D.
Consultant in Anterior Segment and Refractive Surgery

Assistant Professor of Ophthalmology
Damascus University

Senior Lecturer
Al Mouasat University Hospital
Damascus

Founder and Attending Surgeon
Al Zahra Medical Group in Syria

Director of Research
Elite Medical Center
Al Riyadh, KSA

Notification

The information provided via this book is intended for general information purposes.

The information provided via this book is published to assist you, but it is not to be relied upon as authoritative.

The author accepts no liability whatsoever for any direct or consequential loss arising from any use of the information contained in this book.

Contents

Acknowledgments

The author would like to express his deep gratitude to Ruba his wife whose unwavering support was critical for this book.

Abbreviations

AB	Asymmetric bowtie
AC	Anterior chamber
ACD	Anterior chamber depth
AS	Angle supported
BFS	Best fit sphere
BFTE	Best fit toric ellipsoid
BSCVA	Best spectacle corrected visual acuity
CK	Conductive Keratoplasty
CL	Contact lens
CxL	Corneal cross linking
DALK	Deep anterior lamellar keratoplasty
dpt.	Diopters(s)
FFKC	Forme fruste keratoconus
ICR	Intracorneal ring
ICRs	Intracorneal rings
IOL	Intraocular lens
IOP	Intraocular pressure
IORL	Intraocular refractive lens
IORLs	Intraocular refractive lenses
IS	Inferior steep
IS	Iris supported
IS	Iris supported
I-S	Inferior–superior difference
KC	Keratoconus
K-max	Maximal K-readings
KPD	Keratometric power deviation
MR	Manifest refraction
NSAIDs	Nonsteroidal anti-inflammatory drugs
OCT	Optical coherence tomography
PC	Posterior chamber
PH	Pin hole
PKP	Penetrating keratoplasty
PLK	Pellucid-like keratoconus
PMD	Pellucid marginal degeneration
PMMA	Polymethylmethacrylate
PRK	Photorefractive keratectomy
RGP	Rigid gas permeable
S.E	Spherical equivalent
SB	Symmetric bowtie
S-I	Superior–inferior difference

SRAX	Skewed steepest radial axis index
SS	Superior steep
TG	Topography guided
UBM	Ultrasound biomicroscopy
UCVA	Uncorrected visual acuity
UV	Ultraviolet
UVA	Ultraviolet A

Introduction

Keratoconus (KC) is a fairly common bilateral, noninflammatory, degenerative axial ectatic condition of the cornea in which the cornea assumes an irregular conical shape. It is one of the most common corneal diseases that refractive surgeons encounter.

KC is a complex condition of multifactorial etiology, but the exact etiology is unknown. Both genetic and environmental factors are associated with KC. The role of heredity is not clear because most patients do not have a positive family history. Offspring appear to be affected in only about 10% of cases. An autosomal dominant transmission with incomplete penetrance has been proposed. On the other hand, evidence of genetic etiology includes familial inheritance, discordance between dizygotic twins, and association with other known genetic disorders. Several loci responsible for a familial form of KC have been mapped; however, no mutations in any genes have been identified for any of these loci. There are an increasing data suggesting that the environment might also play a role in the development of the condition; the disease is common in dry, cold climates. Reactive oxygen species (i.e., free radicals) are one of the proposed mechanisms of KC development. They include ultraviolet light, atopy, mechanical eye rubbing, and poorly fitted contact lenses.

KC occurs with increased frequency with systemic and ocular conditions:

1. Systemic disorders:

   Down's syndrome, Turner syndrome, Ehlers-Dunlos syndrome, Marfan syndrome, atopy, osteogenesis imperfecta, and mitral valve prolapse.

2. Ocular associations:

   Vernal disease, retinitis pigmentosa, blue sclera, aniridia, and ectopia lentis.

The onset of the disease is at around puberty and progresses slowly thereafter, although it may become stationary at any time.

The hallmark of KC is central or paracentral stromal thinning, apical protrusion, and irregular astigmatism. This usually results in significant impairment in both the quantity and quality of vision because of the progressive nature of the disease.

In advanced KC with corneal opacities, corneal grafting can be the only surgical alternative, in spite of its technical, biological, and refractive complications. Therefore, modern managements have been developed either to stop the progression of the disease or to rehabilitate vision or to achieve both.

There are so many good books in the market talking about this disease, but the purpose of this book is to build a step by step systematic approach for the management of the disease. Personally, I find this strategy practical in handling such hot topics. This book will cover the theoretical aspects of the disease; it will concentrate on the practical aspects including important parameters that affect the decision of the proper managements.

1 Diagnosis of Keratoconus

1.1 Clinical Findings

1.1.1 External Signs

Munson's sign: When the patient is asked to look downward toward the floor, a V-shaped profile of the lower lid margin can be seen (Fig. 1.1). Moderate-to-severe KC tends to produce Munson's sign, while mild cases of KC will not produce this sign since corneal bulging is more subtle.

Rizzuti's sign: This sign is observed by seeing a light on the nasal anterior sclera when the light is directed into the cornea from the temporal direction (Fig. 1.2). This is because of the total internal reflection of light due to the optical properties of the cone. As with Munson's sign, this Rizzuti's sign is more reliable for screening moderate-to-severe cones and is less sensitive for mild KC.

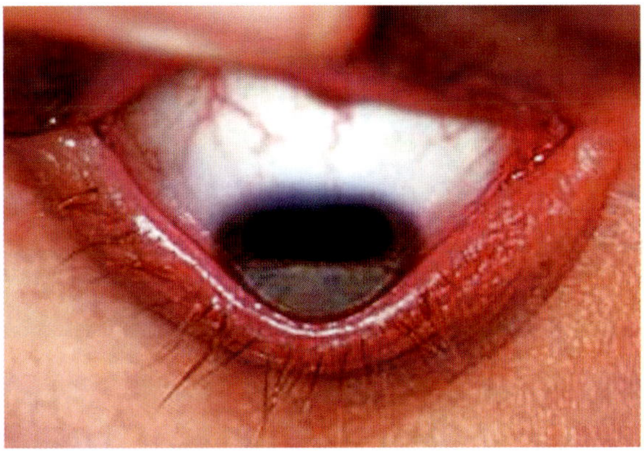

Fig. 1.1 Munson's sign: V-shape of the lower lid when the patient looks down

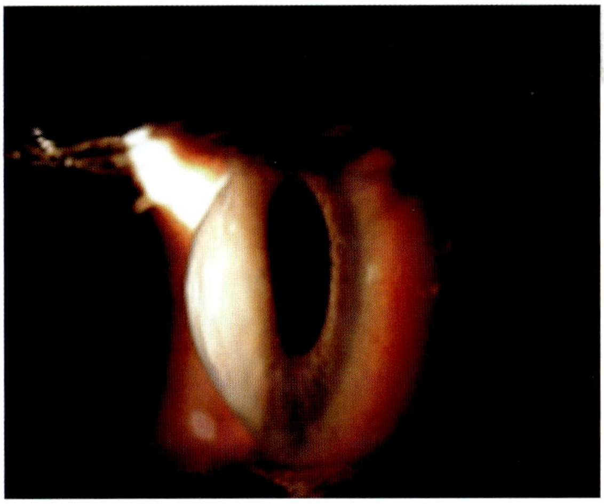

Fig. 1.2 Rizzuti's sign: When the cornea is illuminated from the temporal direction, an illuminated nasal sclera can be seen

1.1.2 Retinoscopy Signs

The scissoring effect of the retinal reflex seen with retinoscopy is highly diagnostic of KC (and of all forms of irregular astigmatism). It is best seen when the pupils are dilated. Unlike Munson's sign, the scissoring effect is considered to be sensitive to even mild forms of KC.

1.1.3 Slit Lamp Biomicroscopy Signs

Focal thinning: focal thinning occurs at the cone apex, which is usually located inferior to the center of the cornea; in pellucid marginal degeneration (PMD), this focal thinning is located in the lower third of the cornea. This sign is better seen under high magnification (Figs. 1.3–1.5a, b).

M.M. Sinjab, *Quick Guide to the Management of Keratoconus*,
DOI 10.1007/978-3-642-21840-8_1, © Springer-Verlag Berlin Heidelberg 2012

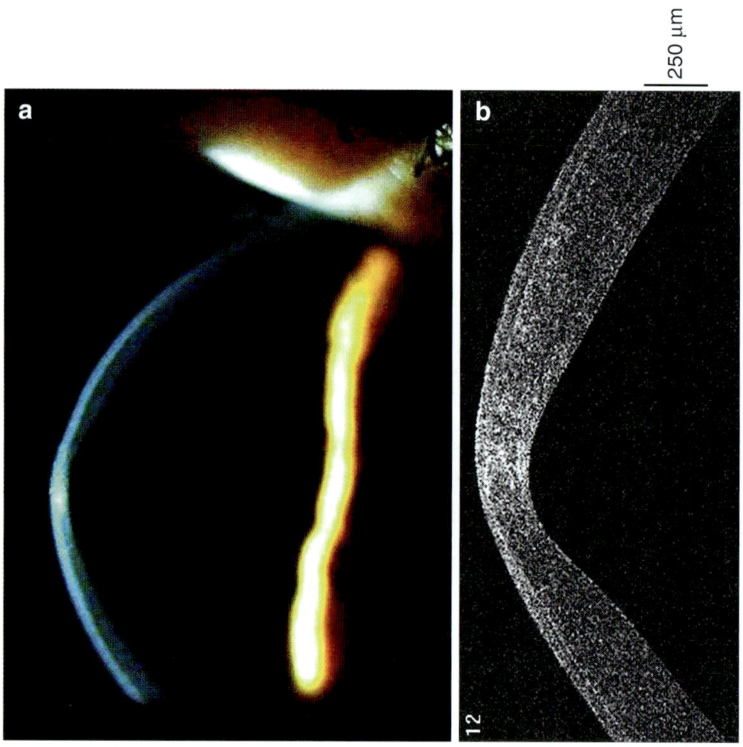

Fig. 1.3 Focal thinning. It is located at the apex of the cone in keratoconus. (**a**) is the slitlamp view; (**b**) is the OCT view

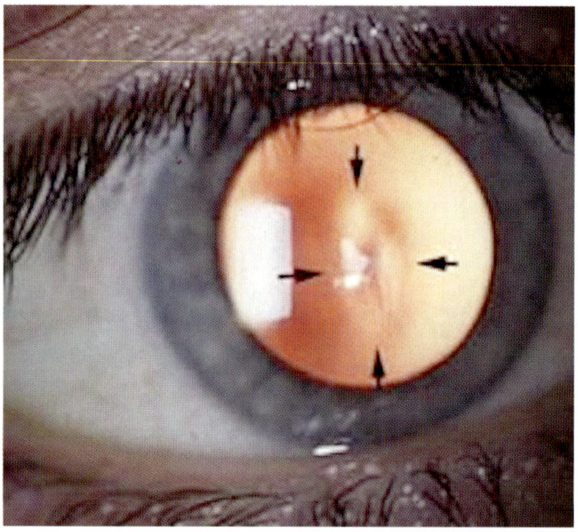

Fig. 1.4 Focal thinning. It appears by retro illumination as an oil drop within the red reflex after dilating the pupil

Fleischer's iron ring: It is due to accumulation of ferritin particles in corneal basal epithelial cells. It partially or completely encircles the base of the cone.

1. *Vogt's striae, hydrops cornea, and corneal scaring*: As the cornea continues to thin and bulge out, "stretch marks" may develop in the form of thin, bright lines located deep in the stroma adjacent to Descemets' membrane called Vogt's striae (Fig. 1.6). Vogt's striae are a sign of corneal stretching and protrusion. When the cornea is depressed, Vogt's striae often disappear. These striae are sometimes called "stress lines."
2. Anterior stromal scars may develop due to continuous protrusion of the cornea. These scars may be small or large (Fig. 1.7). The size and location of the scars determines its impact on visual function.
3. If stretching becomes excessive, the cornea may eventually tear in the Descemets' membrane leading to fluid accumulation within the stroma and therefore to hydrops cornea (Figs. 1.8 and 1.9). This intense stromal edema often results in an acutely blurred vision since the tears often occur centrally. When the endothelium migrates to cover the tear, edema resolves and a posterior scar may form. Tears can occur in the corneal periphery which may have minimal impact on vision.

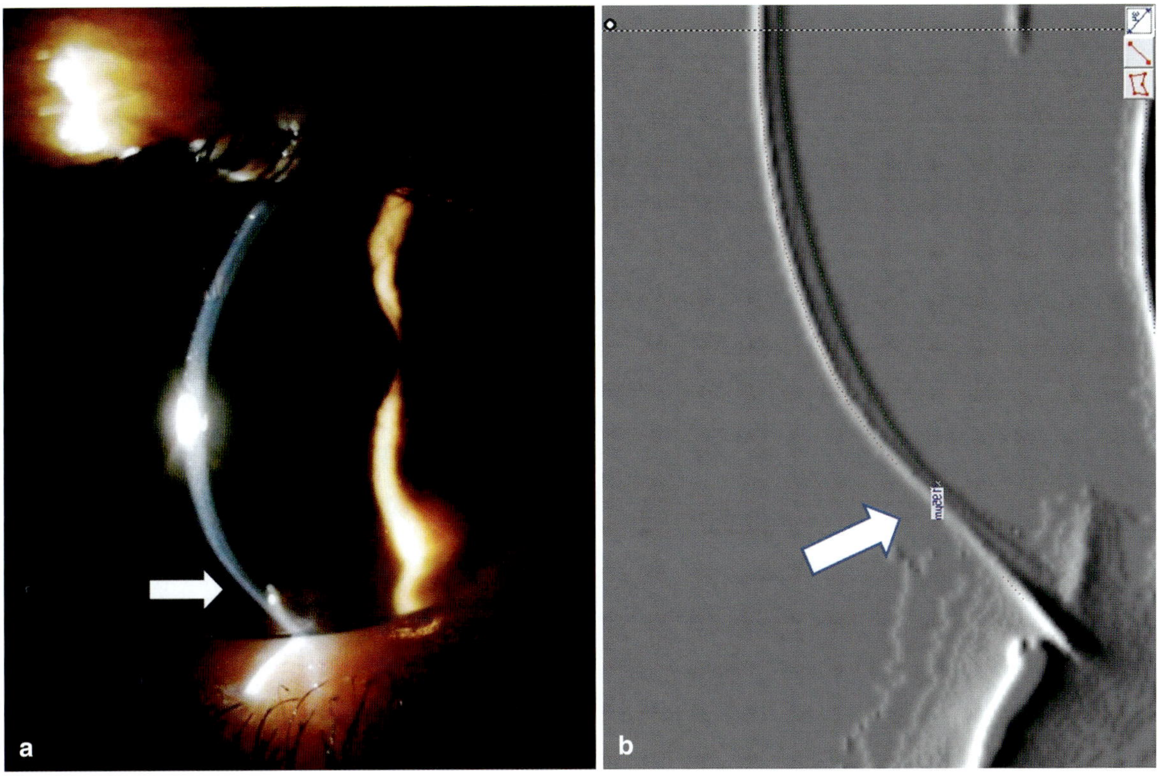

Fig. 1.5 Focal thinning. It is located just below the apex of the cone in pellucid marginal degeneration. (**a**) Slit-lamp view. (**b**) Scheimpflug view. The *white arrows* point at the thinnest location, note that the apex of the cone is above

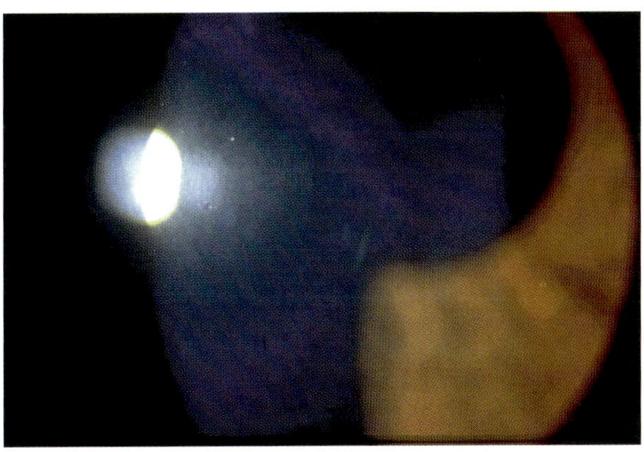

Fig. 1.6 Vogt's striae or stress lines. Fine bright lines in deep stroma adjacent to Descemet's membrane. They represent stretching of the stroma under the tension of intraocular pressure on a thin and weak cornea

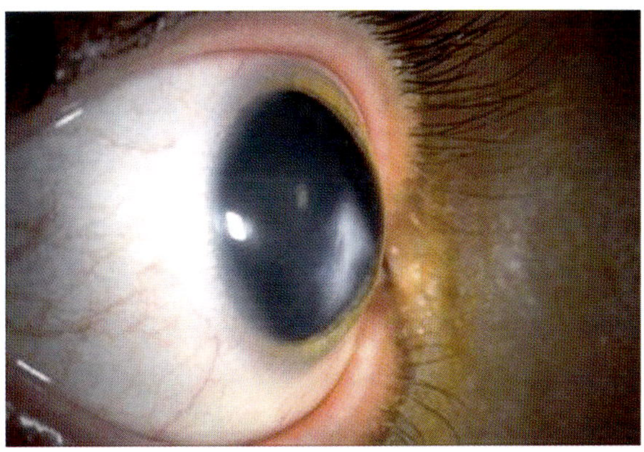

Fig. 1.7 Anterior stroma scars

1.1.4 Keratoscopy and Photokeratoscopy Signs

Keratoscopy is the precursor to modern corneal topography, which still relies – to some extent – on keratoscopy principles. Keratoscopy uses a pattern of concentric rings (mires) called a Placido disk with approximately nine alternating bright and dark rings. The rings are reflected off the anterior cornea surface via Purkinje image number one and viewed directly by the clinician. The Placido disk is nothing more than a simple, inexpensive hand-held device with a central

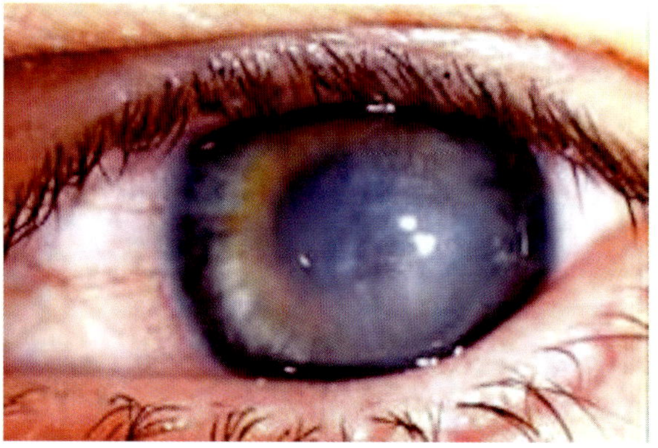

Fig. 1.8 Hydrops cornea. An intensive and abrupt stromal edema due to a tear in Descemet's membrane. The cornea is hazy and grayish

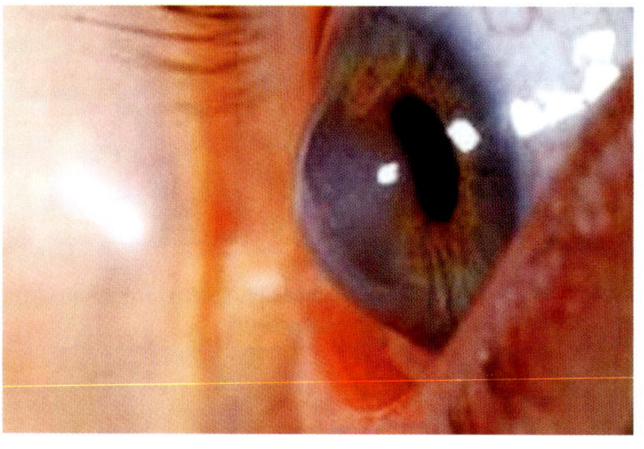

Fig. 1.9 Hydrops cornea. Stromal edema is occasionally confined to cone leaving corneal periphery intact

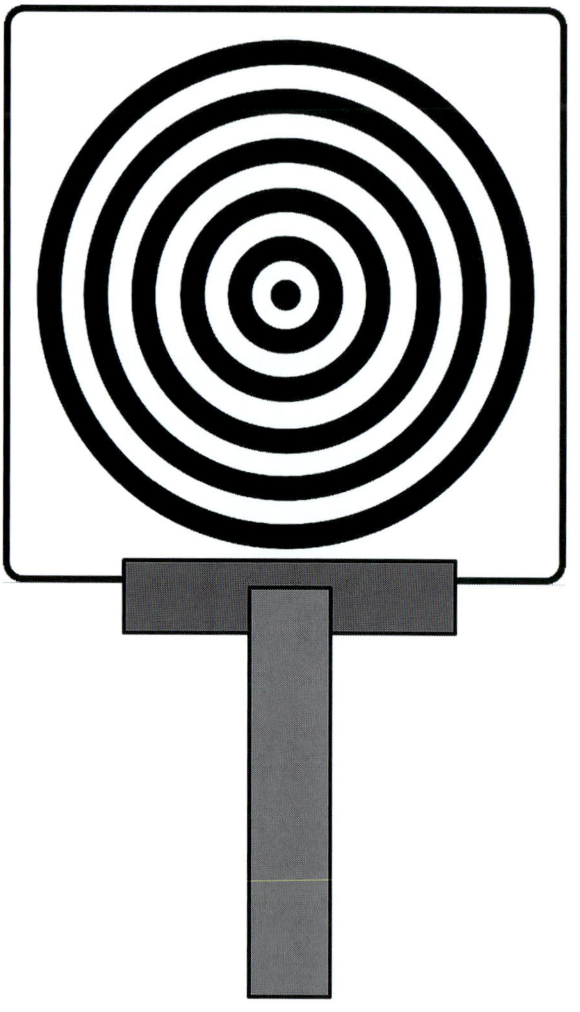

Fig. 1.10 Placido disk. Alternating concentric bright and dark rings reflected off the anterior cornea surface via Purkinje image number one and viewed directly by the clinician through a central hole. This manual device is used to study the anterior corneal curvature

peep-hole for the clinician through which to look (Fig. 1.10). The clinician subjectively analyzes the pattern of the rings to assess if irregular astigmatism or KC exists (Fig. 1.11). Photokeratoscopy has the same principle as the keratoscope except that the Placido disk is back-illuminated with a strobe flash and a camera replaces the clinician's eye at the viewing port that takes a picture of the reflected mire pattern (Fig. 1.12).

When the curved surface of the cornea is viewed with the keratoscope or photokeratoscope, the rings appear to be thin and tightly squeezed together in those regions where the curvature is steep and broadly dispersed wherever the curvature is flat (Figs. 1.13 and 1.14). For a normal spherical cornea, the rings are circular (Fig. 1.15). With corneal astigmatism, the rings are oval with the short axis corresponding to the steep meridian. In KC (Fig. 1.16), the rings are distorted and grouped more closely in the region of the cone (steep curvature). Moderate and severe forms of KC are easy to distinguish using these mires, but subtly compressed rings are difficult to appreciate in mild KC. Central KC detection is also a challenge for keratoscopy as the mires tended to be uniformly tight, which is not as obvious as the asymmetry found in decentered KC. Keratoscopy and photokeratoscopy were replaced by modern corneal topographers, which incorporate their principles. Modern topographers use computer processing of the mires to yield accurate color maps with numerical indices.

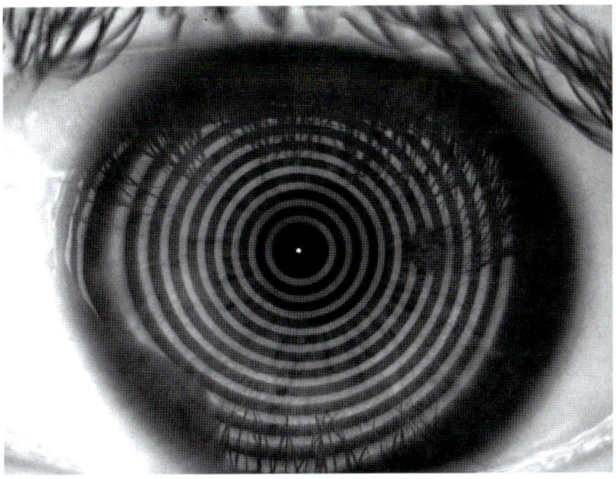

Fig. 1.11 The projection of Placido disk on the anterior surface of the cornea. The shape and the distribution of the mires (*rings*) are affected by any distortion in the anterior part of the cornea

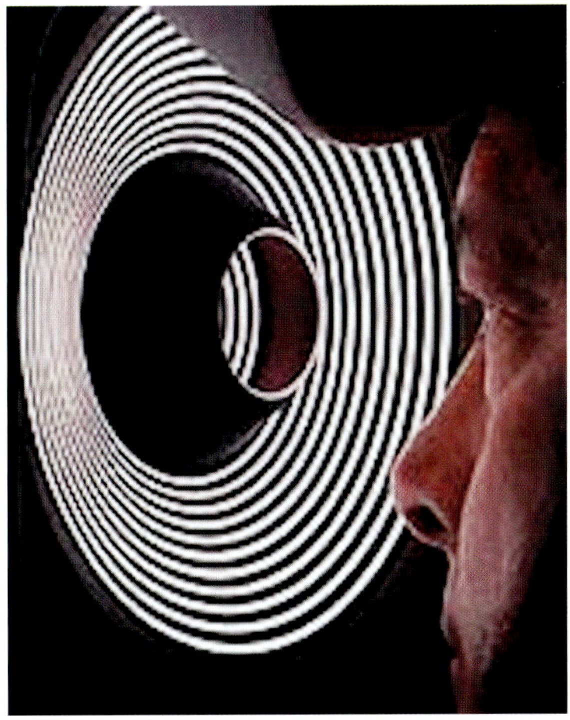

Fig. 1.12 The Photokeratoscope. It depends on the Placido principle except that the Placido disk is back-illuminated with a strobe flash and a camera replaces the clinician's eye at the viewing port that takes a picture of the reflected mire pattern

1.2 Corneal Hysteresis

1.2.1 Principles

"Corneal biomechanics" is a relatively new and increasingly important term in the field of refractive surgery. To understand this term, it is essential to understand

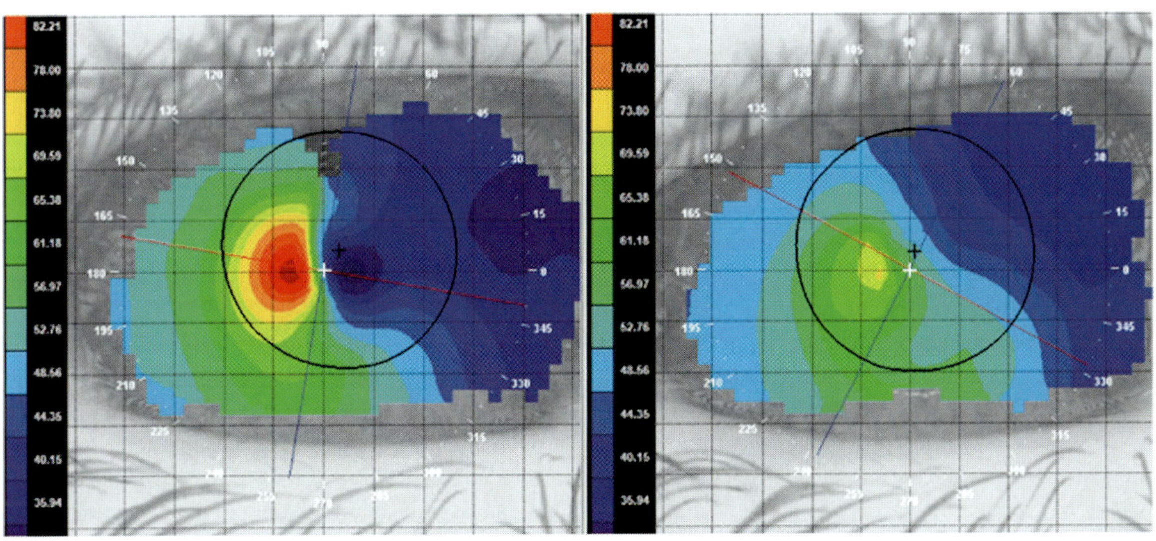

Fig. 1.13 Anterior curvature map showing an irregular surface. The temporal part is steep (*hot colors*), the nasal part is flat (*cold colors*)

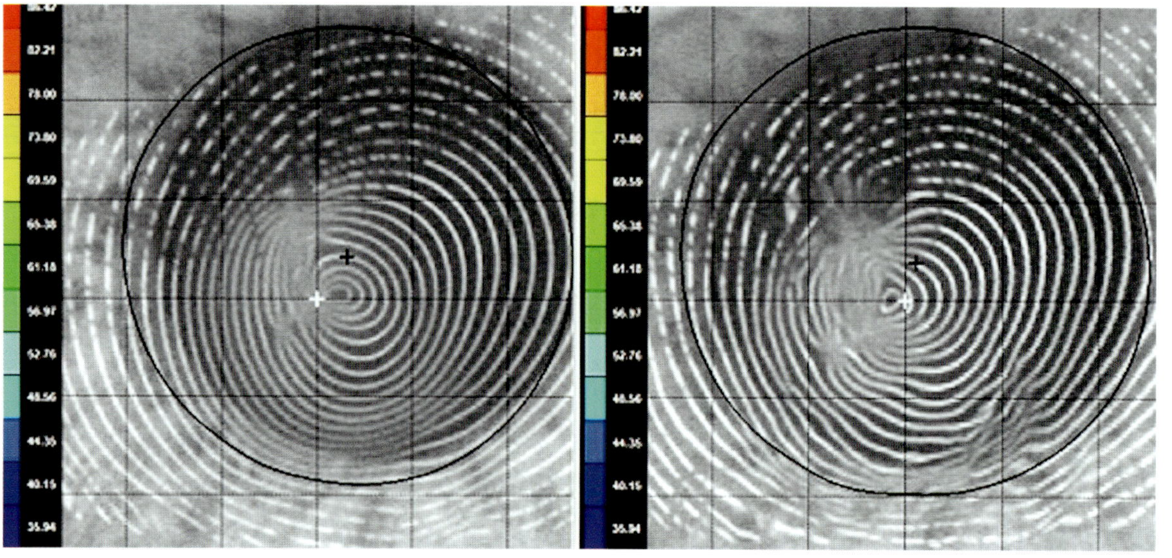

Fig. 1.14 Photokeratoscopy of the same cornea in Fig. 1.13. The rings appear to be thin and tightly squeezed together in those regions where the curvature is steep and broadly dispersed wherever the curvature is flat

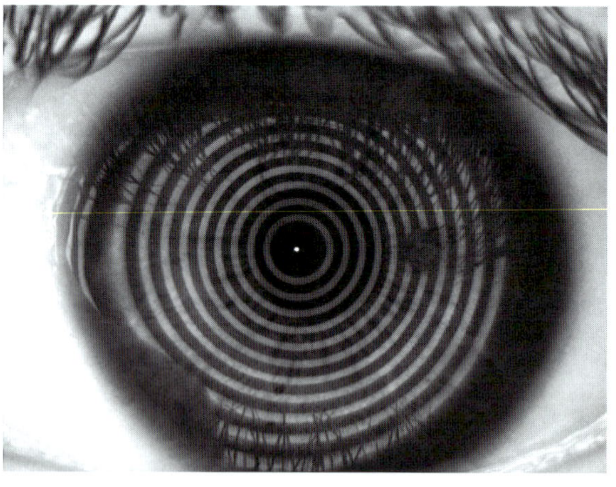

Fig. 1.15 Photokeratoscopy of a normal cornea. The rings are regular and concentric

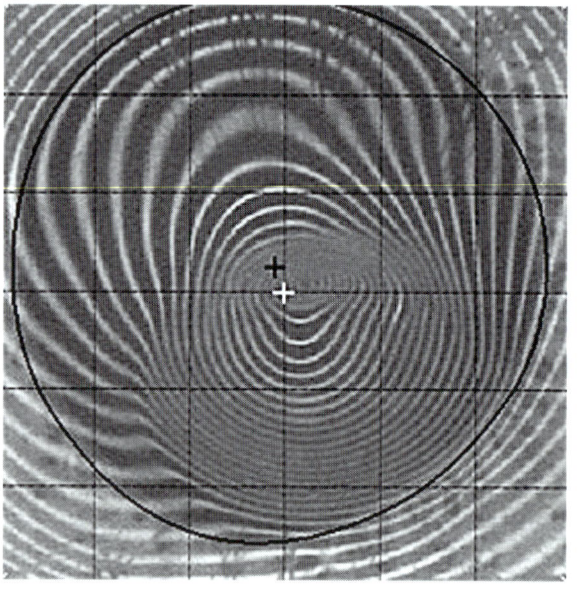

Fig. 1.16 Photokeratoscopy in KC. The rings are distorted and grouped more closely in the region of the cone

the concepts behind, which are elasticity, viscosity, and viscoelasticity.

Elasticity is defined as the tendency of a body to return to its original shape after it has been stretched or compressed. Viscosity is defined as resistance of a liquid to shear forces (and hence to flow). A viscoelastic tissue will deform under the influence of an applied shear stress, but when the stress is removed, the tissue will slowly recover from some of the deformation.

Corneal tissue is a viscoelastic tissue. It is composed mainly of two parts: collagen fibers and the matrix. Collagen fibers are responsible for the elastic properties and the matrix is responsible for the viscous properties of the cornea. Viscoelastic properties of the cornea are responsible for its biomechanical behavior and can explain many of the previously unexplained phenomena such as post-lasik ectasia and undercorrection after myopic correction and others.

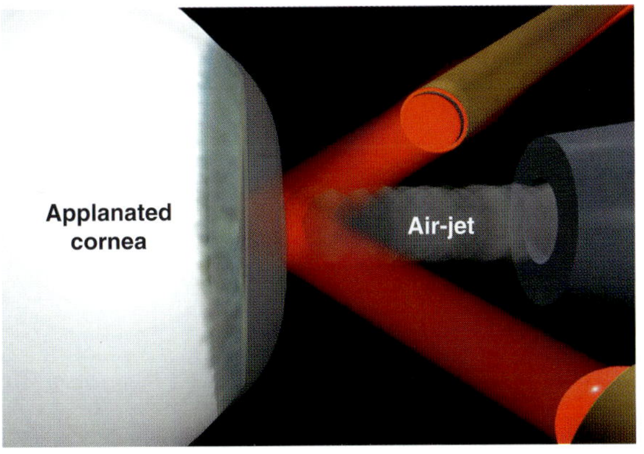

Fig. 1.17 Principle of ocular response analyzer. Applanation pressure is recorded at two points: when the cornea is bending inward and when the cornea is returning to its normal state

The Ocular Response Analyzer (Reichert) is till now the only available machine that measures the biomechanical properties of the cornea. It utilizes a rapid pulse of air to move the cornea inward and outward under the force through a "dynamic bi-directional applanation process." An electro-optical system monitors changes in the shape of the cornea. Applanation pressure is recorded at two points: when the cornea is bending inward and when the cornea is returning to its normal state (Fig. 1.17). Due to bending resistance of the tissue, there are delays in the expected times when the cornea bends and returns to a normal state and the difference in the applanation pressure at these two points is termed corneal hysteresis (Fig. 1.18). Depending on the properties of the cornea for different conditions, one would expect to see different hysteresis values. For example, normal corneas have significantly higher hysteresis values (on average) than do keratoconic corneas (Fig. 1.19a, b).

While the technology looks promising, there is a question as to how extinct the method can distinguish normal corneas from mildly keratoconic and early keratoconic tissue. Data plots of normal and KC corneas show that there is significant overlap in hysteresis values in the two groups (Fig. 1.20). Most recently, new parameters are being developed in the new software of the machine to diagnose corneas that look normal but may develop post-lasik ectasia.

1.3 Confocal Microscopy

The list of confocal microscopy signs associated with KC includes: thinning of the stroma; elongated, exfoliating superficial epithelial cells; enlarged wing and basal epithelial cells; bright reflective material deposited within basal epithelial cells; prominent, thickened sub basal nerves with additional structural changes seen along nerve fibers; increased stromal haze; pronounced reflectivity and an irregular arrangement of the stromal keratocytes; structurally abnormal anterior stromal keratocyte nuclei; lower densities of anterior and posterior stromal keratocytes; Z-shaped folds in the anterior, mid, and posterior stroma; folds in Descemet's membrane; pleomorphism and enlargement of endothelial cells; increased endothelial cell density.

While these signs may occur with KC, most are not specific to KC, and may be also seen with other corneal disorders.

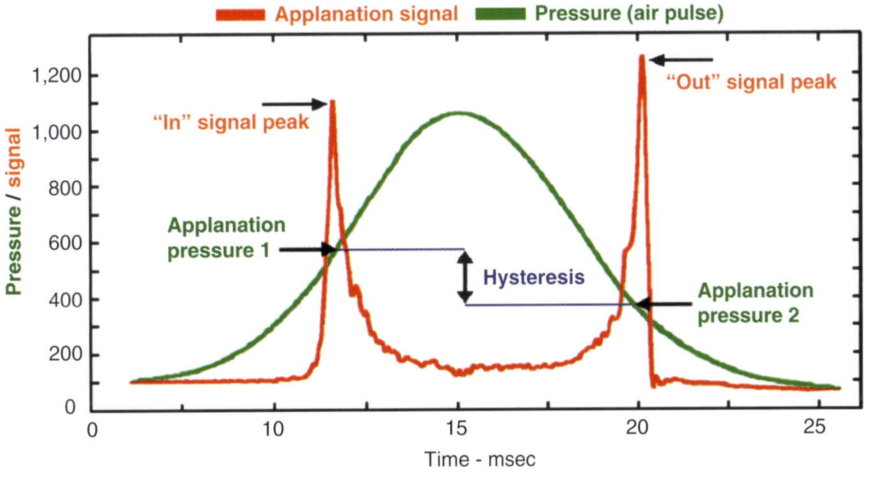

Fig. 1.18 Principle of ocular response analyzer. Due to bending resistance of the tissue, there are delays in the expected times when the cornea bends and returns to a normal state and the difference in the applanation pressure at these two points is termed corneal hysteresis. Corneal hysteresis with other parameters measured by this machine reflects corneal properties which differ according to corneal conditions and pathologies

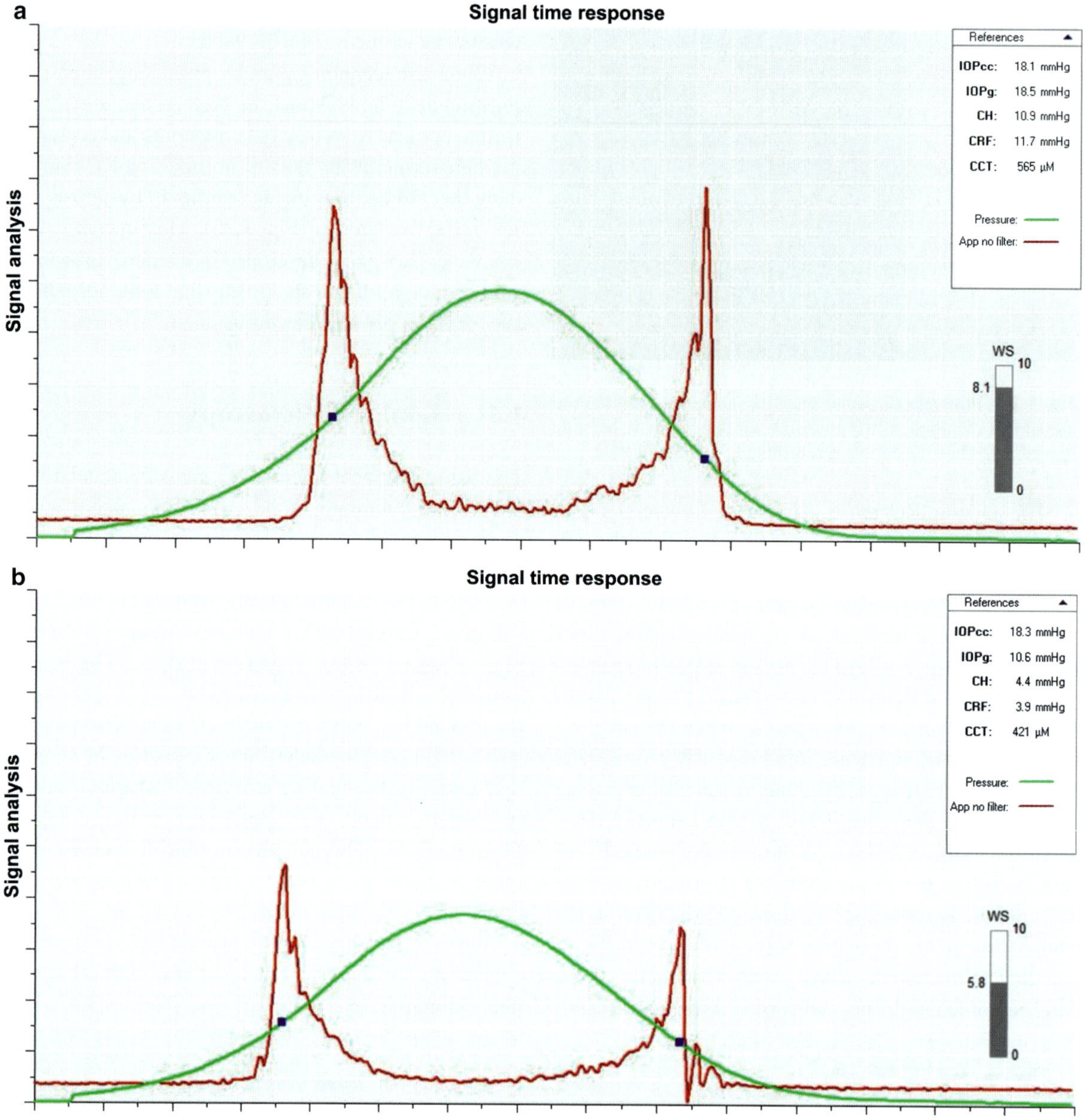

Fig. 1.19 Diagram of the ocular response analyzer: (**a**) in a normal cornea, (**b**) in KC. Note that the amplitudes of the two peaks are lower than normal

1.4 Specular Microscopy

As seen with confocal microscopy, specular microscopy of KC shows signs of altered endothelium cell morphology. There is a significant increase in polymegathism compared with normal controls and a significant decrease in hexagonality in the keratoconic cornea. Higher pleomorphism is seen in KC.

1.5 Corneal Topography

1.5.1 Instruments Measuring Corneal Surface

1.5.1.1 Curvature-Based Instruments

The normal corneal outer surface is smooth; corneal irregularities are neutralized by the tear film layer. The anterior surface acts as an almost transparent convex

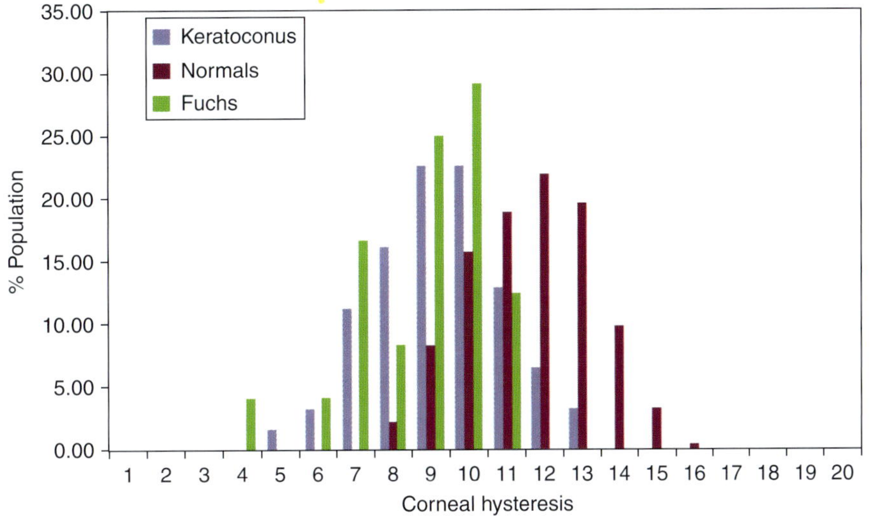

Fig. 1.20 Normative data of corneal hysteresis in normal, keratoconus, and Fuch's endothelial dystrophy patients. Data plots of normal and KC corneas show that there is significant overlap in hysteresis values in the two groups

mirror; it reflects part of the incident light. Many instruments have been developed to assess the anterior surface by measuring the reflected light. These non-contact instruments use light target (in different shapes) and a microscope or other optical systems. The instruments are either quantitative or qualitative, and either reflection-based or projection-based. These instruments are as follows:

The keratometer: It is a quantitative reflection-based instrument.

The photokeratoscope: It is a qualitative reflection-based instrument.

The computerized videokeratoscope: It is a projection-based topographer consisting of a Placido disk with a central camera (Fig. 1.21).

1.5.1.2 Elevation Based Topographers

Placido-based (or curvature-based) systems rely on the data collected from the anterior surface of the cornea either with reflection-based or projection-based systems. Additionally, without the information about the posterior surface, complete evaluation of corneal pachymetry is not possible. Of course, ultrasonic pachymetry can give central and few paracentral measurements, but now we need full pachymetry map. Moreover, the posterior surface of the cornea is being more appreciated as a sensitive indicator of corneal ectasia and can often be abnormal in spite of a normal anterior corneal surface. It is now recognized that while the refractive power of the cornea is mostly determined by the anterior surface, the biomechanical behavior of the cornea is at least equally determined by both surfaces.

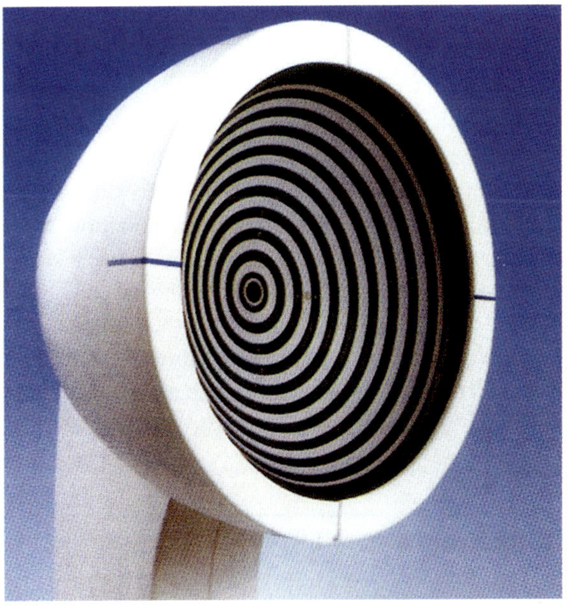

Fig. 1.21 Curvature-based topographer. The computerized videokeratoscopy is a projection-based topographer consisting of a Placido disk with a central camera. The curvature-based topographer evaluates the anterior corneal surface

On the other hand, in the curvature-based systems, the elevation map of the anterior surface is derived from the curvature map, while it is directly calculated in the elevation-based systems.

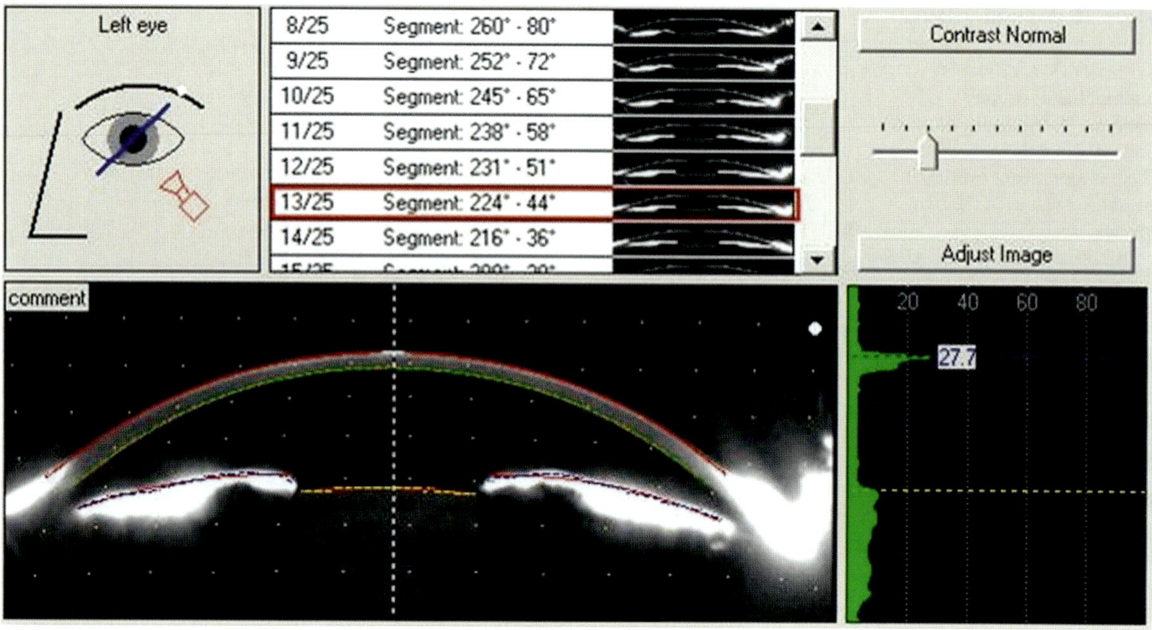

Fig. 1.22 Elevation-based topographer. It depends on the Scheimpflug image and evaluates both corneal surfaces

Although the elevation-based topographers evaluate both corneal surfaces depending on the principle of Scheimpflug image (Fig. 1.22), Placido-based topographers still can give more accurate data about the anterior corneal surface especially in case of corneal scars.

The new topographers combine both techniques to achieve the best corneal topography.

For full discussion of the curvature and elevation maps, please refer to my book "Corneal Topography in Clinical Practice" published by Jaypee Brothers 2009.

Bibliography

Barr JT et al (2006) Estimation of the incidence and factors predictive of corneal scarring in the Collaborative Longitudinal Evaluation of Keratoconus (CLEK) Study. Cornea 25:16–25

Brancati F et al (2004) A locus for autosomal dominant keratoconus maps to human chromosome 3p14-q13. J Med Genet 41:188–192

Caroline P et al (2006) Etiology, diagnosis, and management of keratoconus: new thoughts and new understandings. Pacific University College of Optometry. Retrieved on 2006-03-26

Chwa M et al (2006) Increased stress-induced generation of reactive oxygen species and apoptosis in human keratoconus fibroblasts. Invest Ophthalmol Vis Sci 47(5):1902–1910

Colin J (2006) European clinical evaluation: use of Intacs for the treatment of keratoconus. J Cataract Refract Surg 32: 747–755

Cullen JF, Butler HG (1963) Mongolism (Down's syndrome) and keratoconus. Br J Ophthalmol 47:321–330

Dash DP et al (2010) Mutational screening of VSX1 in keratoconus patients from the European population. Eye (Lond) 24:1085–1092

Elder MJ (1994) Leber congenital amaurosis and its association with keratoconus and keratoglobus. J Pediatr Ophthalmol Strabismus 31:38–40

Fink BA et al (2005) Differences in keratoconus as a function of gender. Am J Ophthalmol 140(3):459–468

Galin MA, Berger R (1958) Atopy and keratoconus. Am J Ophthalmol 45:904

Harrison RJ et al (1989) Association between keratoconus and atopy. Br J Ophthalmol 73:816–822

Haugen OH (1992) Keratoconus in the mentally retarded. Acta Ophthalmol (Copenh) 70:111–114

Hestnes A et al (1991) Ocular findings in Down's syndrome. J Ment Defic Res 35:194–203

Jafri B et al (2004) Asymmetric keratoconus attributed to eye rubbing. Cornea 23:560–564

Kanski JJ (2007) Clinical ophthalmology: a systematic approach. Elsevier, Edinburgh

Krachmer JH et al (1984) Keratoconus and related noninflammatory corneal thinning disorders. Surv Ophthalmol 28:293

Kuming BS, Joffe L (1977) Ehlers-Danlos syndrome associated with keratoconus: a case report. S Afr Med J 52:403–405

Li X et al (2007) Longitudinal study of keratoconus progression. Exp Eye Res 85:502–507

Lichter H et al (2000) Keratoconus and mitral valve prolapse. Am J Ophthalmol 129:667–668

Mazzotta C et al (2008) Confocal microscopy identification of keratoconus associated with posterior polymorphous corneal dystrophy. J Cataract Refract Surg 34:318–321

Nowak DM, Gajecka M (2011a) The genetics of keratoconus. Middle East Afr J Ophthalmol 18:2–6

Nowak DM, Gajecka M (2011b) The genetics of keratoconus. Ophthalmic Genet 18(1):2–6

Olivares JL et al (1997) Keratoconus: age of onset and natural history. Optom Vis Sci 74:147

Rabinowitz YS (1998) Keratoconus. Surv Ophthalmol 42: 297–319

Rahi A et al (1977) Keratoconus and coexisting atopic disease. Br J Ophthalmol 61:761

Shapiro MB, France TD (1985) The ocular features of Down's syndrome. Am J Ophthalmol 99:659–663

Sinjab MM (2009) Corneal topography in clinical practice (pentacam system): basics and clinical interpretation. Jaypee Brothers Medical Publishers, New Delhi

Sinjab MM (2010) Step by step reading pentacam topography (basics and case study series). Jaypee – Highlights Medical Publishers, New Delhi

Wachler BSB (2008) Modern management of keratoconus. Jaypee Brothers Medical Publishers, New Delhi

Weissman BA, Yeung KK (2006) Keratoconus. eMedicine: Keratoconus. Accessed 12 Feb 2006

Yue BY et al (1984) Heterogeneity in keratoconus: possible biochemical basis. Proc Soc Exp Biol Med 175:336

Classifications and Patterns of Keratoconus and Keratectasia

2

Classification of KC is the first step in approaching the disease because the severity of the disease and the stage at which the patient is diagnosed and treated affect treatment results. KC can be classified according to the morphology of the cone and the pattern of corneal topography.

2.1 Morphological Patterns

Morphologically, KC has three types of cones:

(a) Nipple cones, characterized by their small size (5 mm) and steep curvature. The apical center is often either central or paracentral and commonly displaced inferonasally (Fig. 2.1).

(b) Oval cones, which are larger (5–6 mm), ellipsoid, and commonly displaced inferotemporally (Fig. 2.2).

(c) Globus cones, which are the largest (>6 mm) and may involve over 75% of the cornea. Figures 2.3 and 2.4 are the tangential curvature map and the thickness map respectively of a globus cone, note the generalized corneal thinning.

Morphology of the cone is determined according to its size on corneal topography. The best map to evaluate the cone is the tangential map since it is the best to highlight corneal irregularities. In mild cases, cone morphology may be indeterminate.

2.2 Topographical Patterns

Topographically, KC can be classified according to elevation maps, to thickness map or to curvature maps.

2.2.1 Classification According to Elevation Map

Cone location is determined only by the elevation maps. The elevation maps can be displayed either by best fit sphere mode (BFS) as shown in Fig. 2.5, or by best fit toric ellipsoid mode (BFTE) as shown in Fig. 2.6. The best to locate the cone is the BFS, and the best to evaluate the real height of the cone is the BFTE. On the BFS, the cone can be central, paracentral, or peripheral as shown in Figs. 2.7 and 2.8. This classification is important for differentiating KC from PMD and for treatment as will be discussed later in details.

2.2.2 Classification According to Thickness Map

There are two patterns of the thickness map in KC, the conic or dome-like and the "bell" shape. The conic or dome-like shape (Fig. 2.9) is encountered in KC, while the bell shape is encountered in PMD (Fig. 2.10). The bell shape comes from the inferior wide thinning of the cornea found with PMD. When the bell shape is seen, PMD is to be suspected and inserting intracorneal rings carries the risk of perforation, this will be discussed later in details.

2.2.3 Classification According to Curvature Map

Upon studying corneal topography, special attention should be paid to the anterior sagittal curvature map. There are several abnormal signs on these maps that we

M.M. Sinjab, *Quick Guide to the Management of Keratoconus*,
DOI 10.1007/978-3-642-21840-8_2,

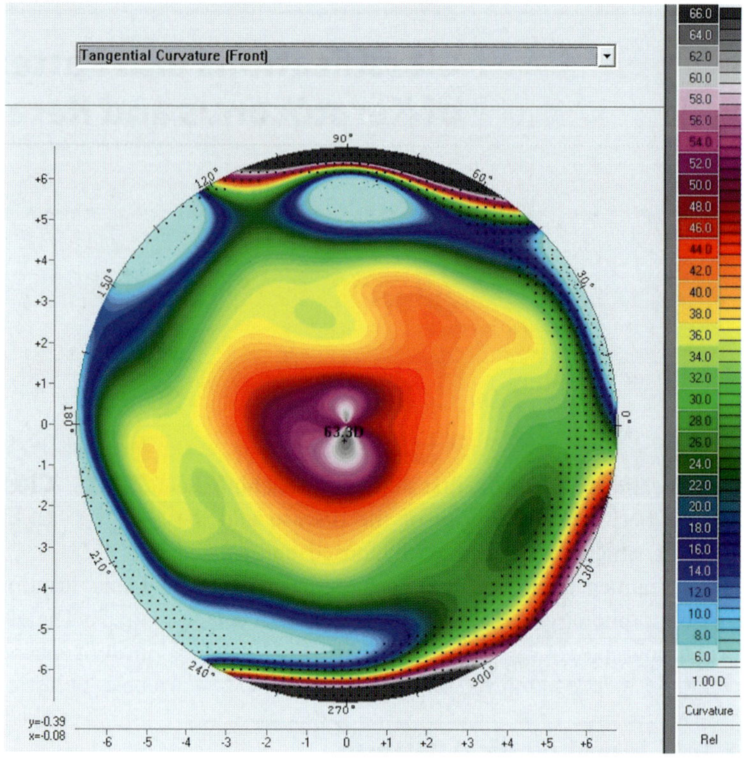

Fig. 2.1 Nipple cone. A small steep central or paracentral cone

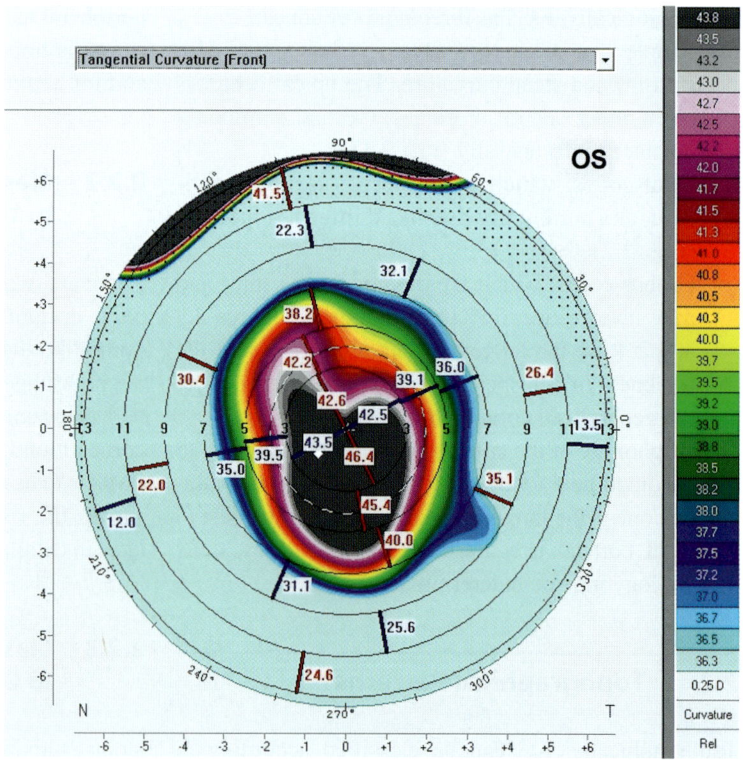

Fig. 2.2 Oval cone. A steep elliptical cone that is commonly displaced inferotemporally

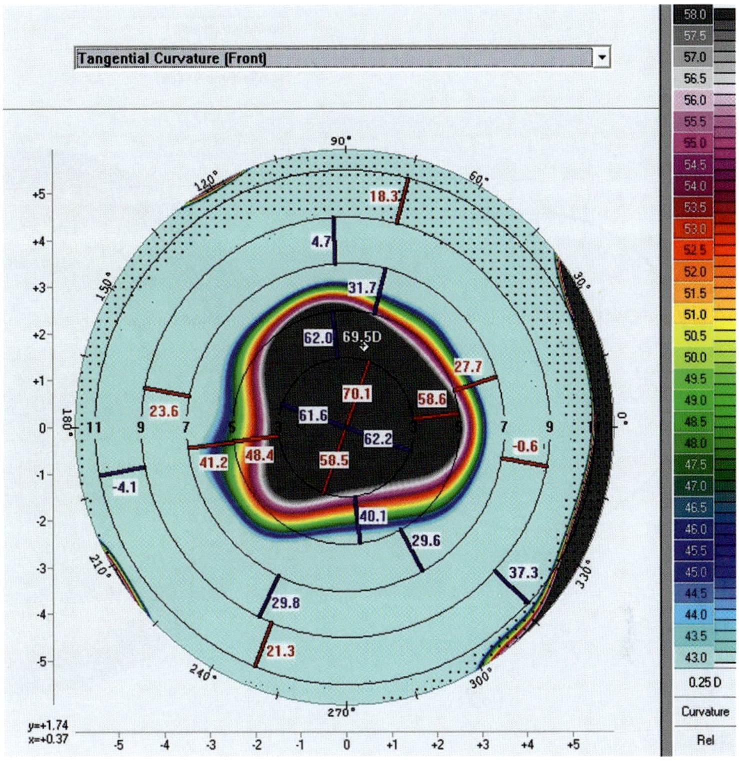

Fig. 2.3 Globus cone. A large steep cone involving over 75% of the cornea

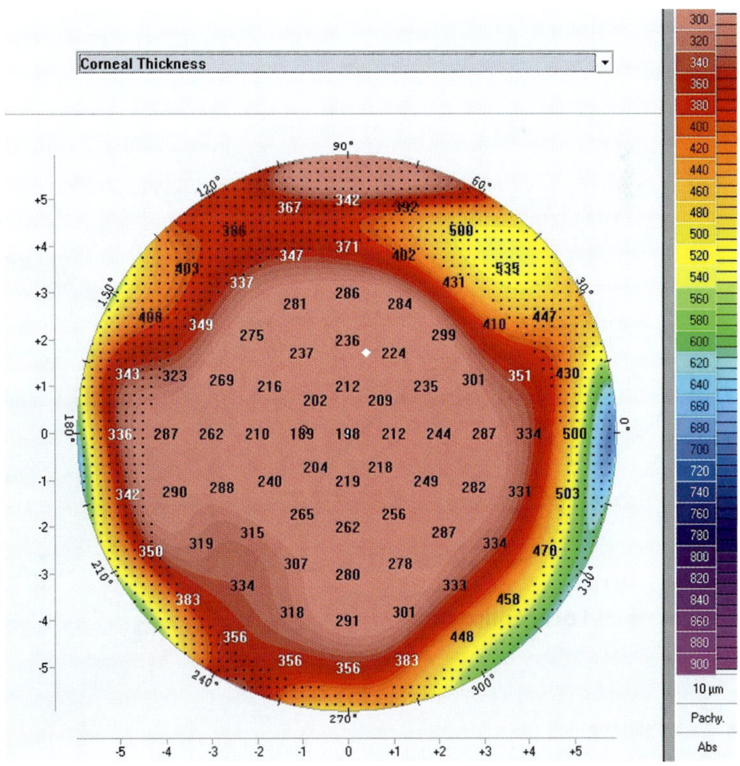

Fig. 2.4 Globus cone. Corneal thickness map: generalized corneal thinning

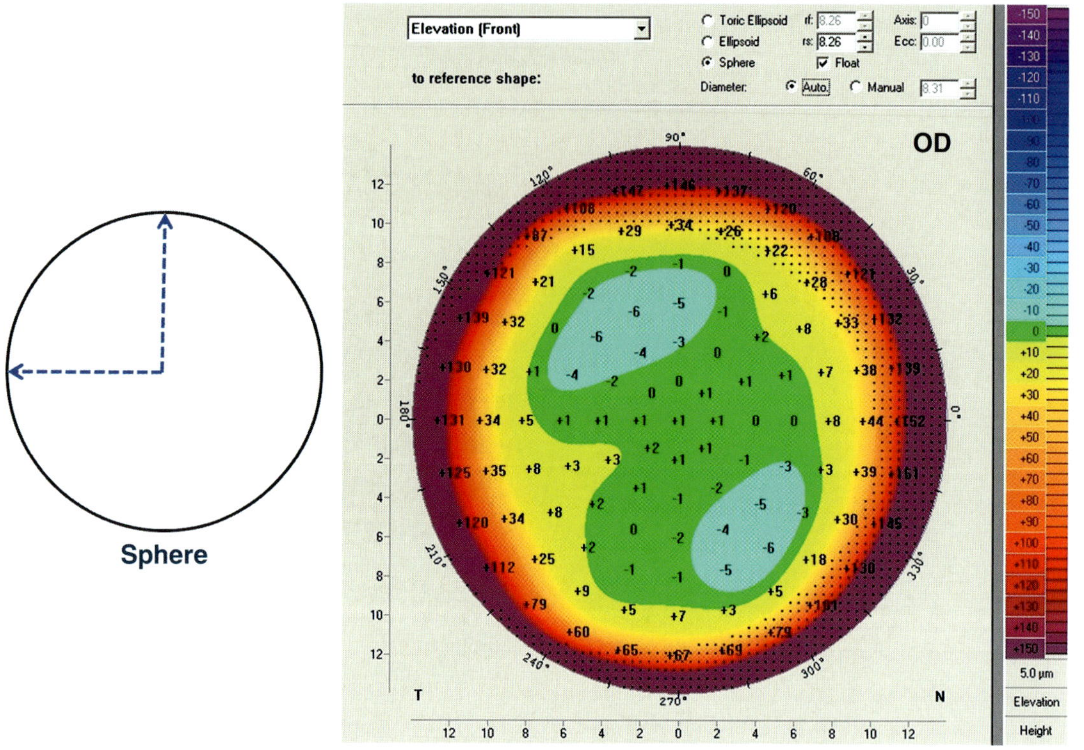

Fig. 2.5 The elevation map displayed in the best fit sphere float mode

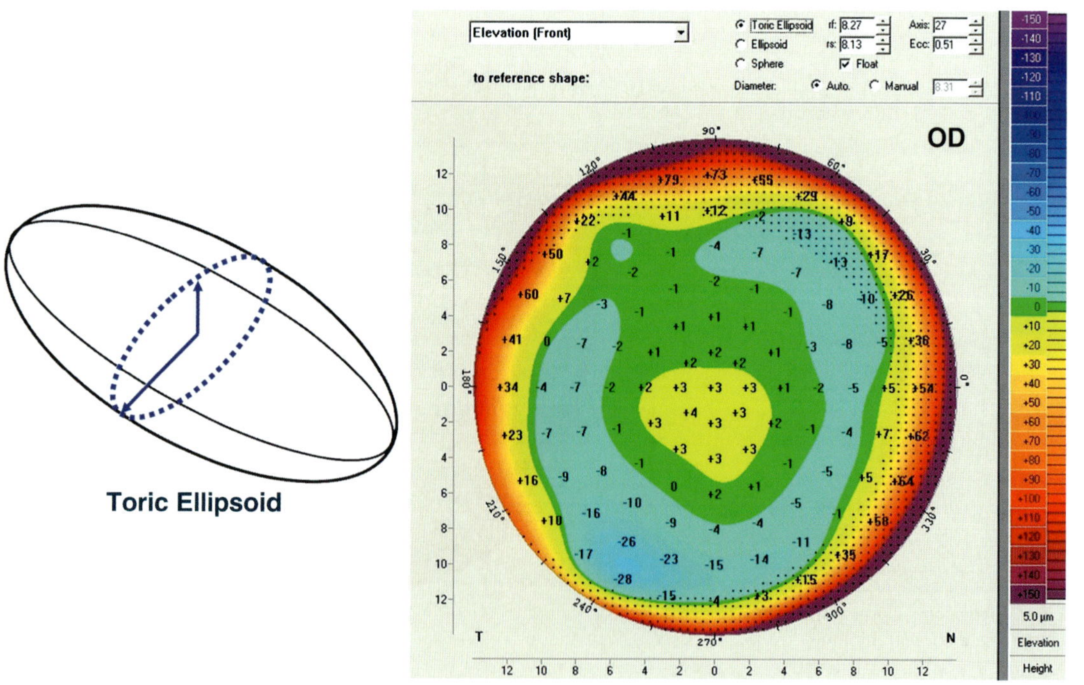

Fig. 2.6 The elevation map displayed in the best fit toric ellipsoid float mode

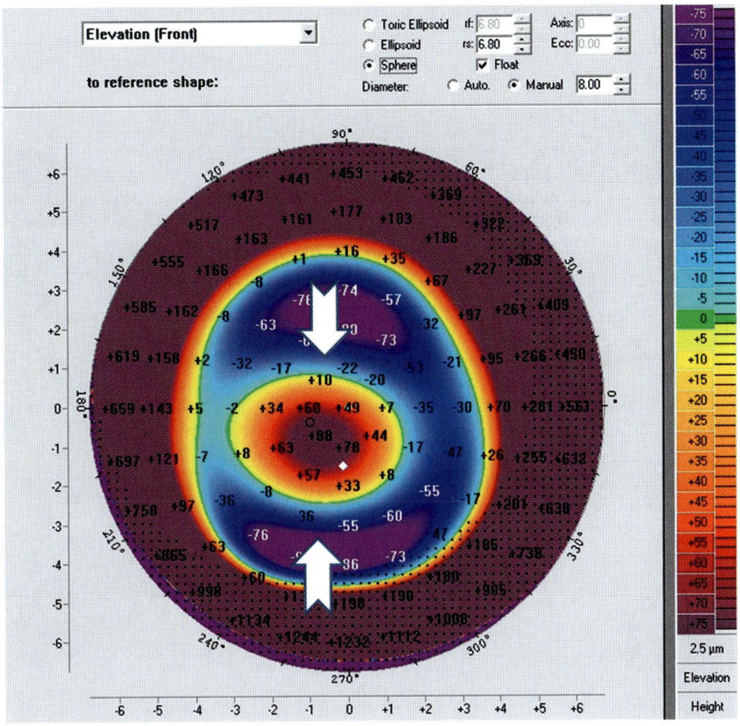

Fig. 2.7 A central cone as shown on the elevation map with the best fit sphere float mode; the white arrows point at the cone

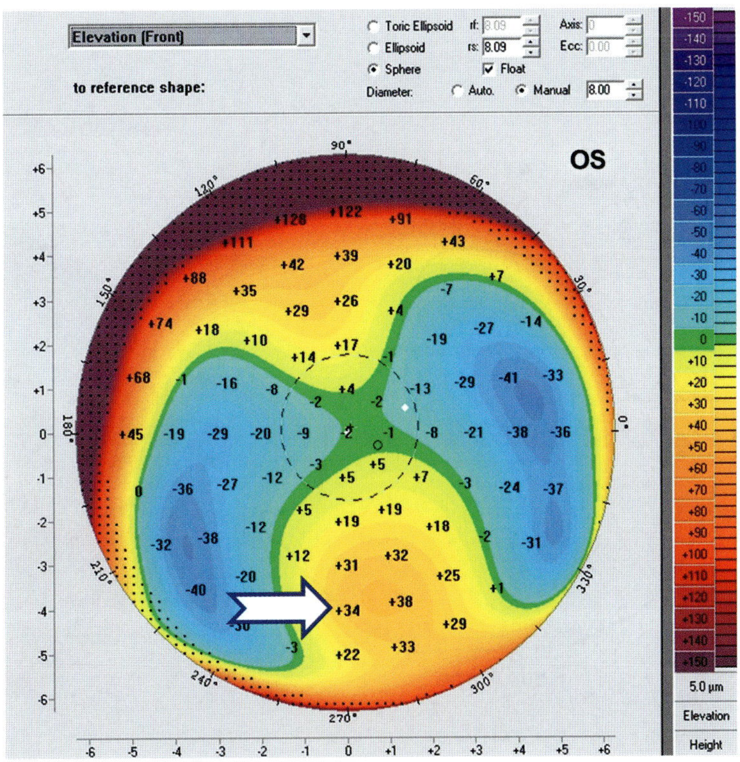

Fig. 2.8 A peripheral cone as shown on the elevation map with the best fit sphere float mode; the white arrow points at the cone

Fig. 2.9 Dome shape of the cone in KC on the corneal thickness map

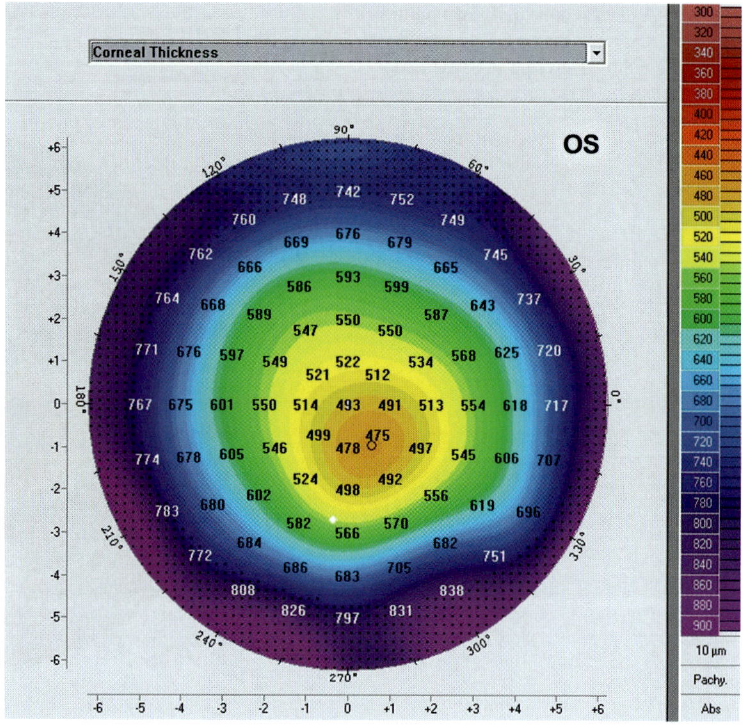

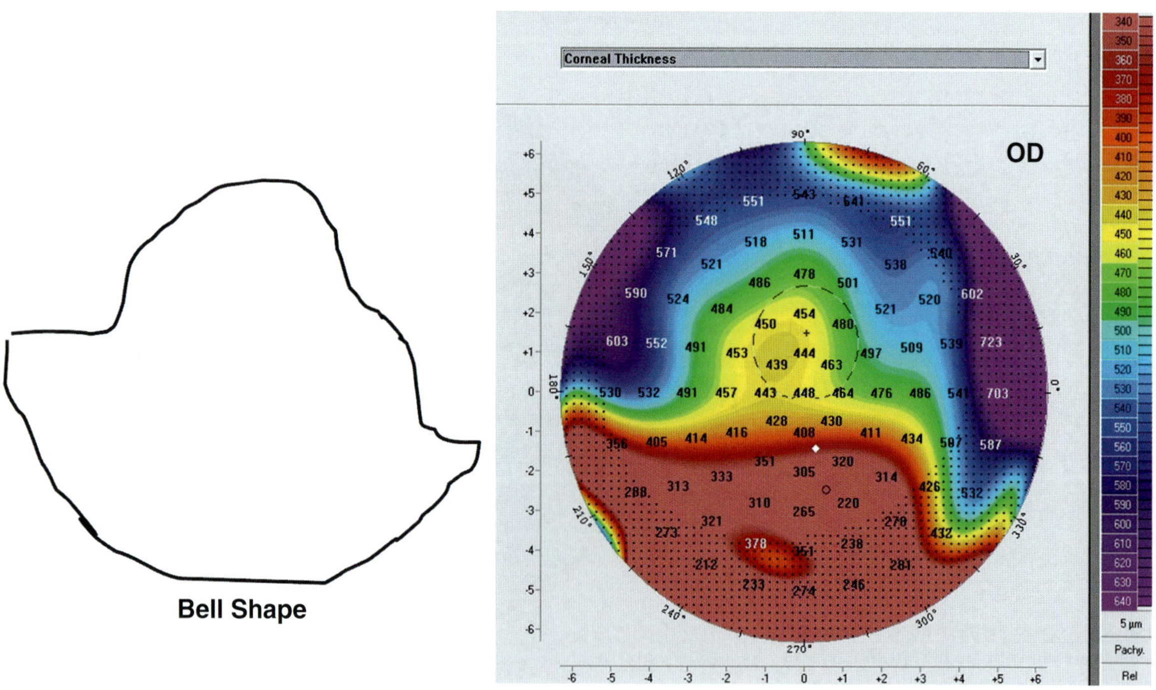

Fig. 2.10 Bell sign on the corneal thickness map in PMD

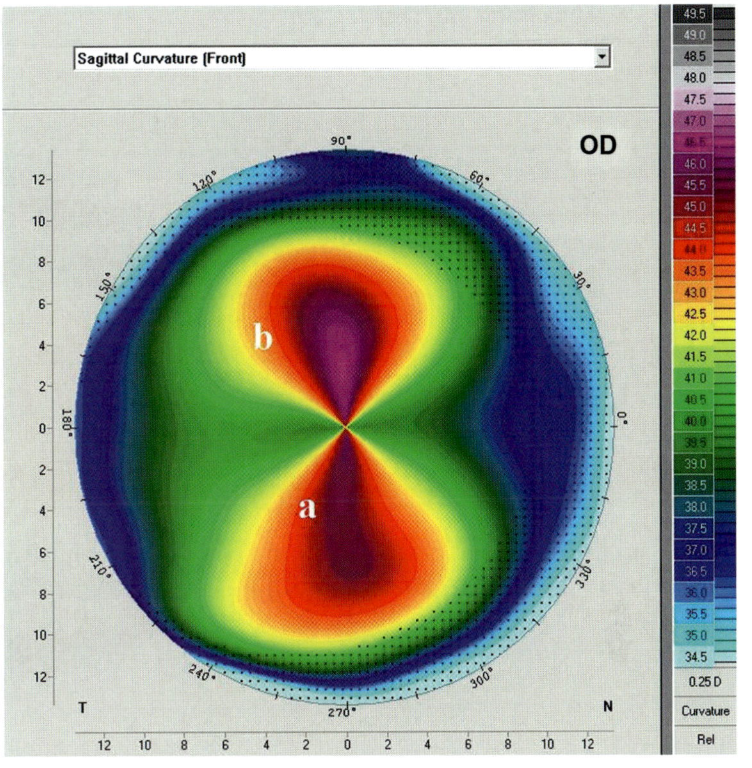

Fig. 2.11 Symmetric bowtie (SB). It has two equal and aligned segments "a" and "b." When the SB is aligned vertically, it represents with-the-rule astigmatism

should be aware of; some of these signs indicate KC and some indicate corneal irregularities, i.e. KC is always considered as corneal irregularity but not every corneal irregularity is a KC! To understand the curvature classification, the normal corneal should be studied.

2.2.3.1 The Normal Cornea

When considering the topography of a normal cornea, we feel the need to remember that there is a wide spectrum of normality. No human cornea demonstrates the kinds of regularity found in the calibration spheres of the topographer: The eye is not molded glass-made. Normal corneal topography can take one of the followings:

Regular astigmatism: Every human being has a certain amount of astigmatism, though minimal. The rule is that the vertical meridian of the cornea is slightly steeper than the horizontal. This is known as with-the-rule astigmatism. Figure 2.11 shows the symmetry between segments "a" and "b." They are also equal in size. That is the normal pattern, it is known as "Symmetric Bowtie (SB)"; see also Fig. 2.16.

If the SB is horizontal, it represents an against-the-rule astigmatism, 90° rotated when compared with a with-the-rule astigmatism (Fig. 2.12).

When the bow tie is diagonal, it represents a cornea having an oblique astigmatism (Fig. 2.13).

In the normal eye, nasal cornea is flatter than temporal. The nasal side of a healthy corneal map becomes blue more quickly, indicating that the nasal cornea is flatter than temporal.

Generally, the two eyes of the same subject are very similar, and present a mirror image of each other (Fig. 2.14). This phenomenon is called enantiomorphism. The knowledge of this fact is useful to decide whether a cornea is normal or not, by comparing with the map of contralateral eye.

P.S. When studying the pattern of corneal curvature, it is important to study the single enlarged map choosing the option of projected circles and the two major axes of curvature; in order to easily compare values in the same eye and between both eyes (Fig. 2.15).

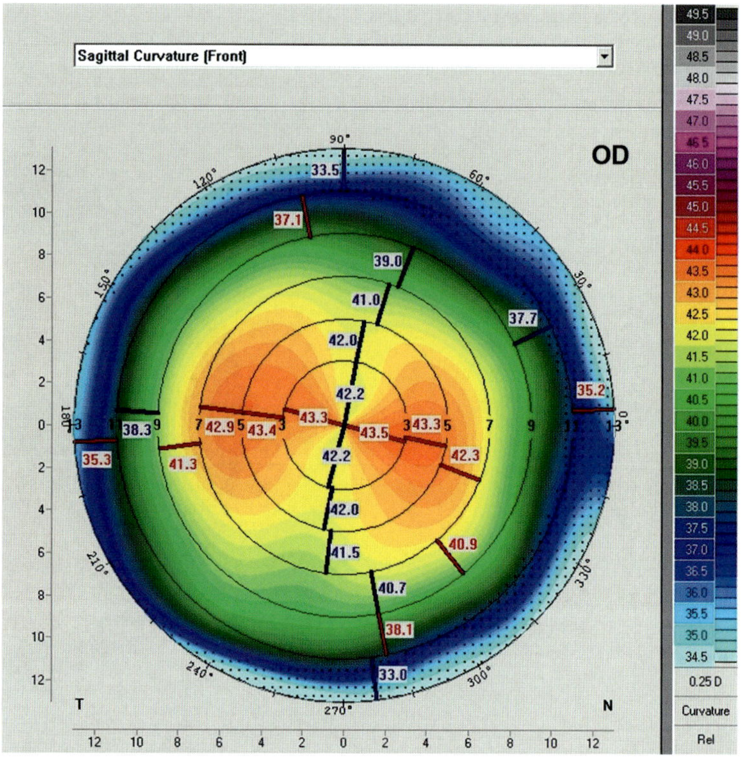

Fig. 2.12 Symmetric bowtie (SB) aligned horizontally representing against-the-rule astigmatism

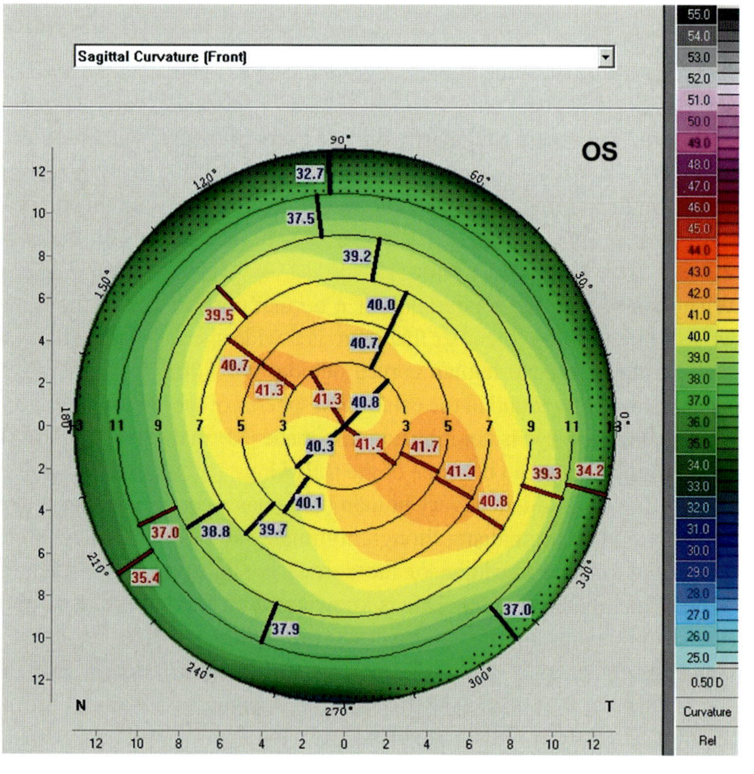

Fig. 2.13 Symmetric bowtie (SB) aligned obliquely representing oblique astigmatism

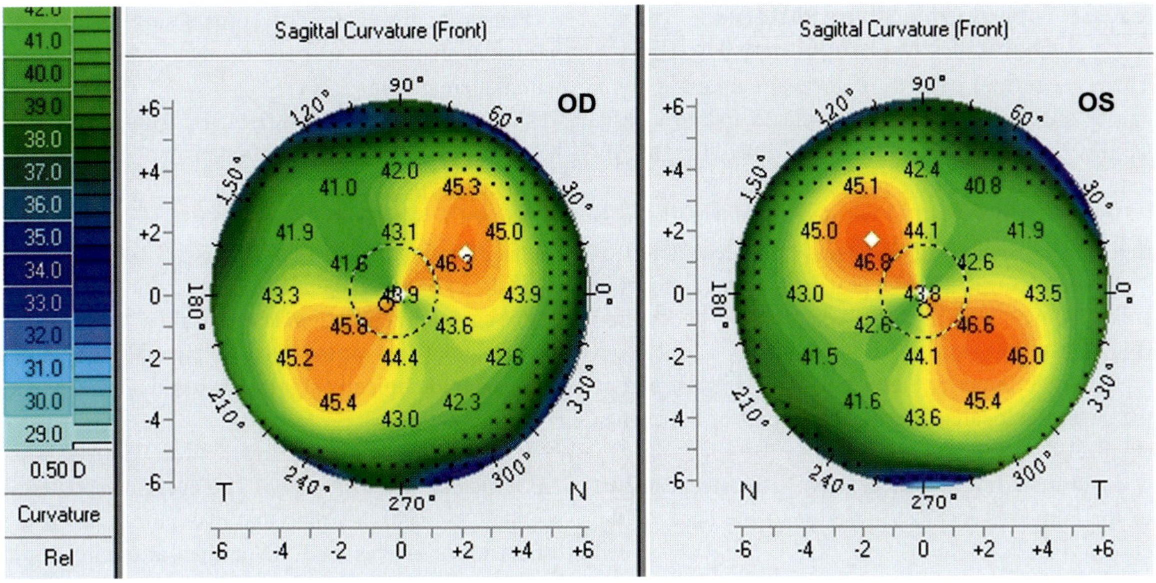

Fig. 2.14 Enantiomorphism. The two eyes of the same subject are very similar, and present a mirror image of each other. The knowledge of this fact is useful to decide whether a cornea is normal or not, by comparing with the map of the contralateral eye

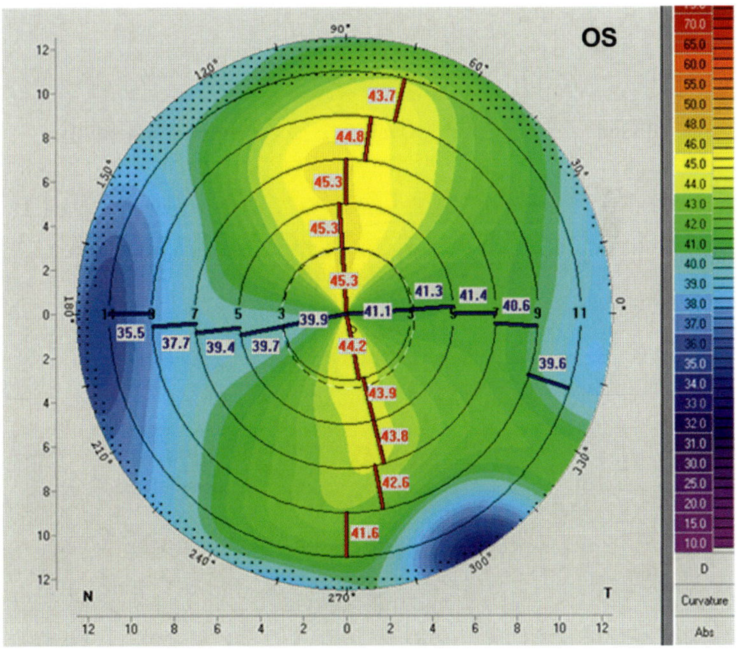

Fig. 2.15 The curvature map as a single enlarged map with projection of circles and the two major axes of curvature. This is important for comparing values in the same eye and between both eyes

2.2.3.2 Topographic Shape Patterns Characterizing Irregularity (Fig. 2.16)

There are several patterns of corneal curvature; some can be accepted, others are considered risky for lasik surgery or even indicators for KC. Corneal irregularity may appear as one of the following patterns:

Pattern 1: Round. The steepest part of the cornea (hot spot) is round (Fig. 2.17) and often decentered.

Pattern 2: Oval. The steepest part of the cornea (hot spot) is oval and may be centered or decentered (Fig. 2.18).

Pattern 3: Superior Steep (SS). The steepest part of the cornea is localized in the upper part of the cornea (Fig. 2.19).

Pattern 4: Inferior Steep (IS). The steepest part of the cornea is localized inferior to the apex of the cornea (Fig. 2.20).

Pattern 5: Irregular. The corneal surface takes no particular shape; in this pattern, steep areas are mixed with flat areas (Fig. 2.21).

Pattern 6: Symmetric bowtie (SB). This pattern may be an indicative of normal astigmatism or occasionally symmetric type of KC (Fig. 2.22).

Pattern 7: Symmetric bowtie (SB)/Skewed Steepest Radial Axis Index (SRAX). That is a SB with angulation (skew) between the axes of segments "b" and "a." In this case, corneal astigmatism is called "non-orthogonal astigmatism," or the "lazy 8" pattern. Angulation is considered clinically significant when it exceeds 22° (Fig. 2.23).

Pattern 8: Asymmetric Bowtie (AB)/IS. That is an AB which is inferiorly steep. The curvature power of segment "a" is higher than that of segment "b." If the difference is more than 1.5D on the 4-mm circle, it is

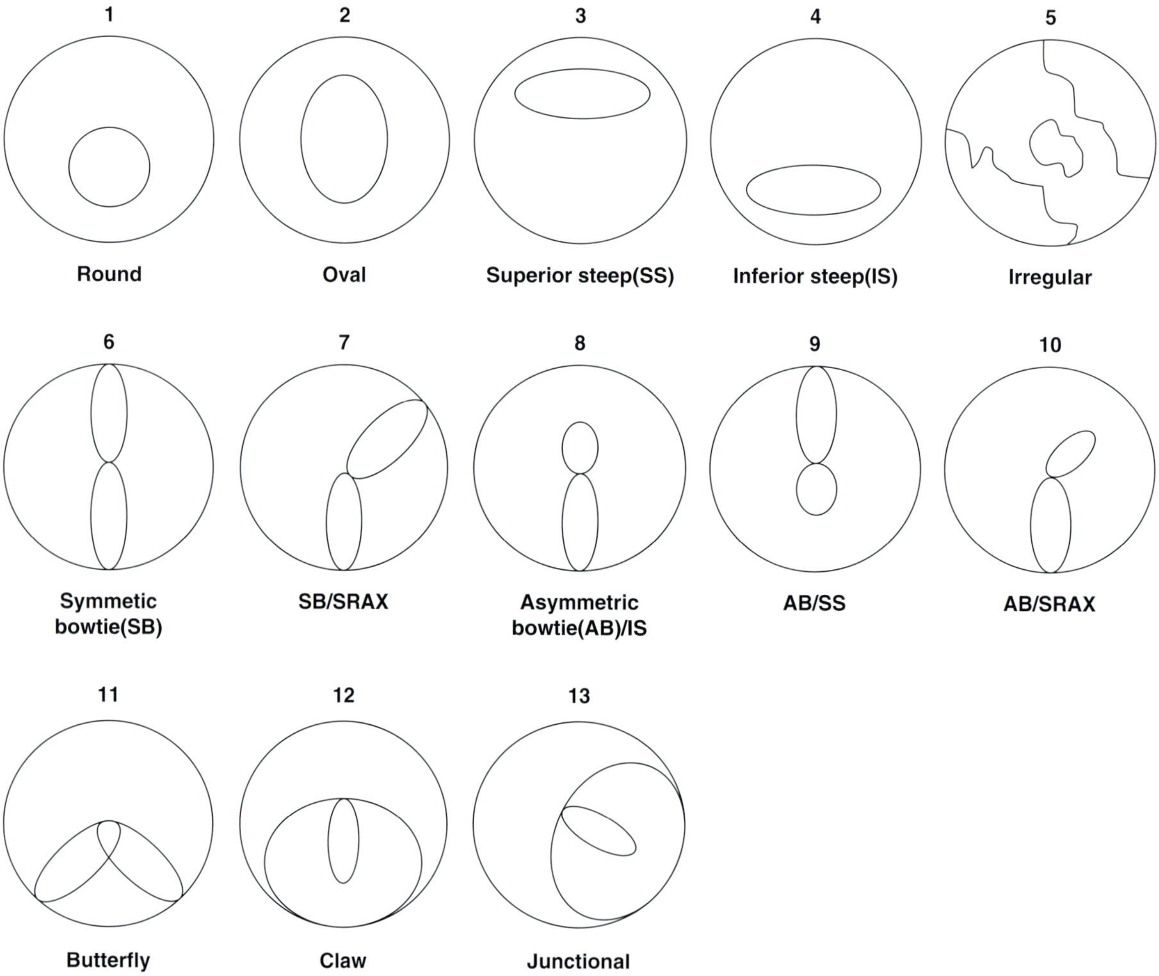

Fig. 2.16 Patterns of the anterior curvature map. The steep part of the curvature map may take a bowtie shape, a hot spot shape, or an irregular shape

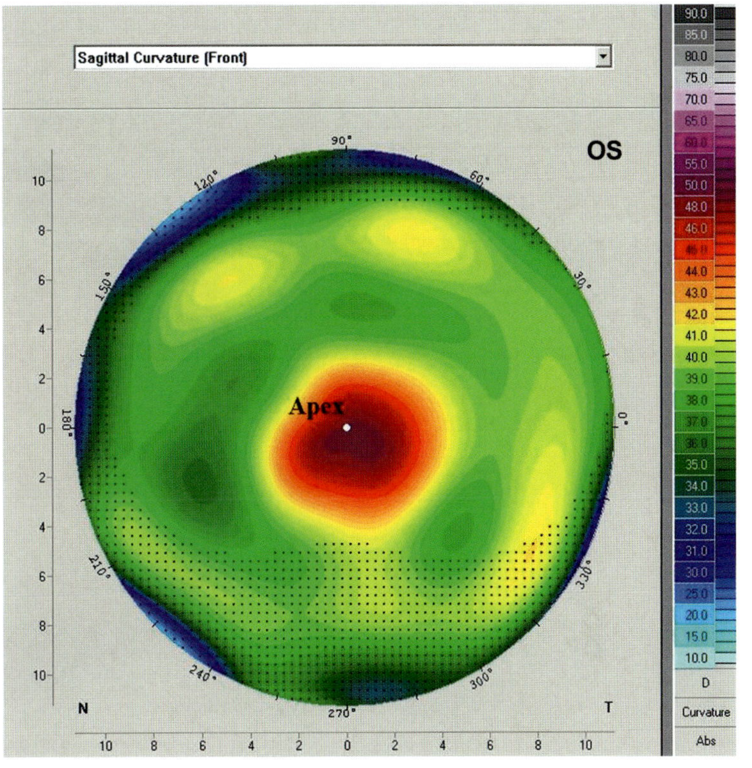

Fig. 2.17 Round hot spot

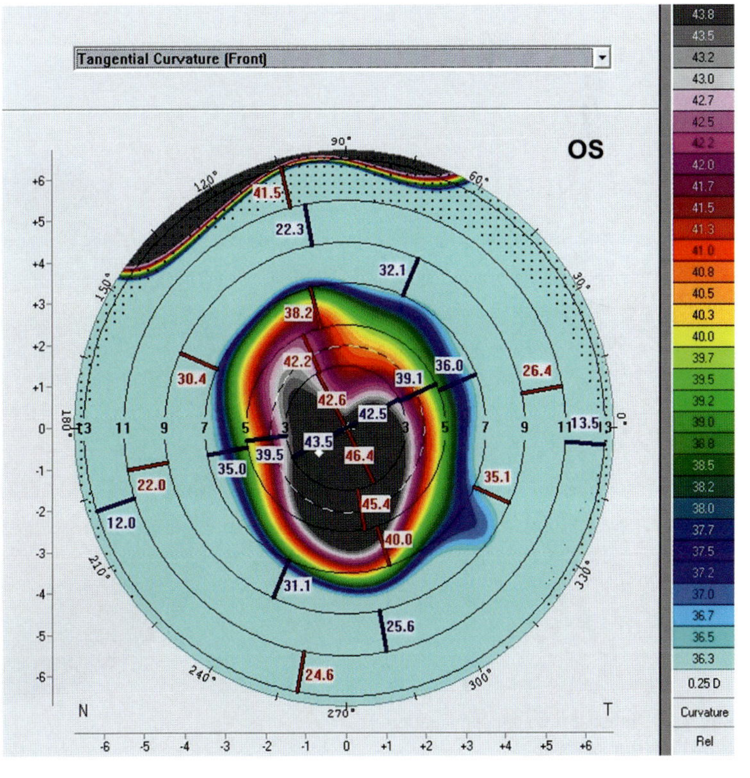

Fig. 2.18 Oval hot spot

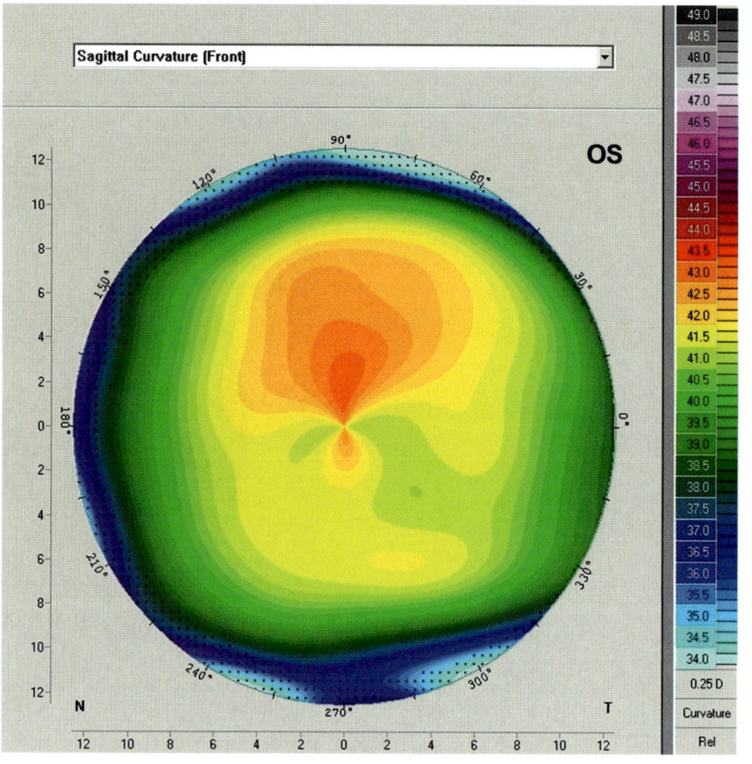

Fig. 2.19 Superior hot spot: This pattern is called superior steep (SS)

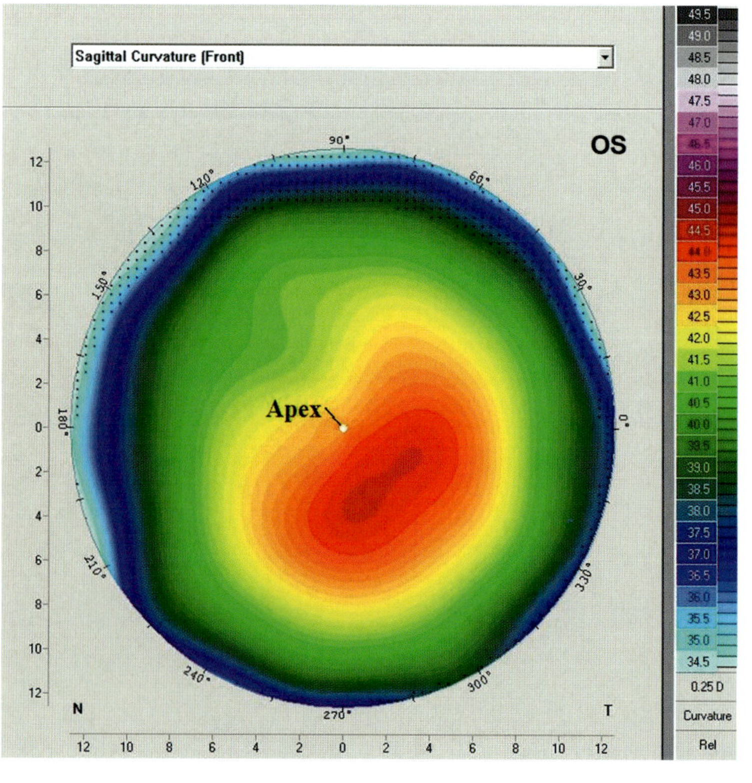

Fig. 2.20 Inferior hot spot: This pattern is called inferior steep (IS)

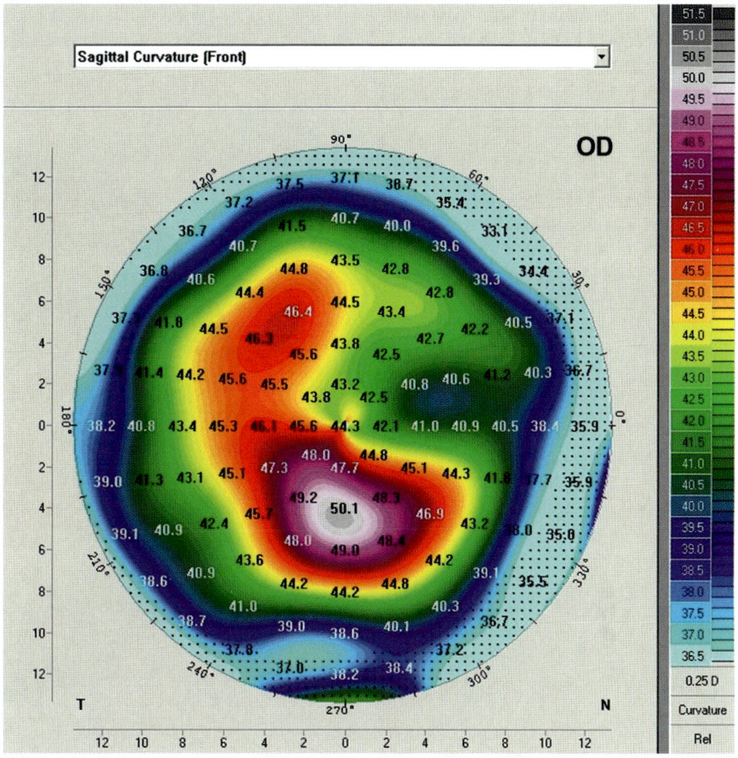

Fig. 2.21 Irregular shape: There is no particular shape where steep areas are mixed with flat areas

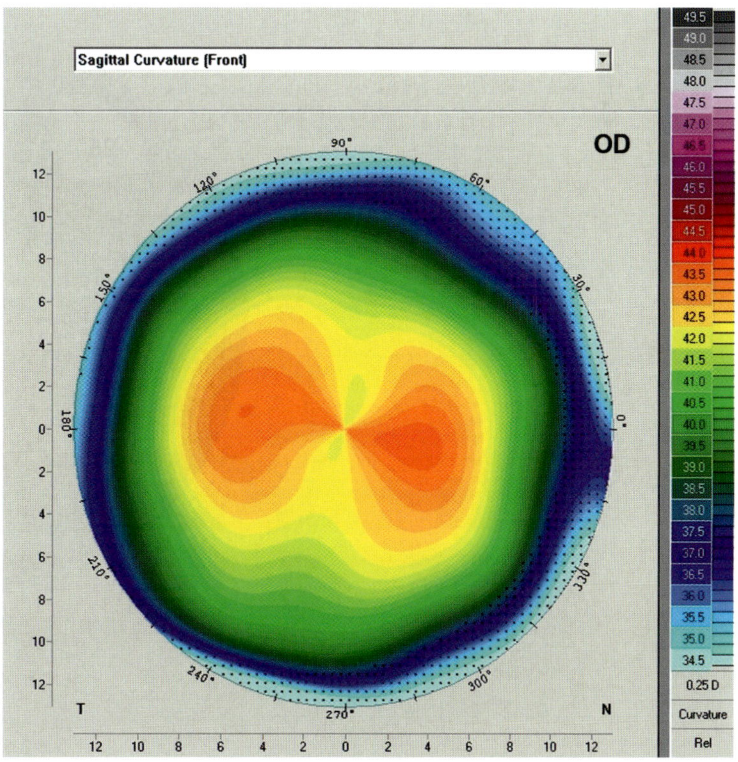

Fig. 2.22 Symmetric bowtie: It may be an indicative of normal astigmatism or occasionally symmetric type of KC

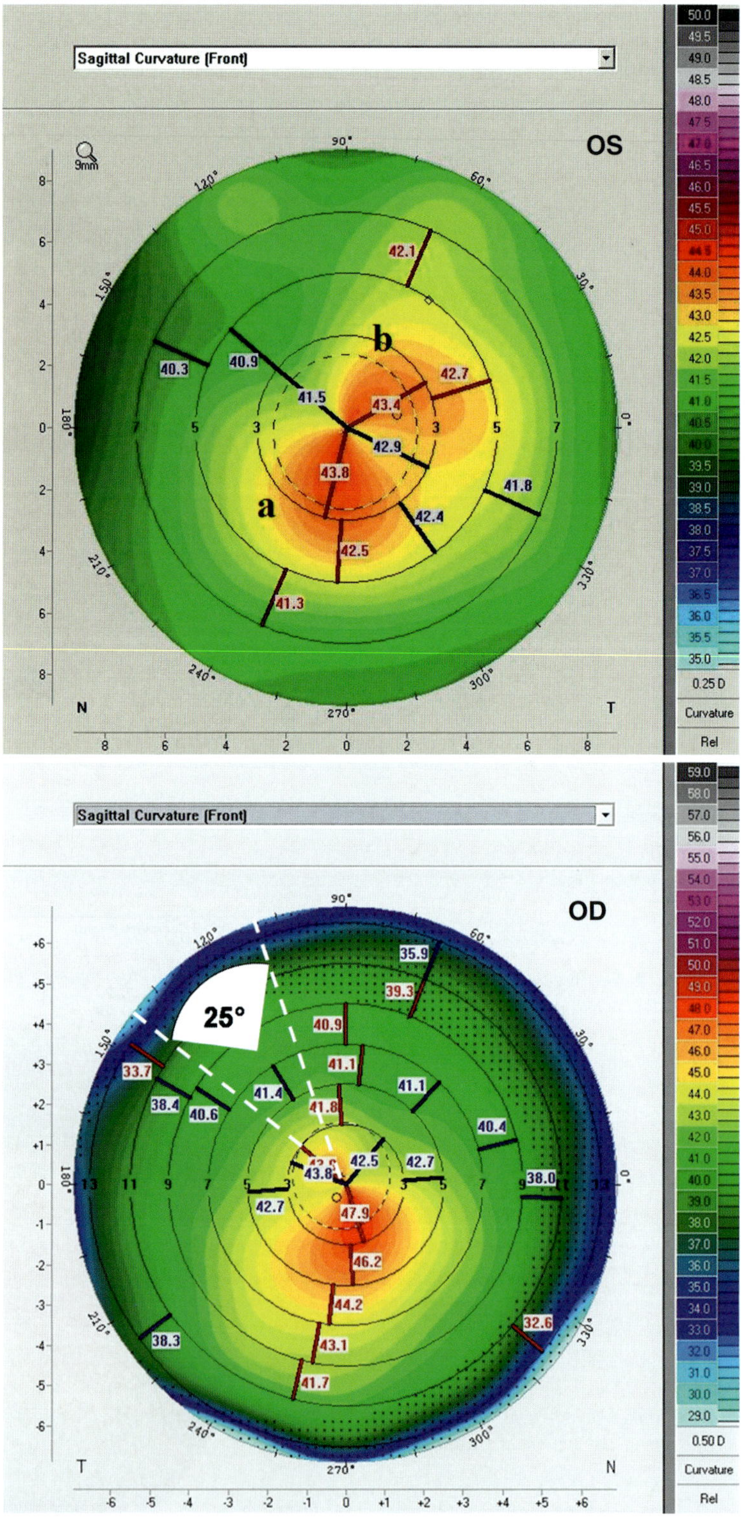

Fig. 2.23 Symmetric bowtie (SB) with Skewed Steepest Radial Axis Index (SRAX): SB/SRAX. There is an angulation between segments' axes. This angulation is clinically significant when it is >22°

considered significant (Fig. 2.24). Corneal apex is located in this type in the direction of the steeper (inferior) segment.

Pattern 9: AB/SS. That is an AB superiorly steep. This pattern is the reverse of pattern 8. If the difference is more than 2.5D, precaution should be taken when taking the decision (Fig. 2.25). In this type, the corneal apex is located in the direction of the steeper (superior) segment.

Pattern 10: AB/SRAX. That is an AB with angulation between the axes of the two segments (Fig. 2.26a, b).

Pattern 11: Butterfly: The bow-tie is horizontally aligned with the lobes inferiorly angulated or wing-like spread just like the wings of a butterfly. The lobes are not necessarily equal in size, therefore it can be considered as horizontal sisterhoods of patterns 7 and 10 (Fig. 2.27).

Pattern 12: Claw pattern: it is also known as "kissing birds": it is like the butterfly pattern added that the wings are joined inferiorly with a central flat area (Fig. 2.28). The vertical meridian of the cornea is flat, on which the K-readings are low, and usually the patient has a hyperopic component. This pattern is encountered in PMD or in PLK.

Pattern 13: Junctional: It is a circular shape, where the two lobes are laterally connected. It can be considered a vertical or oblique type of pattern 12. It is a subject of suspicion (Fig. 2.29a and b).

Pattern 14: Smiling Face: This is certainly risky because it often leads to postoperative ectasia, and might be an indicator of KC (Fig. 2.30) .

Pattern 15: Vortex pattern: It is also known as the "Nazi Logo" (Figures 2.31a to d). This is an indicator of corneal instability, and it may precede KC, (notice the vortex distribution of the red and blue lines).

P.S. The most concerning of the previous parameters are steep K-readings, inferior-superior asymmetry, and skewing of the steep axis.

2.2.4 Summary of Topographic Criteria of Keratoconus

When more than one of the following criteria are found, any of the above mentioned patterns is considered as frank KC, Forme Fruste KC (FFKC), early stage KC, or at least a case of suspicion (according to the severity and amount of signs):

On the sagittal map:

(a) K-readings > 48 dpt.
(b) SRAX > 22°.
(c) Superior–inferior difference (S-I) on the 5 mm circle > 2.5 dpt.
(d) Inferior–Superior difference (I-S) > 1.5 dpt.
(e) Corneal astigmatism on either surface should not be higher than 6D; otherwise, it is a risk factor.
(f) Against the rule, astigmatism is considered suspicious.

On the thickness map:

(a) Cone-like shape.
(b) Superior–inferior at 5 mm circle > 30 μ.
(c) Thinnest location < 470 μ.
(d) Thickness at pachy apex – thickness at thinnest location > 10 μ.
(e) *Y* coordinate value of the thinnest location > –500 μ.
(f) Difference in thickness between both eyes at thinnest locations > 30 μ.

On the elevation maps:

(a) Isolated island or tongue-like extension (BFS mode) on either surface.
(b) Values > 12 μ within the central 5 mm on the anterior elevation map (BFTE mode).
(c) Values > 15 μ within the central 5 mm on the posterior elevation map (BFTE mode).

For further information, please refer to my book: "Corneal Topography in Clinical Practice, Jaypee Brothers 2009."

2.2.5 The Author's New Classification of Topographical Patterns of Keratoconus

Upon revision of the results of the author's first 400 cases of intracorneal rings with at least 6-month follow-up, he could recognize some factors affecting the results. From a topographical point of view, studying the changes that occurred in the sagittal curvature map revealed that there are three factors affecting the response to the rings: (1) the skew between the axes of the bowtie segments, (2) the size of the bowtie segments, and (3) the shape of the map. To understand this, the steep and flat segments should be projected on

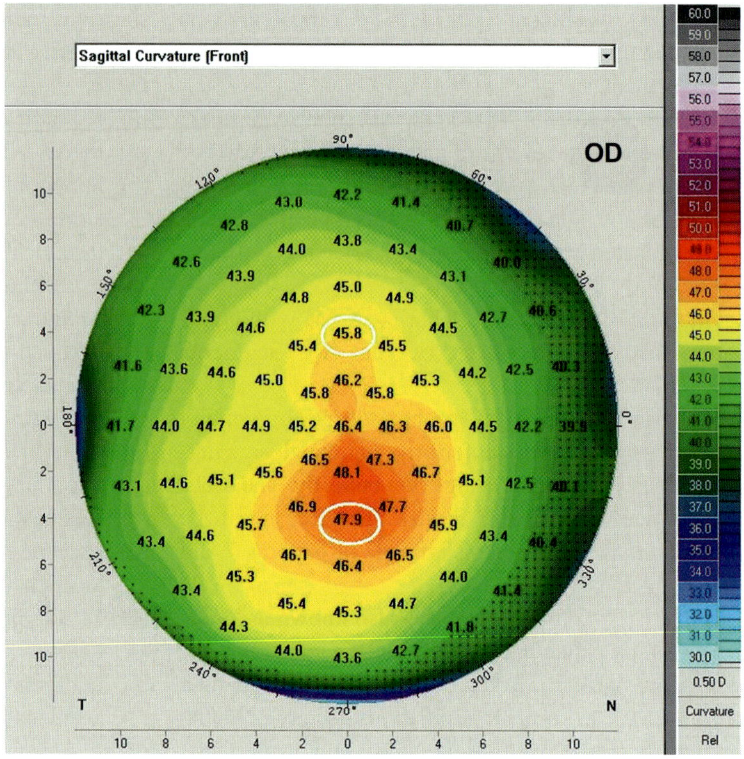

Fig. 2.24 Asymmetric bowtie inferiorly steep: AB/IS. The inferior segment has higher values than the superior one. As shown in *white circles*, the inferior value is higher than the superior by more than 1.5 dpt, which is clinically significant

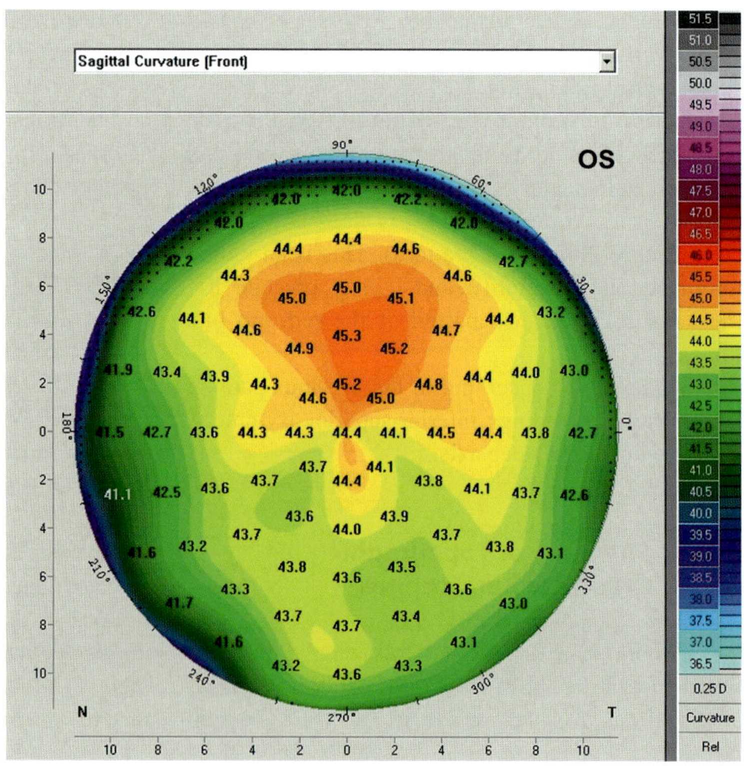

Fig. 2.25 Asymmetric bowtie superiorly steep: AB/SS. It is opposite to the pattern ion Fig. 2.24

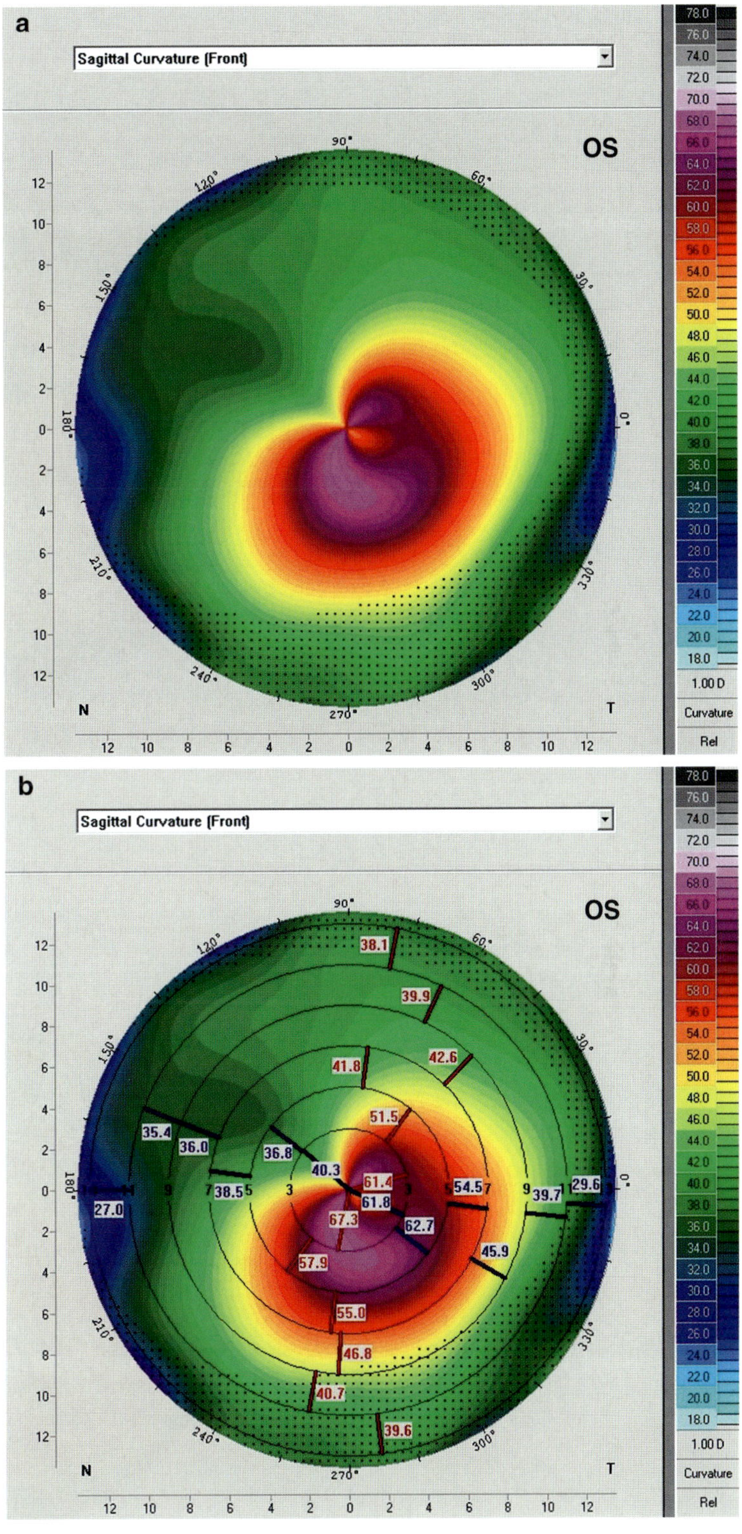

Fig. 2.26 Asymmetric bowtie with Skewed Steepest Radial Axis Index: AB/SRAX. There is an angulation between asymmetric segments. This angulation is clinically significant when it is >22°. (**a**) is the anterior sagital map without projected meridians; (**b**) is the same map with projected meridians to show the skew

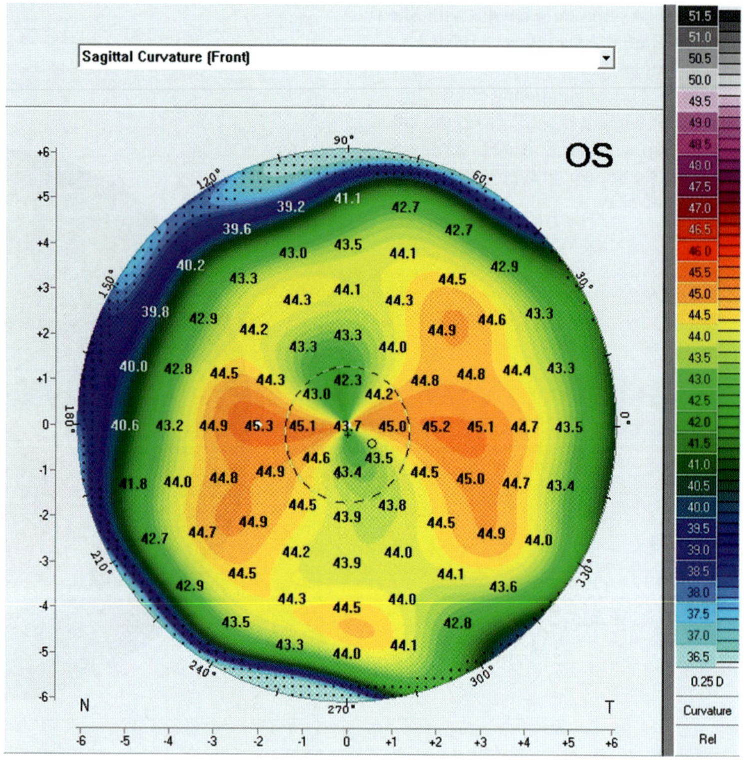

Fig. 2.27 Butterfly. The Bow-tie is horizontally aligned with wing-like spread of the lobes

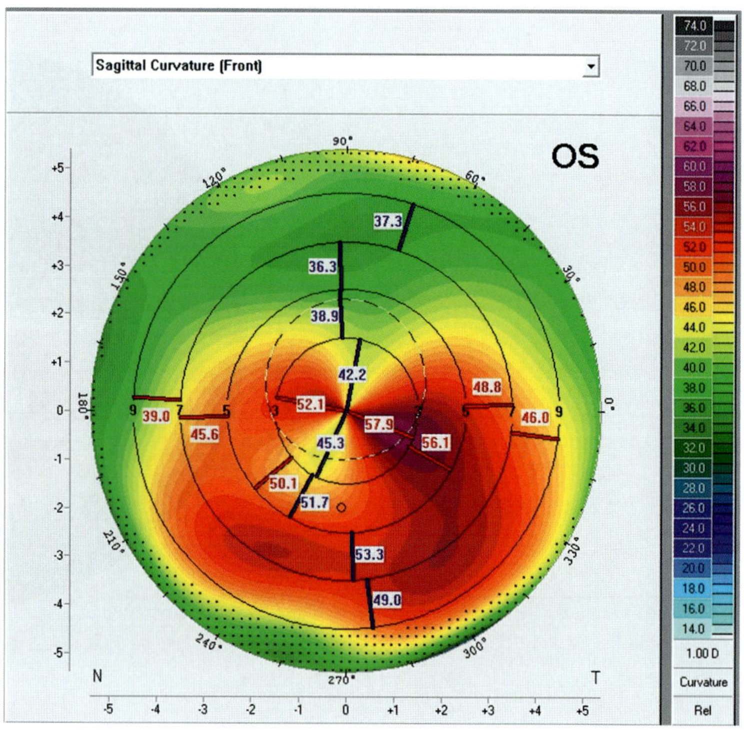

Fig. 2.28 Claw pattern or the kissing birds pattern. The lobes of the bow-tie or the wings of the butterfly are inferiorly joined

Fig. 2.29 Junctional pattern. KC may present with this pattern. Junctional pattern is better seen with the projected circles and curvature segments off. (**a**) With and (**b**) without

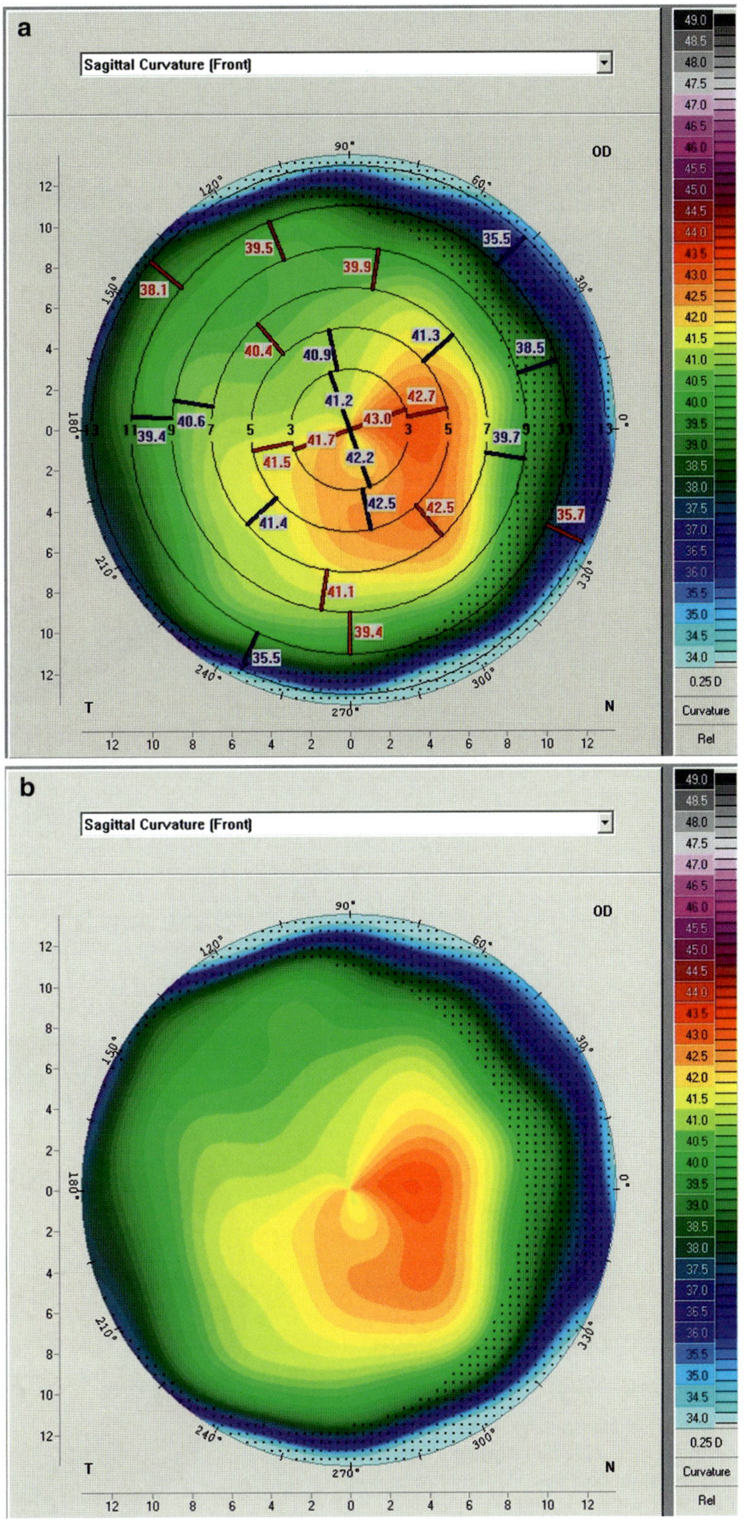

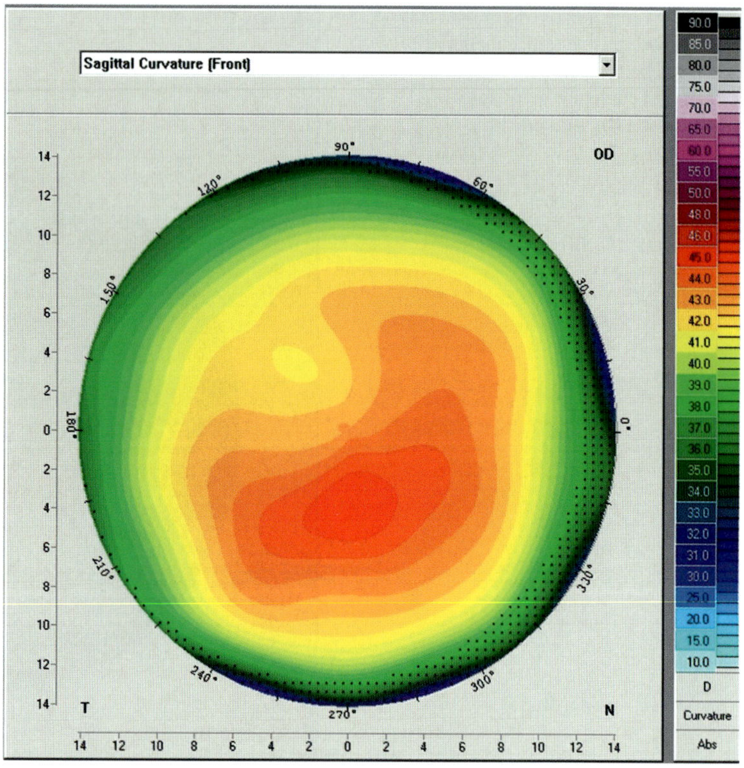

Fig. 2.30 Smiling face. KC may present with this pattern

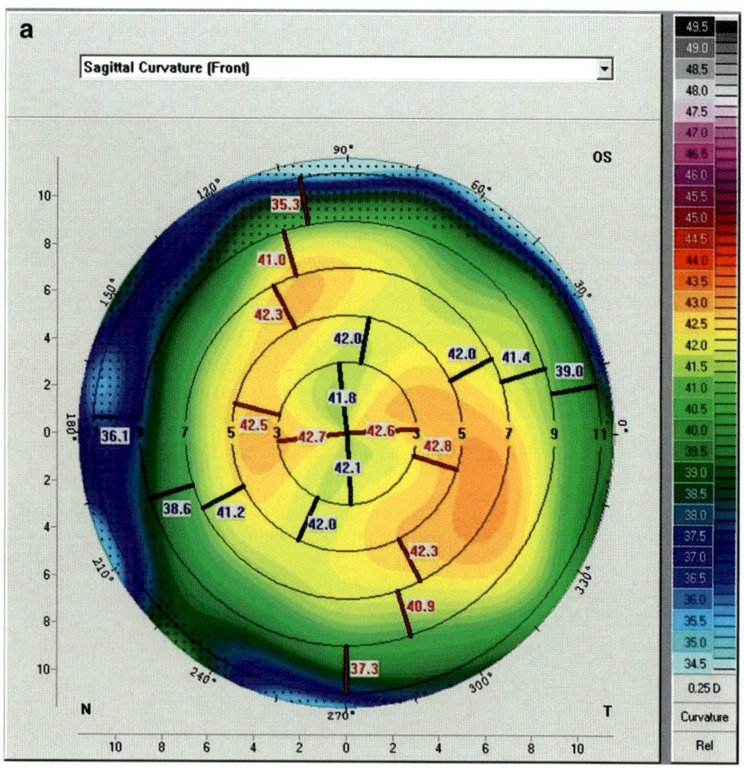

Fig. 2.31 Vortex pattern. The projected curvature (*red and blue*) segments take a vortex distribution. (**a**–**c**) Different shapes of the vortex pattern. Unlike the junctional pattern, the vortex pattern is better recognized with the projected curvature segments on, this can be seen when comparing (**d**) with (**a**–**c**)

Fig. 2.31 (continued)

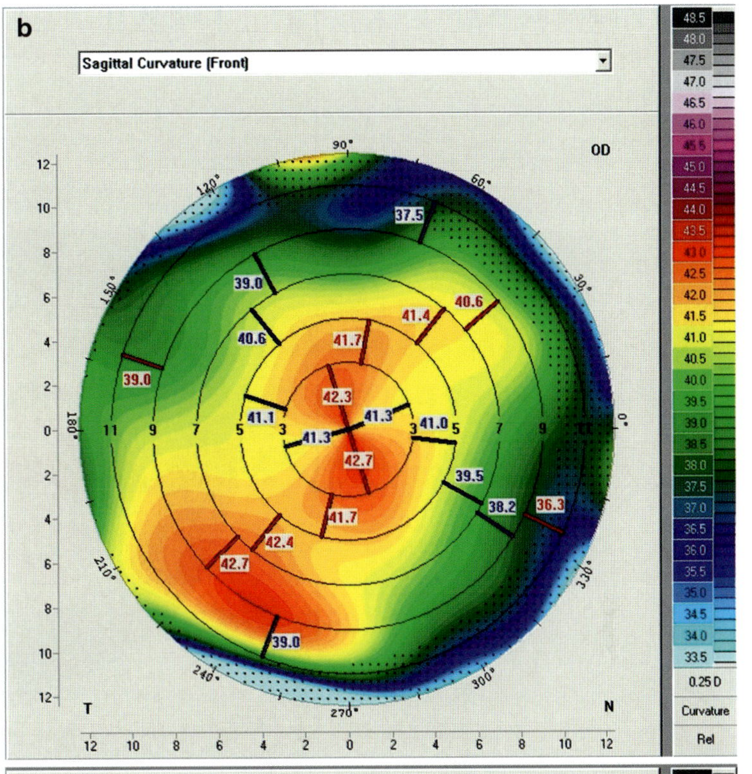

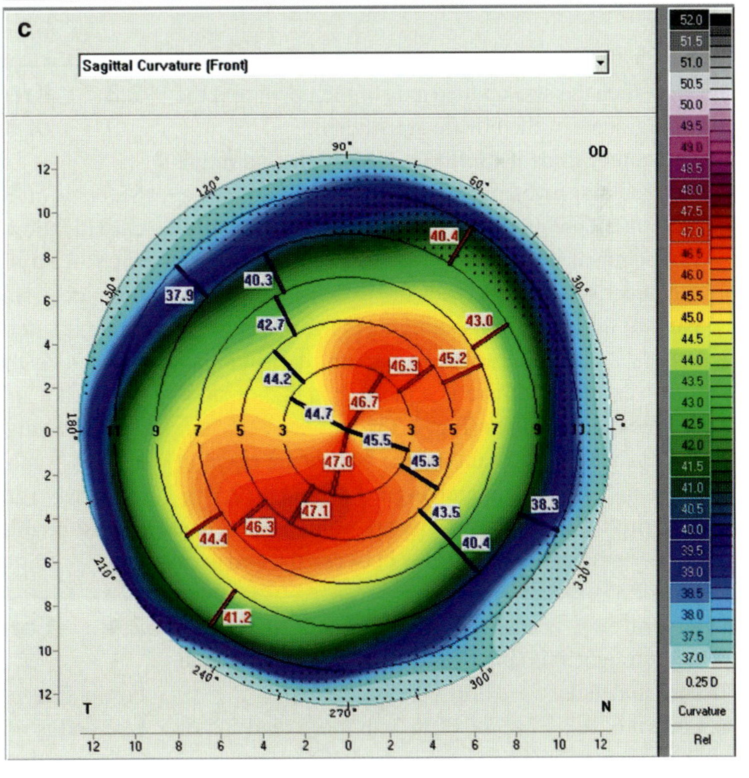

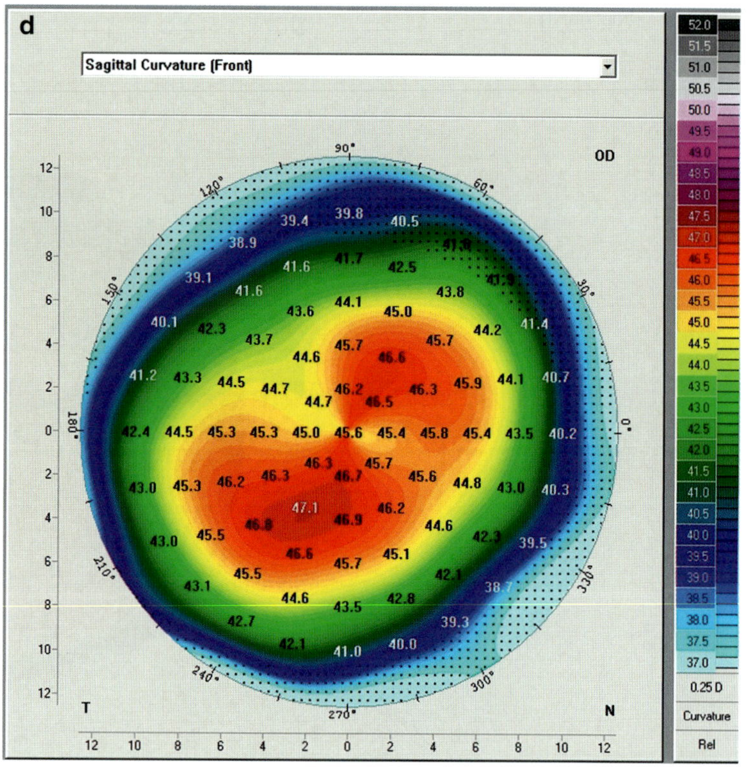

Fig. 2.31 (continued)

the map, then the size and the axis of the upper and the lower segments of the bowtie are studied.

The author finds it useful to classify the curvature map of KC into seven patterns as follows:

1. Pattern 1: The inferior steep pattern, where the inferior segment of the bowtie is steeper (larger) than the superior segment, with the axes of the central parts of these segments straight (Fig. 2.32).
2. Pattern 2: The inferior steep pattern, it is like pattern 1 except that there is a more than 22° of skew between the two axes (Fig. 2.33).
3. Pattern 3: Both segments of the bowtie are equal in size and have straight and aligned axes (Fig. 2.34).
4. Pattern 4: The two segments are equal in size but there is more than 22° of skew between the two axes (Fig. 2.35).
5. Pattern 5: It is PMD or Pellucid-like KC (PLK) with straight axis (Fig. 2.36). PLK will be discussed later in details.
6. Pattern 6: It is PMD or PLK with more than 22° of skew between the two axes (Fig. 2.37).
7. Pattern 7: Where the cone is eccentric and the steep and flat axes are difficult to identify (Fig. 2.38a, b).

The importance of this classification will be clear when talking about the intracorneal rings.

2.3 Krumeich Classification of Keratoconus

Severity of KC is also classified by Krumeich. This classification depends on mean K-readings on the anterior curvature sagittal map, thickness at the thinnest location, and the refractive error of the patient. Table 2.1 demonstrates grading of KC severity, where grade 4 is the worst. This classification is useful; it helps choosing the best approach for KC.

There might be some intersection between the categories, such as > 55 dpt of Km (grade 4) and 400 μ thickness (grade 2). In such cases, a full judgment should be followed, which is the aim of this book.

2.4 Forme Fruste Keratoconus

Forme Fruste Keratoconus (FFKC) is a subclinical disease and is not a variant of KC. Although clinicians use many other terms such as mild KC, early KC, and subclinical KC, their exact meanings and applications are less certain. These terms are not universally accepted. The diagnosis of KC is a clinical one that is aided by topography, while the diagnosis of FFKC is topographic.

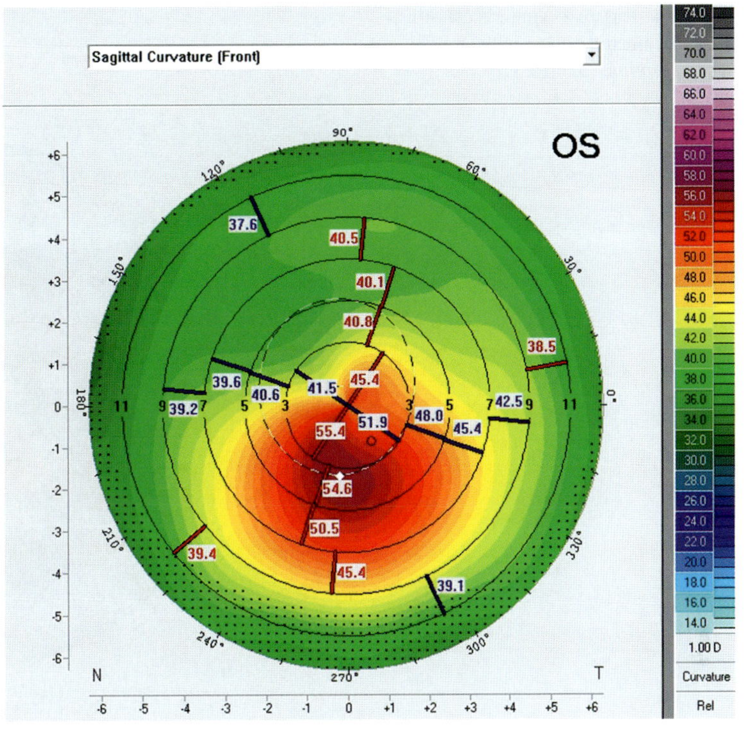

Fig. 2.32 Pattern 1 (author's classification). Inferior steep with straight *central red line* (steep axis)

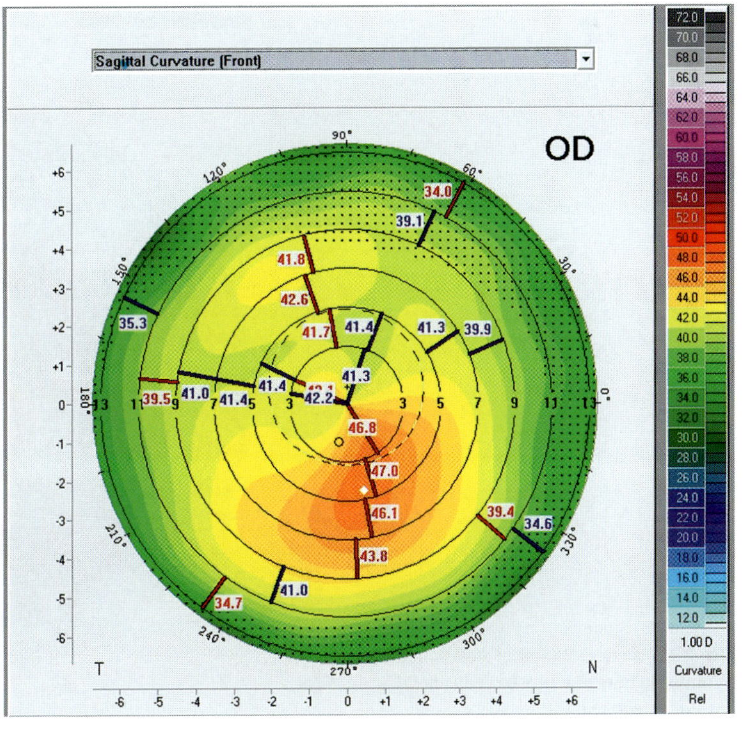

Fig. 2.33 Pattern 2 (author's classification). Inferior steep with skewed *central red line* (steep axis)

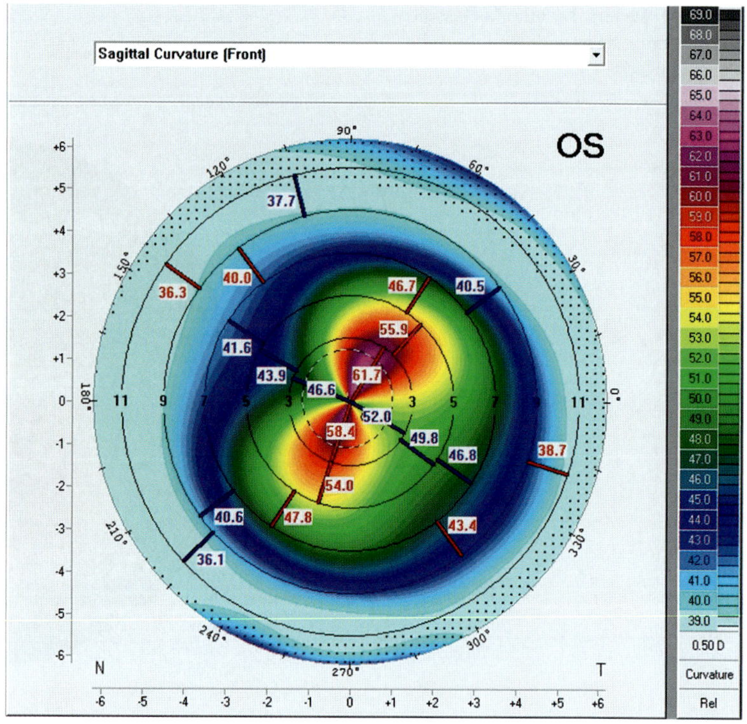

Fig. 2.34 Pattern 3 (author's classification). Symmetric bowtie with straight *central red line* (steep axis)

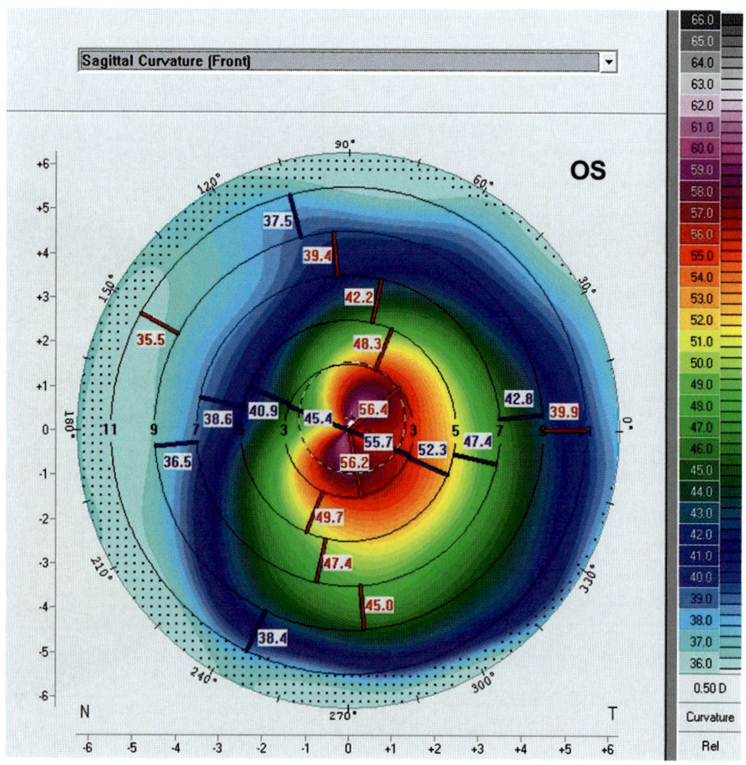

Fig. 2.35 Pattern 4 (author's classification). Symmetric bowtie with skewed *central red line* (steep axis)

Fig. 2.36 Pattern 5 (author's classification). PMD or Pellucid-like keratoconus with straight *central red line* (steep axis)

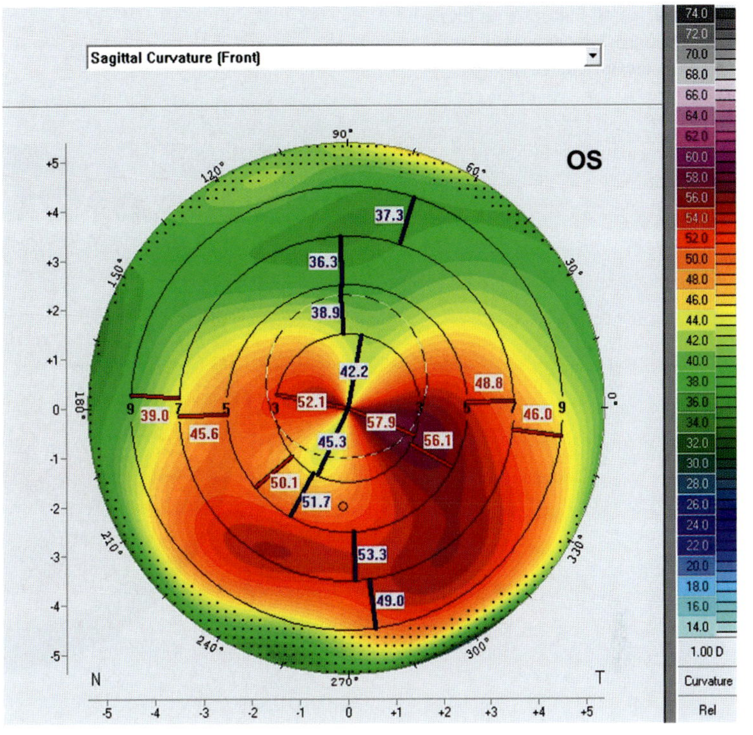

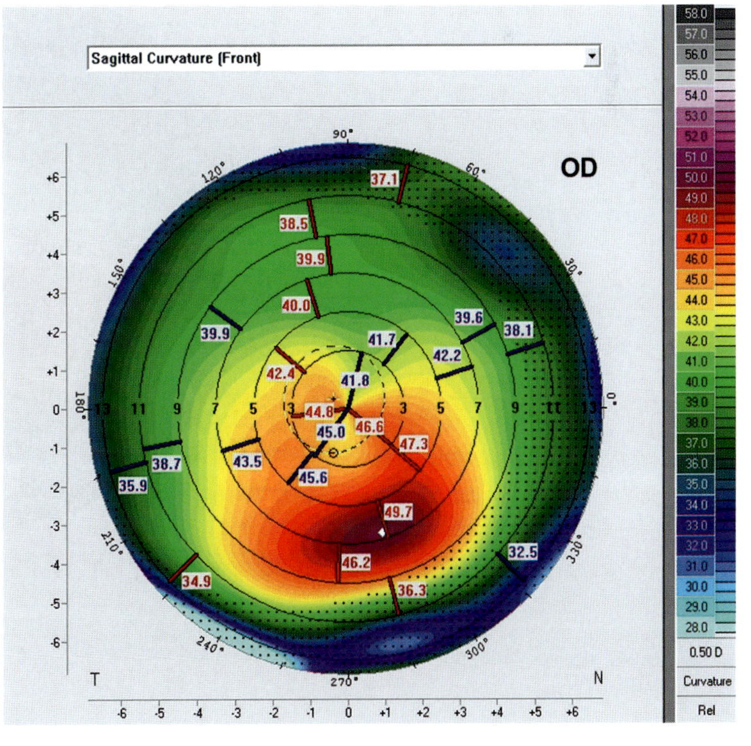

Fig. 2.37 Pattern 6 (author's classification). PMD or Pellucid-like keratoconus with skewed central *red line* (steep axis)

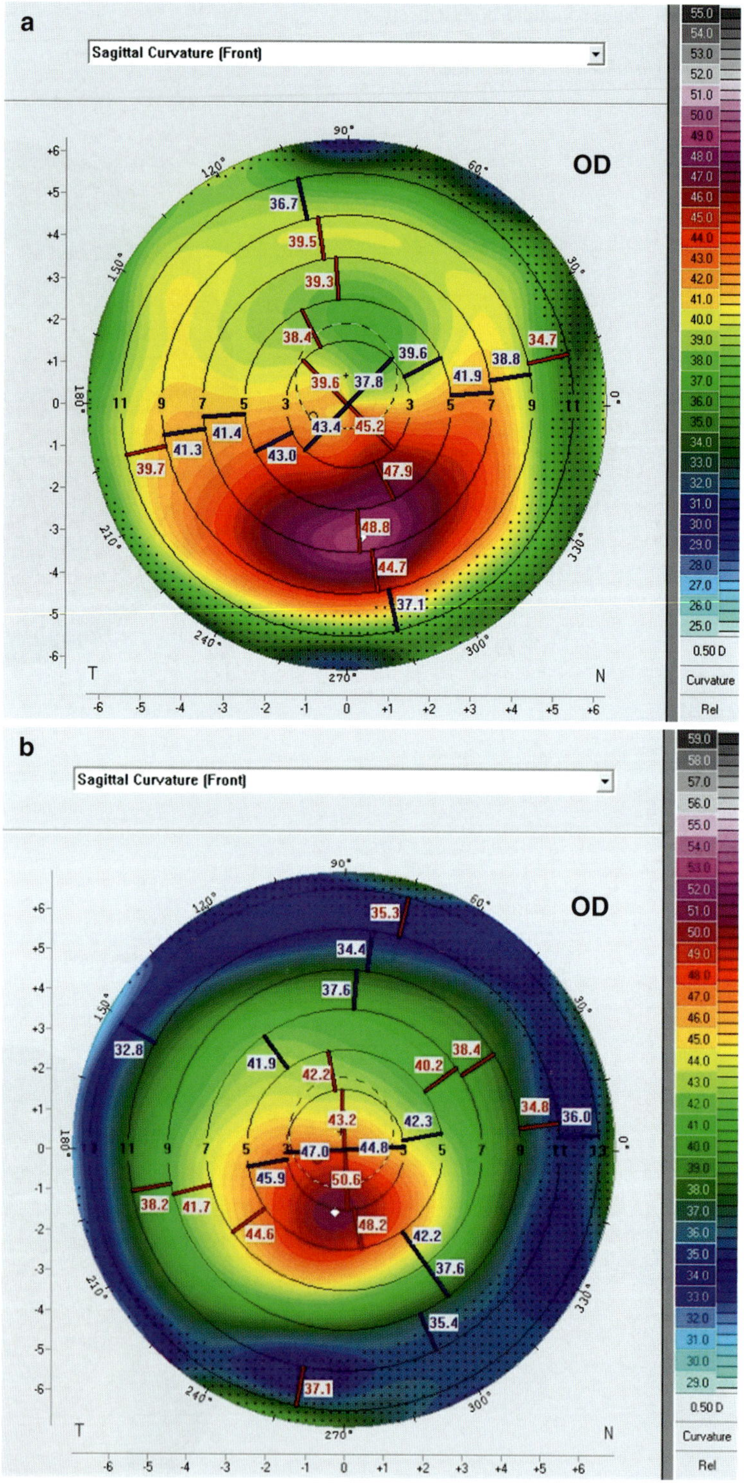

Fig. 2.38 (**a**, **b**) Pattern 7 (author's classification). Eccentric cone with the steep and flat axes difficult to identify

Table 2.1 Krumeich classification of keratoconus

Severity	Km (sim K)	Thickness (μ)	Spherical equivalent	Cornea
4	>55	<200	Not measurable	Central scars
3	54–55	200–400	>−8D	No central scars
2	48–53	400–500	[−5,−8]D	No central scars
1	<48	>500	<−5	No central scars

Recently, there are two opinions regarding the definition of this disease:

1. FFKC is a completely normal cornea with neither clinical nor topographical risk factors, but this cornea is able to develop KC when treated by laser. The fellow eye may be keratoconic or there may be a family history of KC as shown in Fig. 2.39a–c. Figure 2.39a represents a relatively normal corneal topography of the left eye. Figure 2.39b represents

a

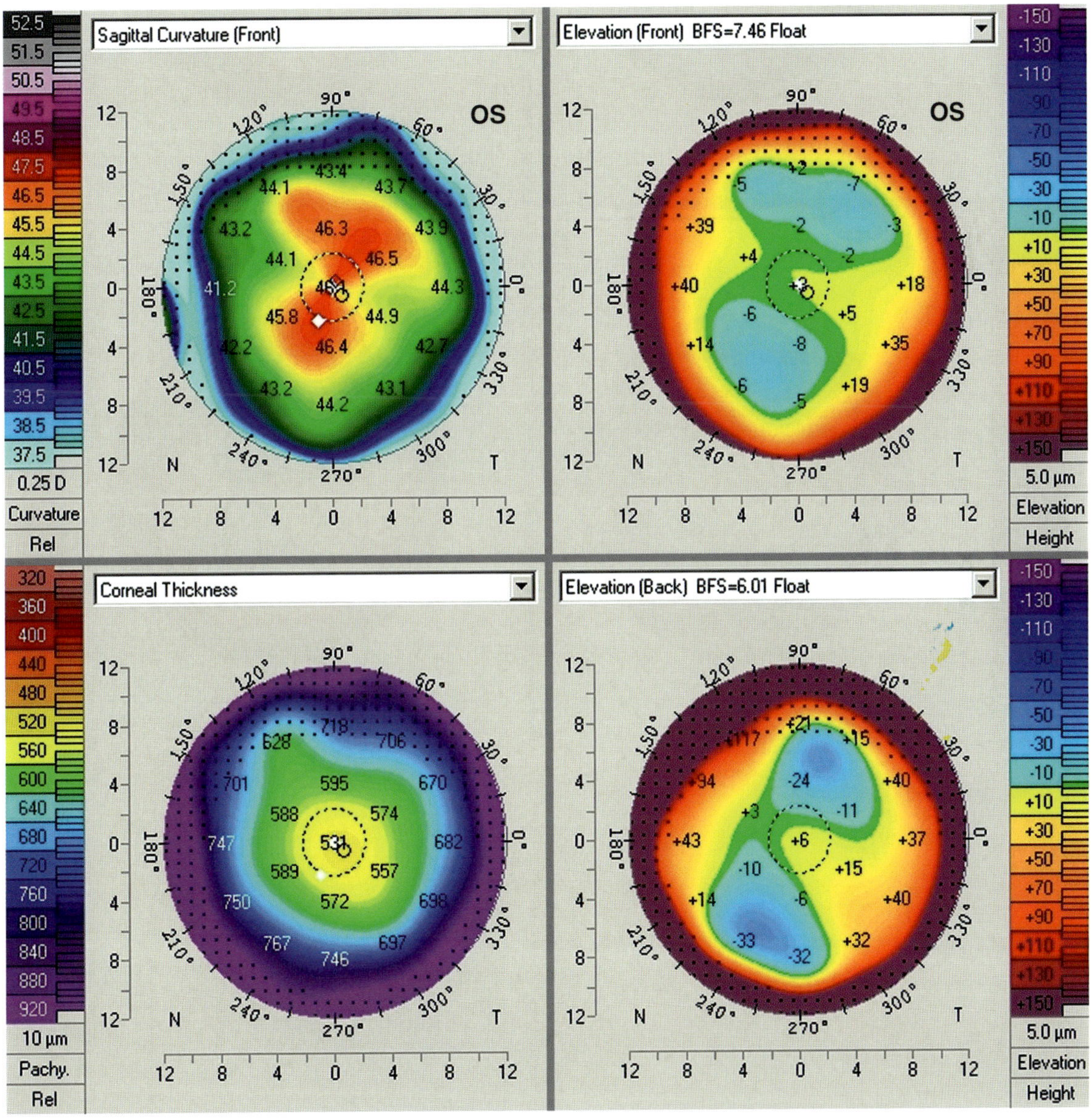

Fig. 2.39 Corneal topography of FFKC. (**a**) corneal topography of the left eye which is defined as having FFKC, (**b**) corneal topography of the right eye of the same patient, it is very irregular and can be considered KC, (**c**) corneal topography of the patient's brother who has frank KC

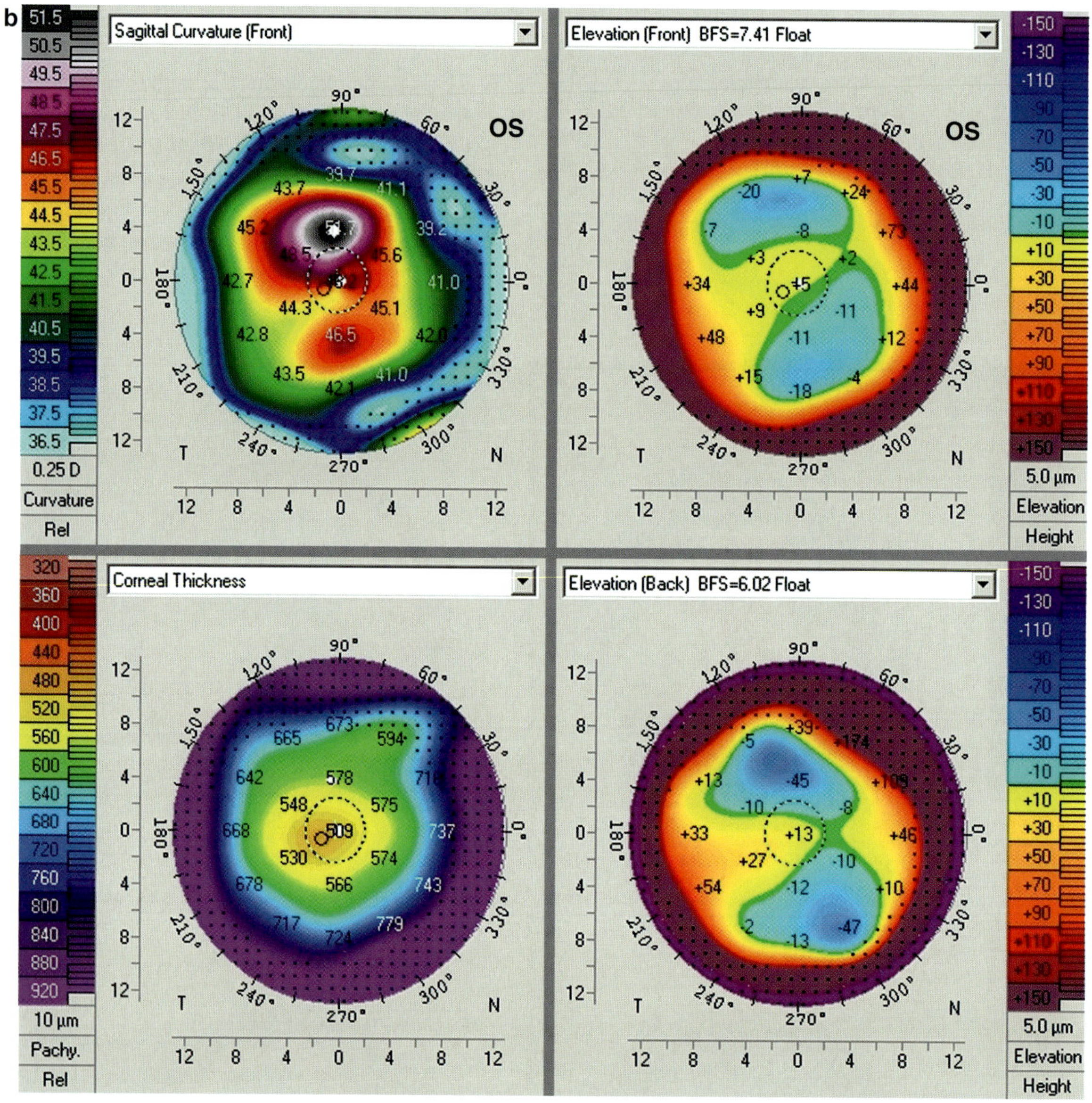

Fig. 2.39 (continued)

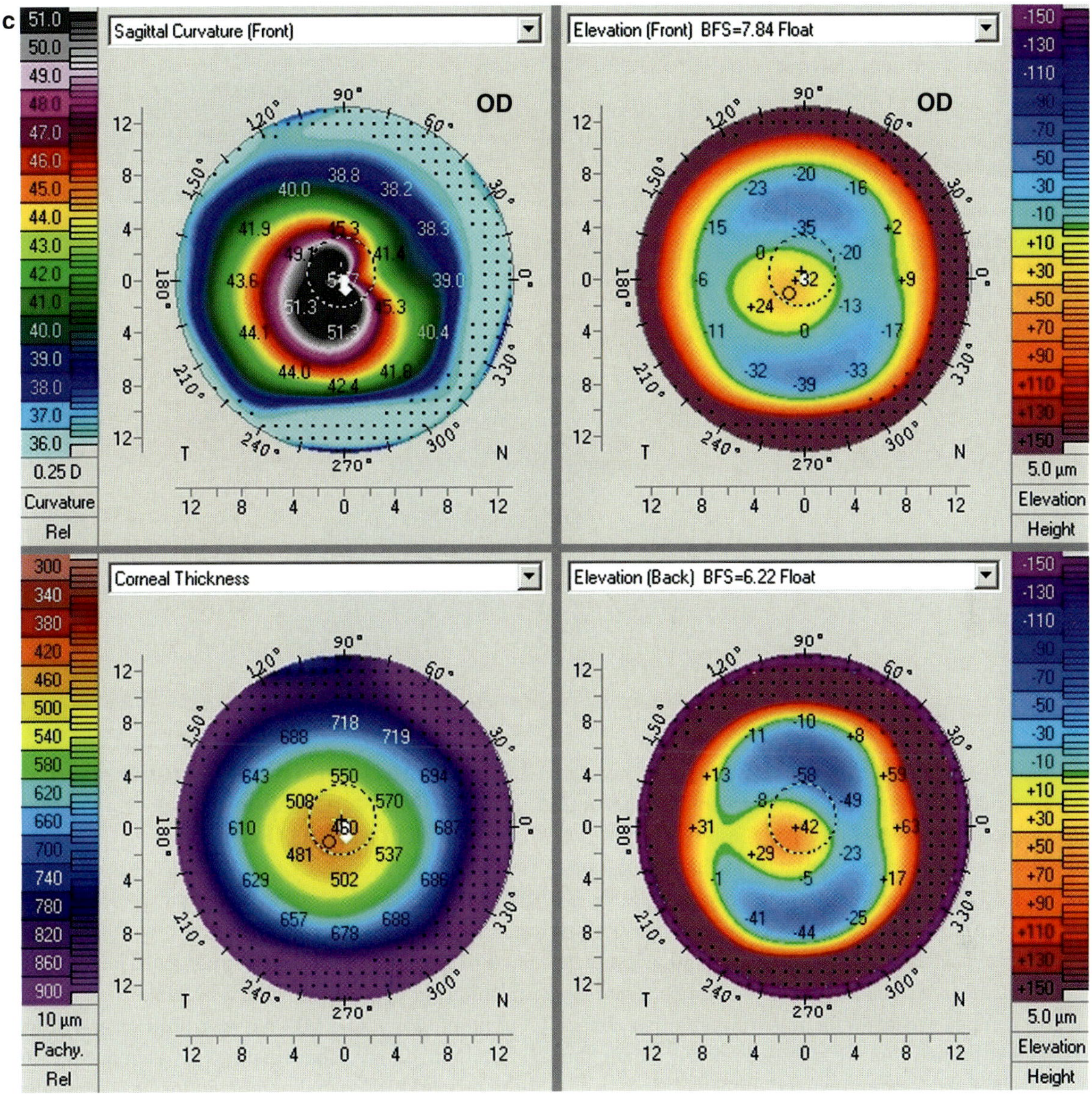

Fig. 2.39 (continued)

the right eye of the same patient, please note the abnormal and irregular cornea which can be considered as KC. Figure 2.39c is corneal topography of the right eye of the patient's brother, it is a frank KC. According to this definition, the left eye of the patient is FFKC.

2. FFKC is an abnormal cornea. Corneal topography or corneal hysteresis or both are abnormal; i.e., there are risk factors but the case is still not a clinically obvious KC. There are also two opinions regarding this definition:
   (a) The numerical values of topography and/or corneal hysteresis are in the suspected field (neither normal nor risky). Readers can refer to author's two books in corneal topography by Jaypee Highlight.
   (b) The shape of corneal topography is taken into consideration. Anterior tangential curvature map, relative pachymetry map, and posterior elevation maps are the key. The tangential map is the most sensitive for determining the geometry of the cornea. Unlike the sagittal map, curvatures on the tangential map are relative to the surface, not to the axial center of the surface. Thus, it shows the exact location of the nipple of the cone. The relative pachymetry map gives the thickness of the

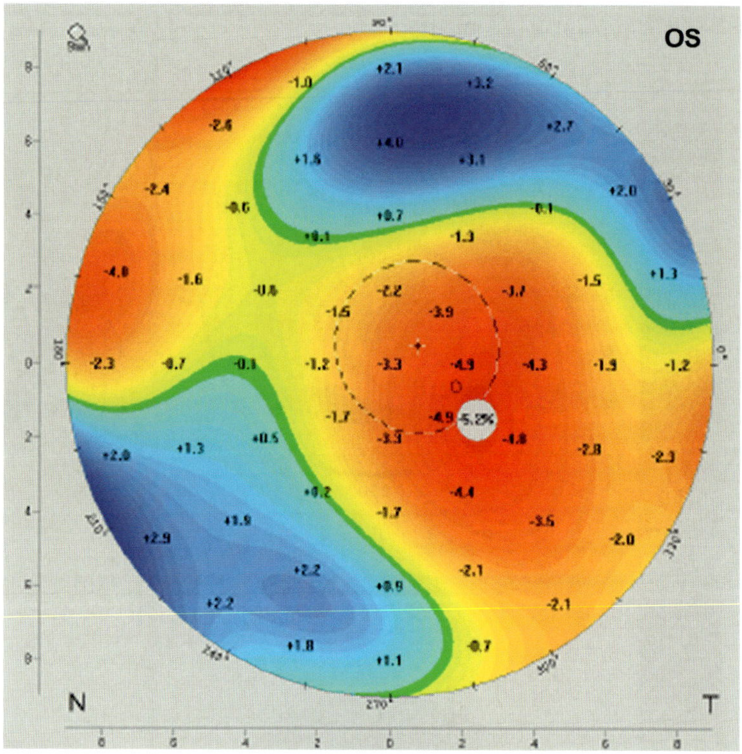

Fig. 2.40 The relative thickness map. Zero values mean that such points match those in the reference normative map. Positive values mean that such points are thicker than those in the reference normative map. Negative values mean that such points are thinner than those in the reference normative map. When the most negative point corresponds with the K-max point on the anterior tangential map and the highest point on the posterior elevation map (BFTE mode), it is FFKC

cornea at a given point relative to the normal thickness at that point as a percentage. For example: +5 and +8 points, i.e., these two points are thicker than the zero point by 5% and 8% respectively, and vice versa when the values are negative. A standard value study was carried out on untreated corneas to adopt the normal average values as a standard reference map. So, when the computer matches the relative map of an abnormal cornea with the standard reference map, the abnormal locations can be immediately noticed, especially when the cornea is keratoconic. A normal map would be 0% at all points. When there is an abnormal point, it appears with minus value on this map as shown in Fig. 2.40. The back elevation map values are more accurate when using the BFTE reference body rather than the BFS. It is of interest to note that the epithelium of the corneal anterior surface thins over the nipple, reducing the sensitivity of the diagnosis from the front surface alone. When the hot spot on the anterior tangential curvature map, relative pachymetry, and posterior elevation map using the toric ellipsoid are all at the same point, the diagnosis of FFKC is confirmed.

2.5 Pellucid Marginal Degeneration (PMD) and Pellucid-like Keratoconus (PLK)

PMD is a bilateral, non-inflammatory, peripheral corneal thinning disorder characterized by a peripheral band of thinning of the inferior cornea. The cornea in and adjacent to the thinned area is ectatic.

The etiology of PMD has not been clearly established, but collagen abnormalities, as seen in KC, have been reported. No racial preponderance has been identified. An equal distribution exists between the sexes. Patients usually are aged 20–40 years at the time of clinical presentation.

2.5.1 Clinical Findings

PMD is usually asymptomatic, except for the progressive deterioration in uncorrected and spectacle-corrected visual acuity caused by the irregular astigmatism induced by the corneal ectasia.

The thinned and presumably weakened cornea may protrude as a result of the positive intraocular pressure.

Episodes of corneal hydrops with resultant pain, as seen in KC, have been reported, but they occur only rarely.

Uncorrected visual acuity is often severely reduced. Visual acuity, as measured by using a pinhole, is close to normal. Refraction and keratometry show against-the-rule astigmatism. Visual acuity typically cannot be restored by using a spherocylindrical combination of lenses. Using rigid gas permeable (RGP) contact lenses are often required to achieve good Snellen acuity, but patients often experience glare and decreased contrast sensitivity despite this. It is unclear if this condition is due to the corneal disease or the contact lens wear.

Both eyes are usually affected, but the degree of involvement may be asymmetric.

Results of slitlamp examination are characterized by:

1. A peripheral band of thinning of the inferior cornea from the 4 o'clock position to the 8 o'clock position. This thinning is accompanied by 1–2 mm of normal cornea between the limbus and the area of thinning.
2. Corneal ectasia is most marked just central to the band of thinning. The central cornea is usually of normal thickness, and the epithelium overlying the area of thinning is intact.
3. The area of thinning typically is epithelialized, clear, avascular, and without lipid deposits.
4. On careful slitlamp evaluation, prominent lymphatics often are detected at the inferior limbus parallel to the area of thinning.
5. Vertical striations at the level of the Descemets' membrane (similar to the Vogt striae) may be seen in rare instances.
6. The light slit becomes very narrow abruptly in the inferior part of the cornea which is the hallmark of the disease (Fig. 2.41).
7. Fluorescein pattern with the RGP lens: there is an inferior touch between the cornea and the lens as shown in Fig. 2.42. In the same figure, the Placido rings are distributed in a vertically oriented oval due to the against-the-rule astigmatism. Note that the rings become very thin and close to each other in the inferior cornea while they are relatively broader and not crowded in the superior part of the cornea, this is due to the inferiorly displaced cone characterizing PMD.

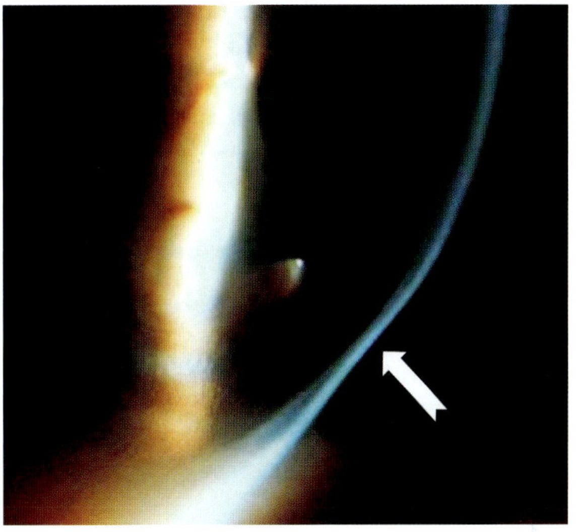

Fig. 2.41 Slitlamp view of PMD, the light slit becomes very narrow abruptly in the inferior part of the cornea (*white arrow*) which is the hallmark of the disease

2.5.2 Topographical Findings

Identifying features of PMD on corneal topography is very important. That is because there is some similarity between PMD and PLK on corneal topography especially in early stages of PMD. This similarity leads doctors to misinterpret PLK as PMD. Careful studying of the topography reveals many differences between these two entities. Features are mainly seen on the curvature, elevation and thickness maps, and on the keratoconus curve diagram.

- Curvature map: The anterior sagittal curvature map is extremely useful in detecting and diagnosing early disease, which may not be readily detectable on slitlamp evaluation. It shows low corneal power along the central vertical axis, increased power as the inferior cornea is approached, and high corneal power along the inferior oblique meridians. This topographical pattern takes a butterfly appearance, as shown in Fig. 2.43. These features are seen in both PMD and PLK.
- Elevation maps: There are two important things related to each others that can be identified on the elevation maps, mainly the anterior elevation map, the location of the cone and the "kissing birds" sign. Figure 2.44 shows the "kissing birds" sign. When the cone is peripheral, this sign is present; when the cone is central or paracentral, this sign is absent (Figs 2.44 and 2.45). This sign appears when the

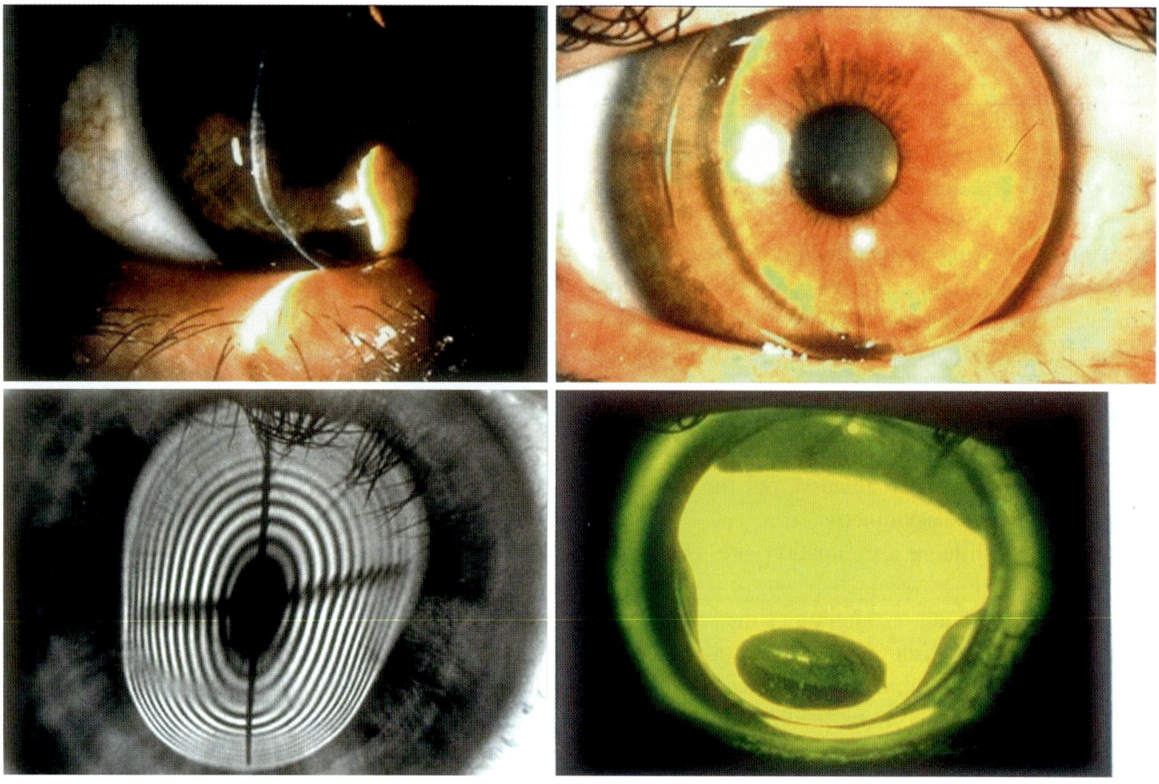

Fig. 2.42 PMD. The *upper left image* is the slitlamp view demonstrating the inferior thinning. The *upper right image* is an RGP lens. The *lower right image* is the fluorescein pattern, note the inferior touch. The *lower left image* is Placido image; note the vertical oval distribution of the mires

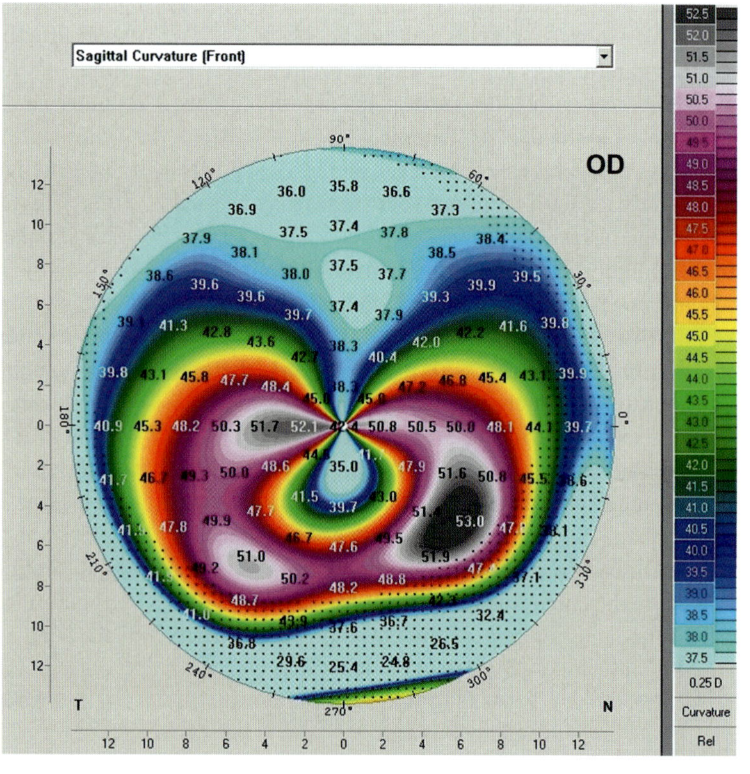

Fig. 2.43 Butterfly appearance of PMD and PLK on the anterior sagital curvature map. Corneal power is low along the central vertical axis, but it increases as the inferior cornea is approached

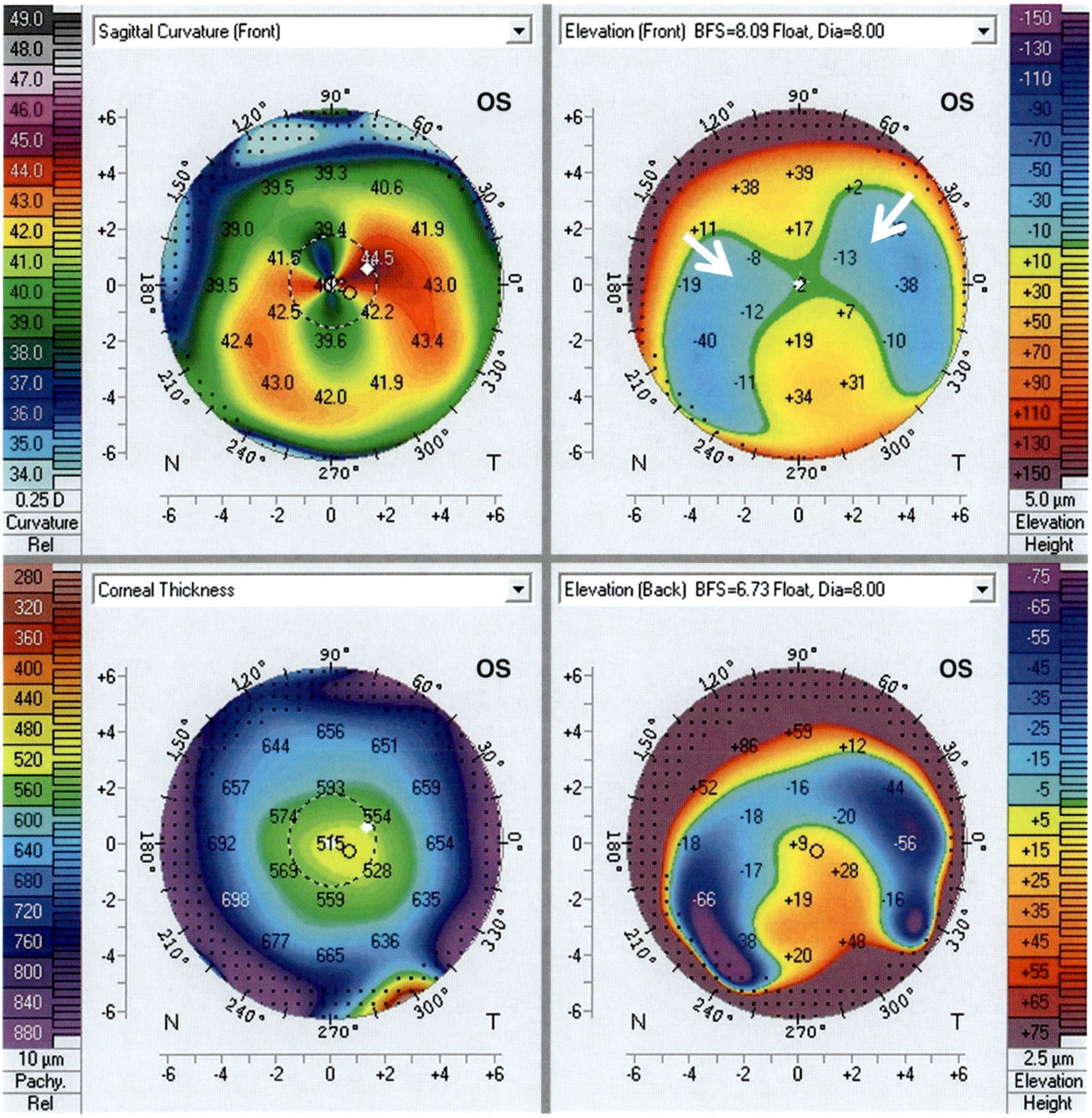

Fig. 2.44 The kissing birds sign on the anterior elevation map (*arrow heads*). This sign exists when the cone is peripheral

BFS float mode is used (Fig. 2.46), while it disappears when switching to the BFTE float mode (Fig. 2.47). On the other hand, there is no correlation between the cone location and the differentiation between PMD and PLK, i.e., the cone can be central, paracentral, or peripheral in both entities. Therefore, neither the kissing birds sign nor the peripheral cone is a hallmark of PMD. Figure 2.48 is a PMD case without the kissing birds sign; Fig. 2.49 is a PLK case with this sign.

- Corneal thickness map: Corneal thinning is a reversal of the typical pattern in which the cornea thickens from the center to the periphery. If any part of the peripheral cornea is thinner than the center, this is a cause for concern. In PMD, the corneal thickness map reveals a thinning of the inferior cornea. This thinning is characterized by a special sign that can be called "bell" shape (Fig. 2.50). This sign is a hallmark of PMD; it is absent in PLK. In regard with the location of the thinnest point of the cornea, theoretically, the thinnest point should be inferiorly displaced in PMD and in KC, but the amount of displacement on *Y* coordinate is much bigger in PMD especially in advanced cases (Figs. 2.51 and

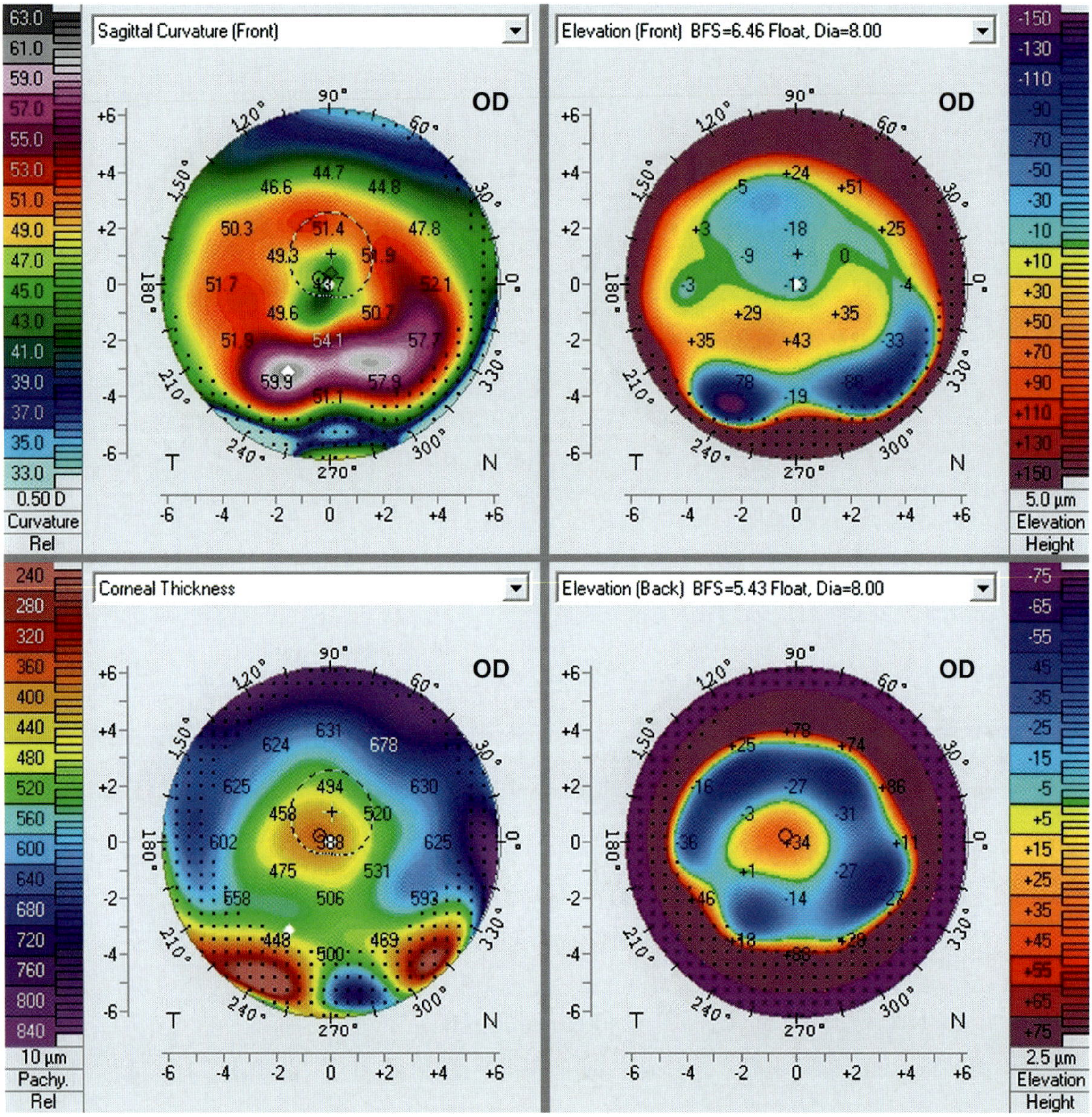

Fig. 2.45 The kissing birds sign. It does not exist when the cone is central or paracentral

2.52: white arrows). This is not always true. In very advanced PMD, the cornea is severely distorted, and the topographers may miss many data from the inferior part of the cornea and may display a proposed plotting with dark dots indicating that an important part of the data is missing in this area. Figure 2.53 is a PMD case as it appears on the slit lamp; notice the very thin area in the inferior cornea and the bulging above. Figure 2.54a and b are the vertical sector of the Scheimpflug image of the same cornea; notice the very thin inferior part (white arrow). Figure 2.55 is the topography of the case; surprisingly, the thinnest location is relatively not displaced (red arrows), but if we look at the inferior part of the thickness map (black arrow), relatively black dots are present. This point is very important when concerning intracorneal rings or corneal grafts as will be discussed later in details.

- Keratoconus Curve Diagram: This curve is an indicator of the gradual change in thickness beginning

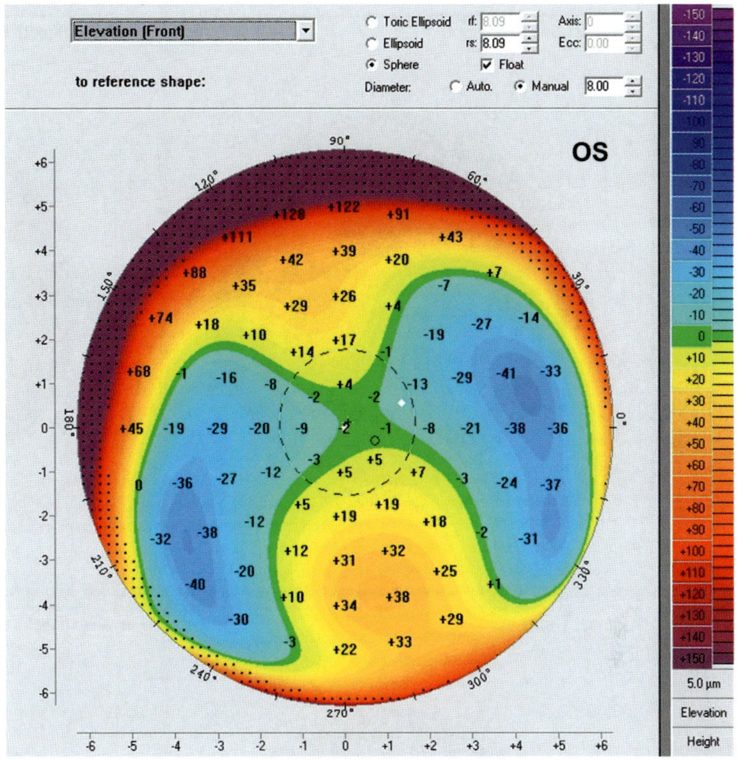

Fig. 2.46 The kissing birds sign. It can be seen when the BFS mode is used

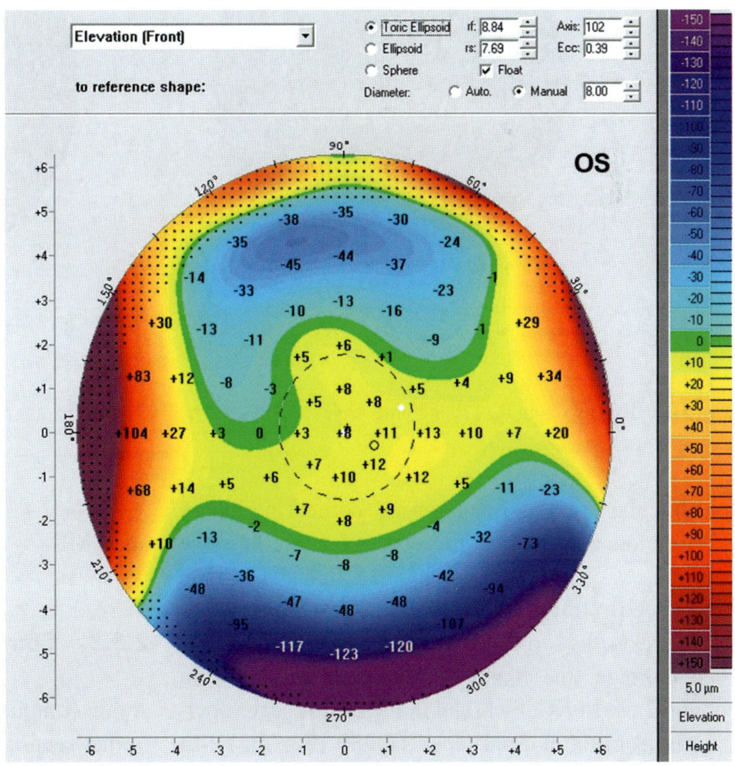

Fig. 2.47 The kissing birds sign. It cannot be seen when the BFTE mode is used

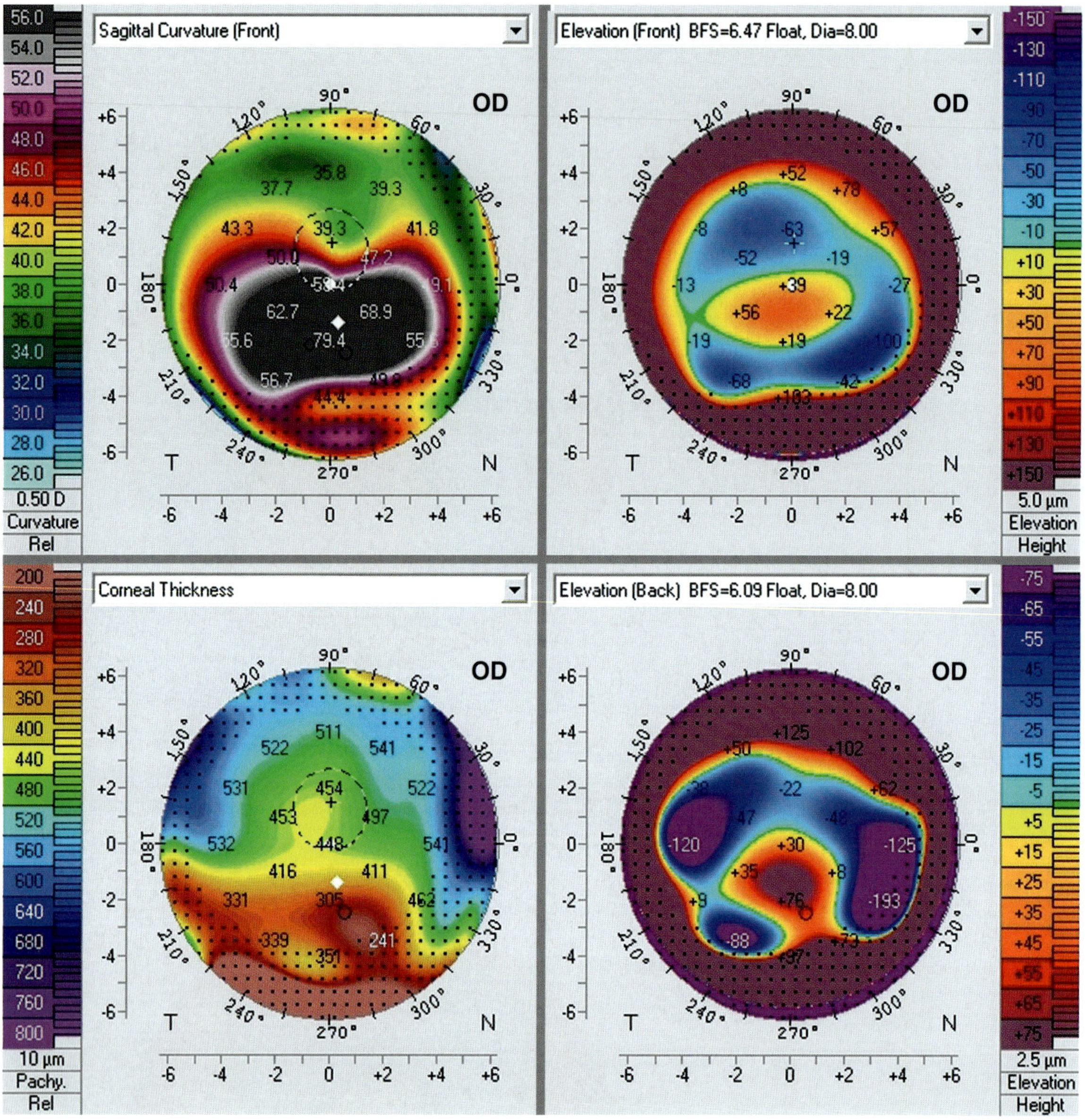

Fig. 2.48 PMD without the kissing birds sign

from the thinnest point toward corneal periphery (for more details about this curve please refer to the book: "Corneal Topography in Clinical Practice, Jaypee Brothers, 2009). In normal corneas, the red line takes the same slope of and lies within the normal range (the black dotted lines) as shown in Fig. 2.56. In KC, PLK and in PMD, this curve deviates from the normal range rapidly (Fig. 2.57). In advanced cases of PMD, the curve usually takes an inverted passage (Fig. 2.58).

Table 2.2 summarizes the difference between PLK and PMD.

2.5.3 Complications

A rare complication in PMD is corneal hydrops similar to that seen in KC, with disruption of the endothelial basement membrane and hydration of the adjacent corneal stroma.

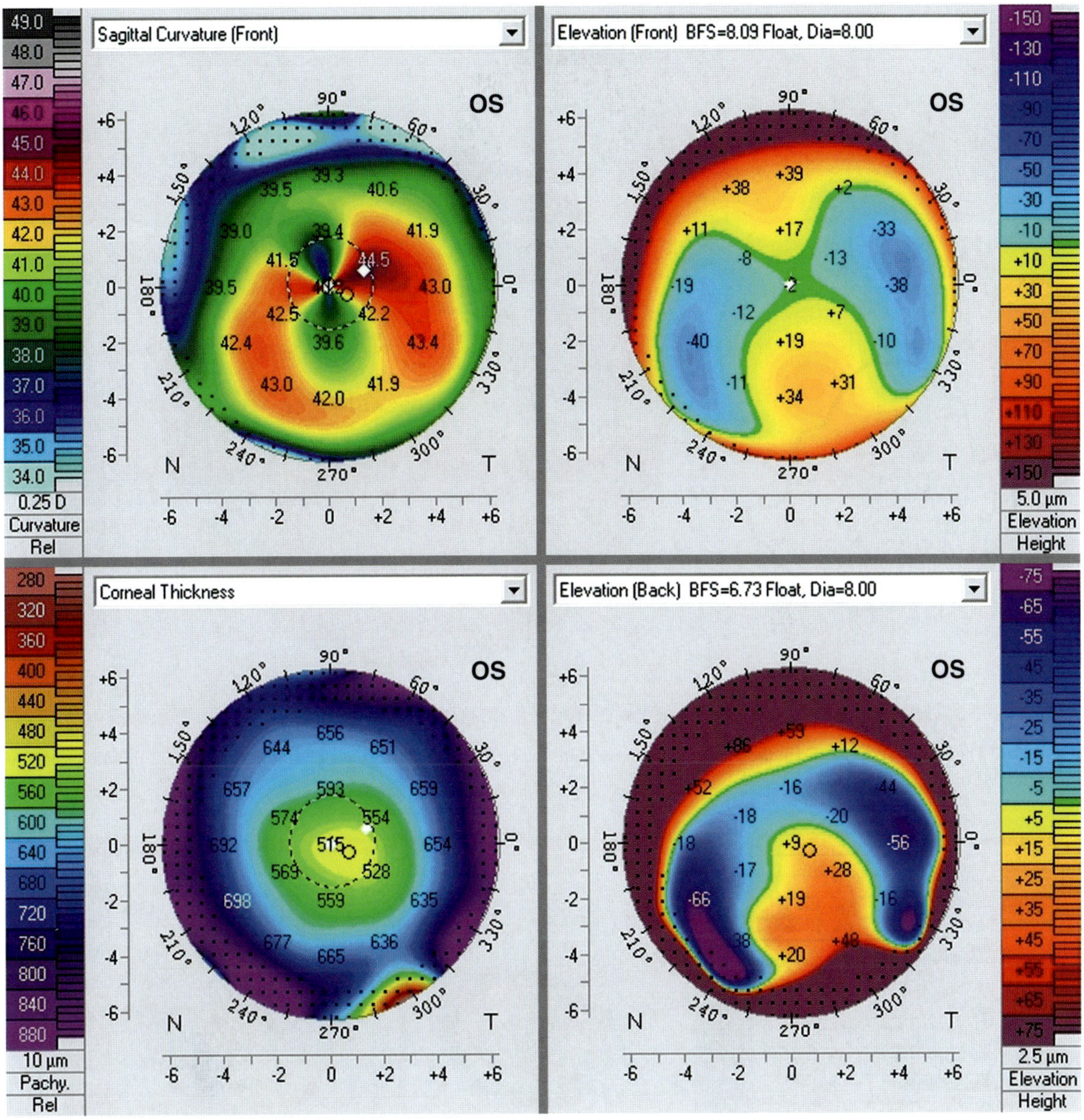

Fig. 2.49 PLK with the kissing birds sign

2.5.4 Differential Diagnosis

1. Keratoglobus: It is a generalized thinning of the cornea (Figs. 2.59 and 2.60).
   - The thinning is most marked at the limbus, extending circumferentially for 360°; this makes it different from the globus morphological pattern of the KC.
   - The whole cornea protrudes, in contrast to the regional thinning seen in KC and the inferior paralimbal thinning in PMD.
2. Terrien marginal degeneration: It affects an age group similar to that affected by PMD (Fig. 2.61).
   - Terrien marginal degeneration can be bilateral.
   - Although this condition can be associated with large amounts of astigmatism, it can be differentiated from PMD because the superior cornea is predominantly affected and because the area of thinning is often associated with vascularization and lipid deposition.

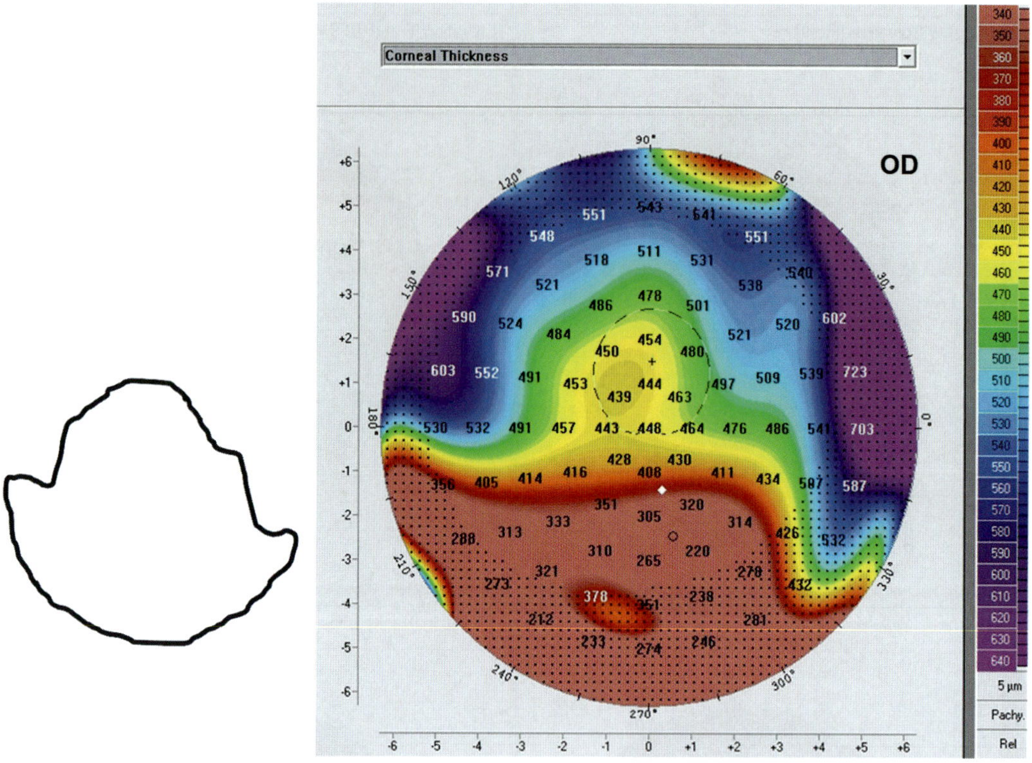

Fig. 2.50 The hallmark of PMD on the corneal thickness map: the bell sign. This sign is due to inferior corneal thinning encountered in PMD

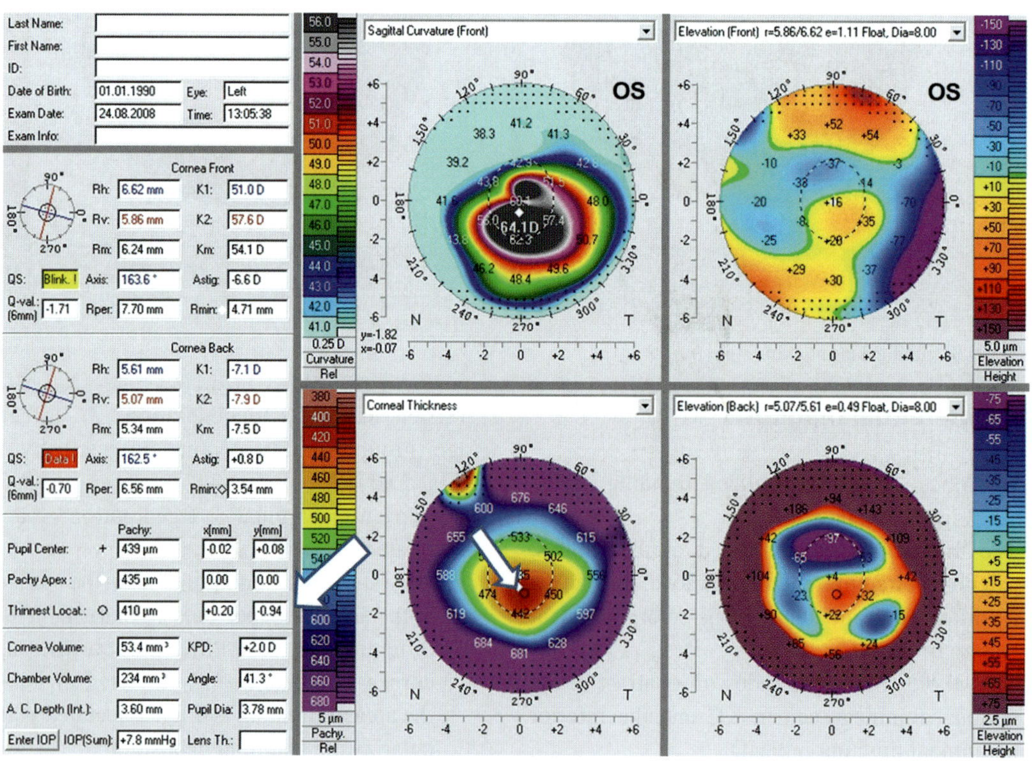

Fig. 2.51 Vertical displacement of the thinnest point on the corneal thickness map in KC. The *white arrows* point at the symbol of the thinnest location and at the value of displacement on the *Y* axis

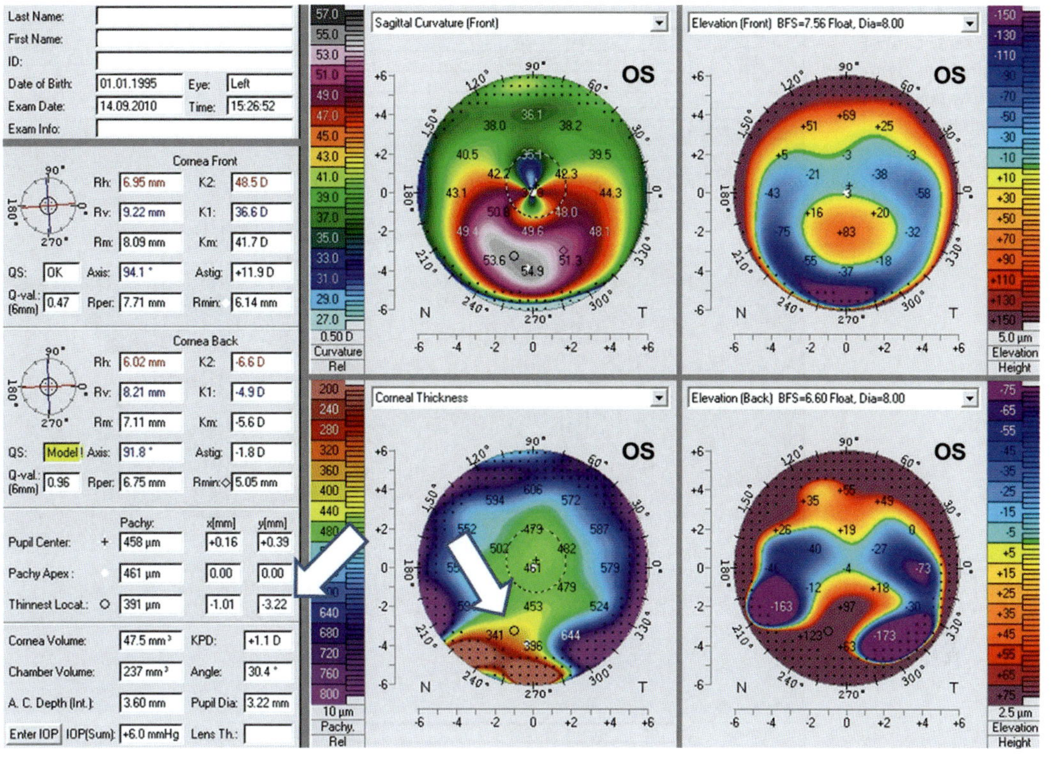

Fig. 2.52 Vertical displacement of the thinnest point on the corneal thickness map in PMD. The *white arrows* point at the symbol of the thinnest location and at the value of displacement on the *Y* axis

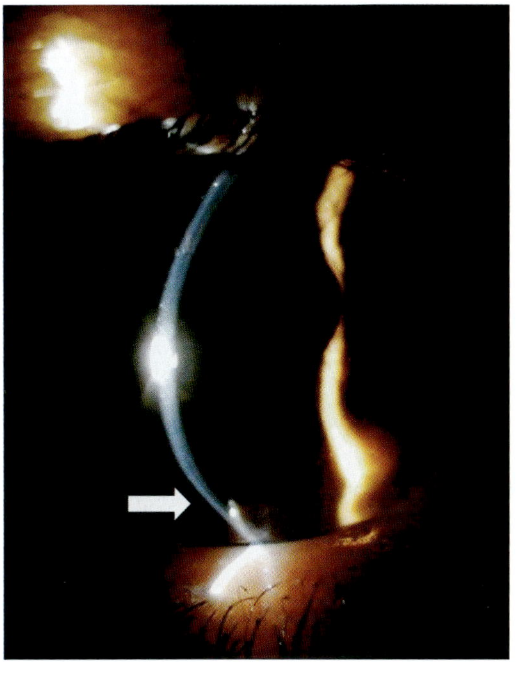

Fig. 2.53 Slitlamp view of a case of PMD. The *white arrow* points at the inferior thin area

3. Furrow degeneration: It has some features of PMD (Fig. 2.62).
   - An intact epithelium is present, and the area of corneal thinning is not vascularized, at least in the acute phase.
   - The differentiating feature is that the area of thinning is closer to the limbus with virtually no intervening zone of normal cornea, unlike the findings in PMD.
   - Furrow degeneration occasionally involves the superior cornea, and an associated adjacent area of scleritis may be present.
   - Edges of the furrow are steeper than the gradual attenuation seen in PMD.
   - Furrow degeneration occurs adjacent to the lipid deposition in arcus senilis, which is typically observed in elderly patients.
   - May be associated with systemic diseases such as rheumatoid arthritis, systemic lupus erythematosus, polyarteritis nodosa, or other collagen vascular diseases.

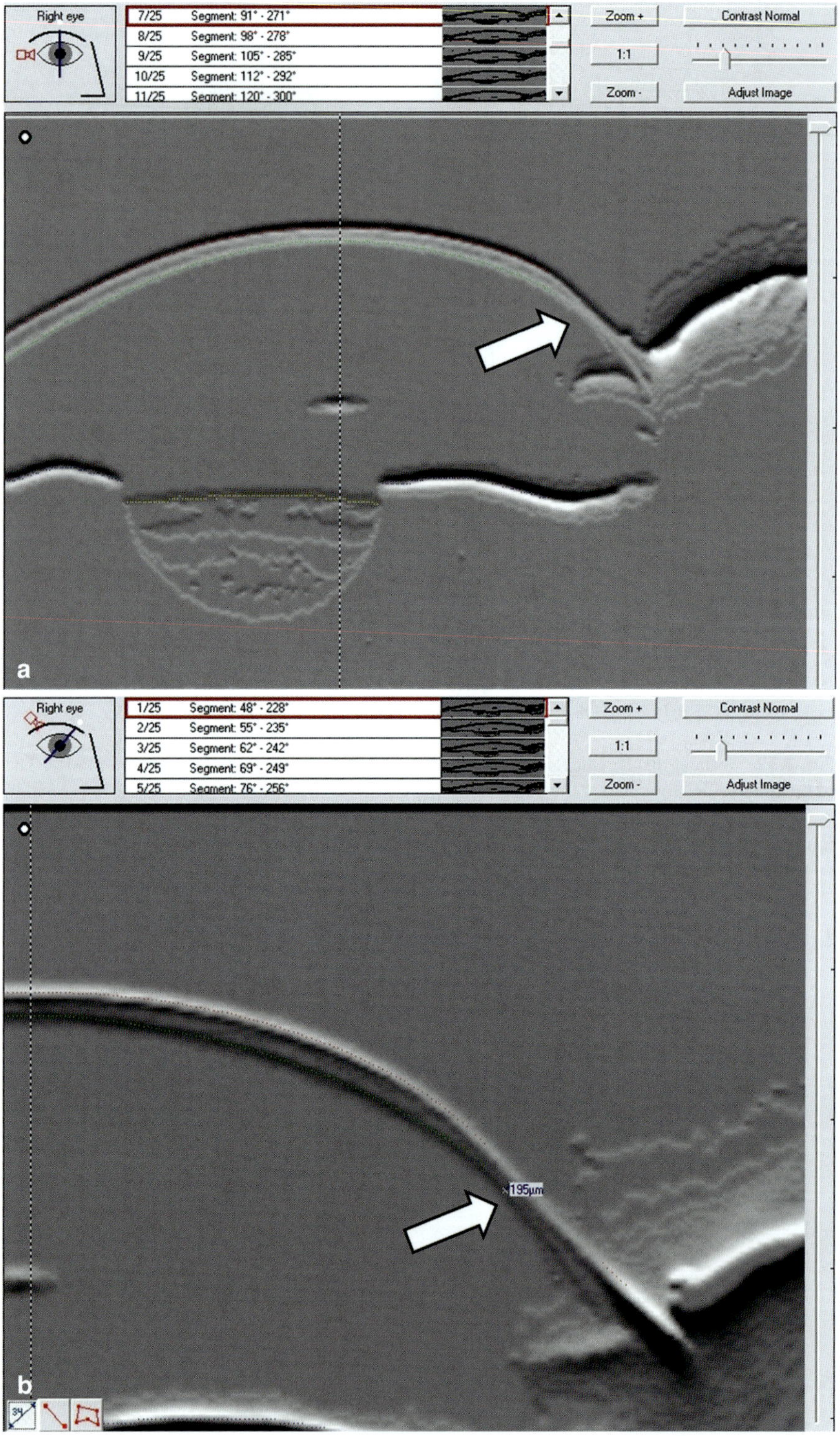

Fig. 2.54 (**a**, **b**) Scheimpflug images of the same case of PMD in the previous figure. The white arrow points at the inferior thin area

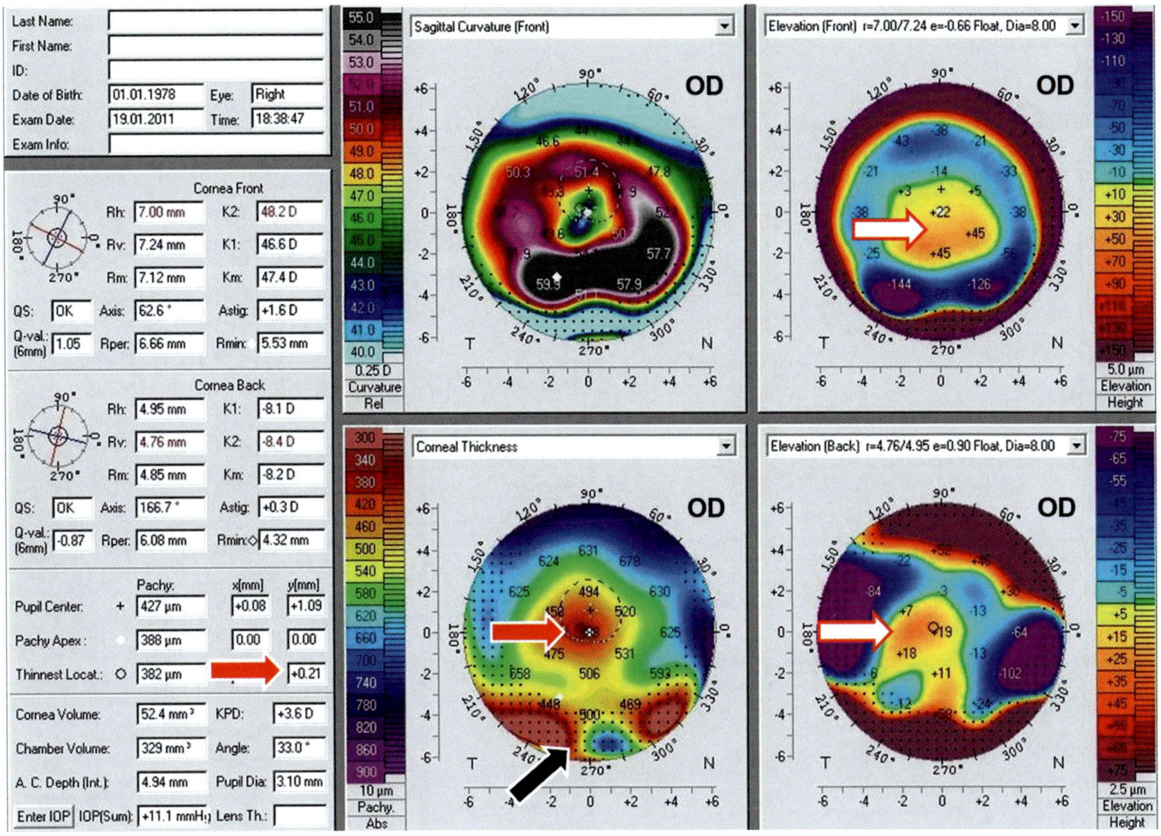

Fig. 2.55 Corneal topography of the same case in the previous figures. Although there is an inferior thin area, the thinnest point is plotted centrally (*red arrows*). The *black arrow* points at the proposed dotted inferior area. Note the bell sign

4. Peripheral corneal melting disorders, such as Mooren ulcer, or peripheral melting secondary to rheumatologic disorders are characterized by pain.
   - This pain may be severe in cases of Mooren ulcer.
   - Associated findings include an epithelial defect over the area of thinning and corneal vascularization adjacent to the area of thinning in the acute phase.
5. Contact lens-induced warping of the cornea can mimic the appearance of PMD and PLK on corneal topography. History of prolonged usage of contact lenses and recapturing corneal topography after proper stop of usage will retain corneal regularity and hence differentiates the case from PMD and PLK.

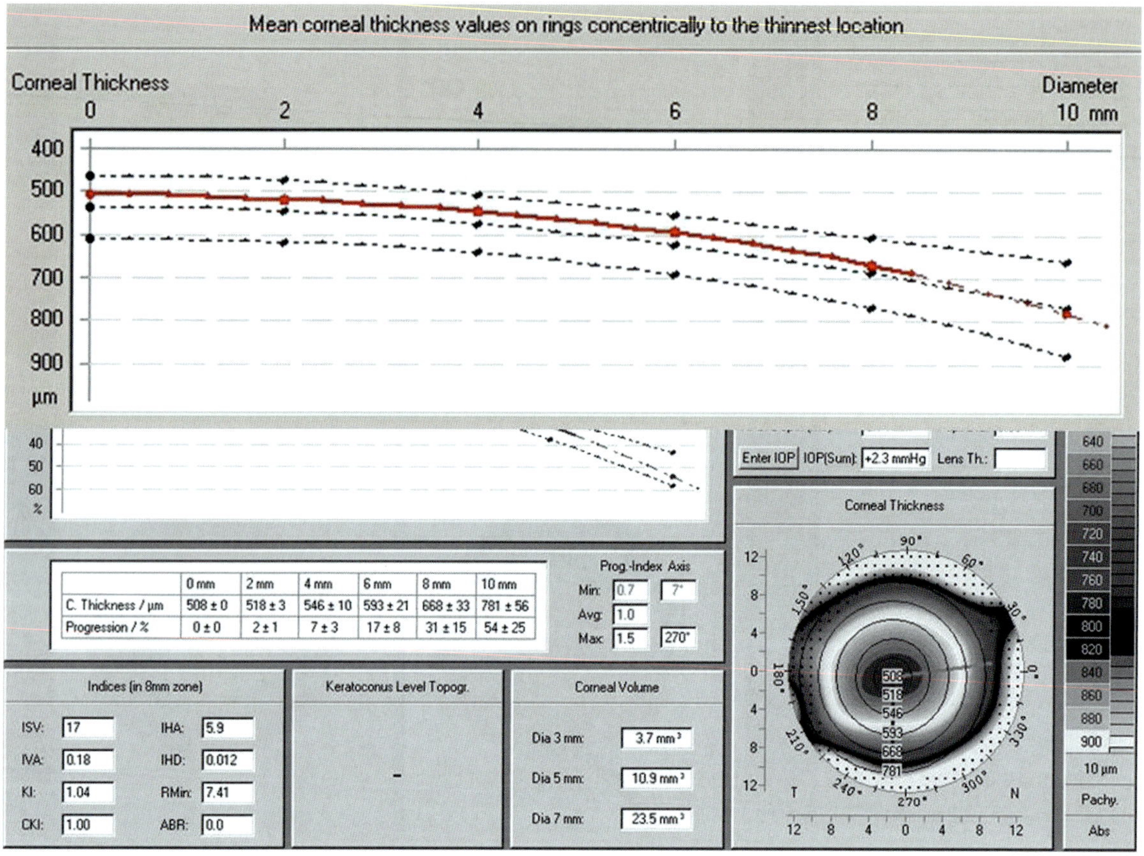

Fig. 2.56 Normal keratoconus curve diagram. The *red line* (patient's data) is consistent with and lies within the normative data range

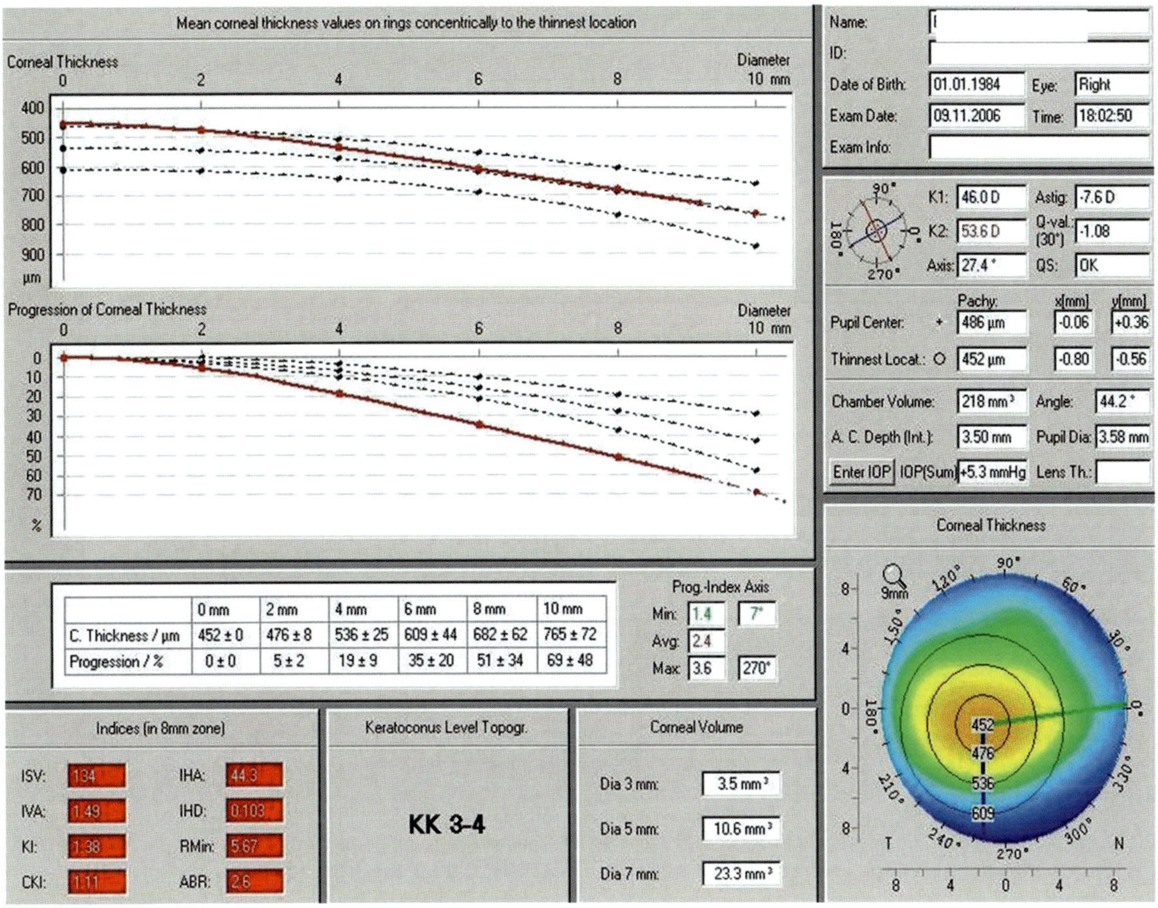

	0 mm	2 mm	4 mm	6 mm	8 mm	10 mm
C. Thickness / µm	452 ± 0	476 ± 8	536 ± 25	609 ± 44	682 ± 62	765 ± 72
Progression / %	0 ± 0	5 ± 2	19 ± 9	35 ± 20	51 ± 34	69 ± 48

Fig. 2.57 Keratoconus curve diagram in a KC case. The *red line* is out of the normal range and does not take the same slope of it

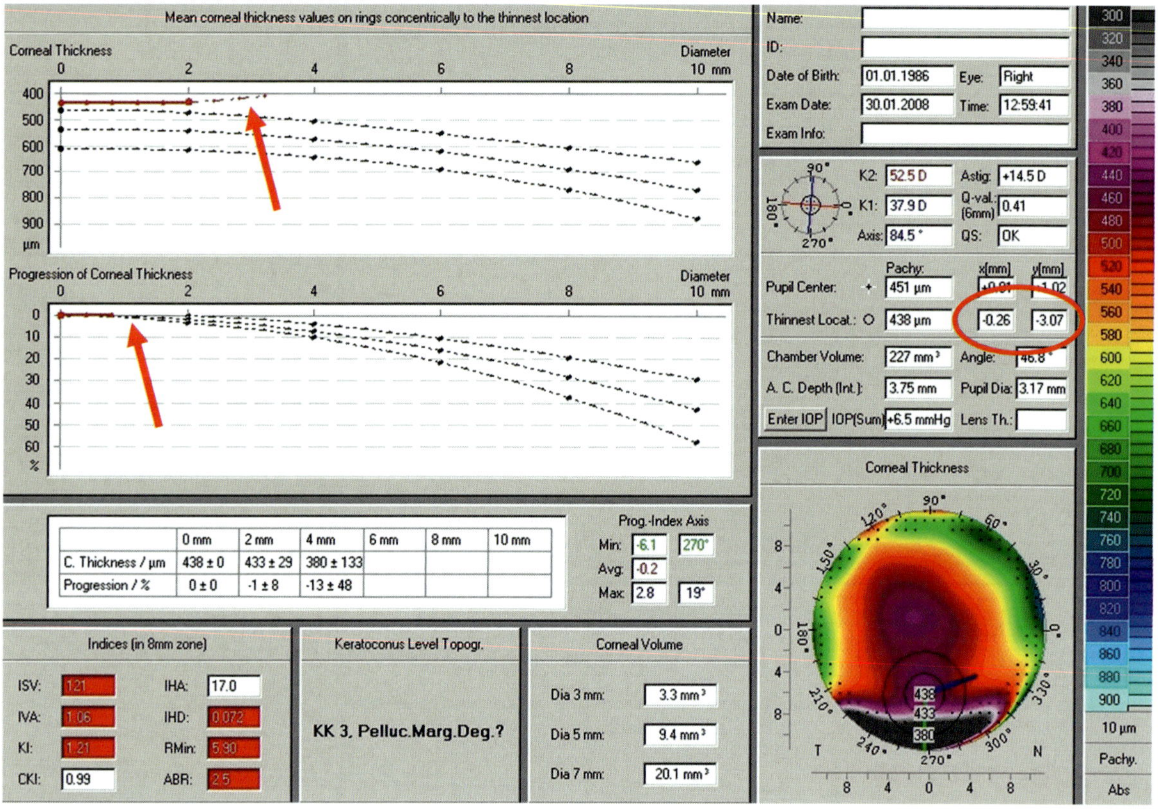

Fig. 2.58 Keratoconus curve diagram in an advanced case of PMD. The *red line* is out of the normal range and inverted superiorly (*red arrows*). Notice the big displacement of the thinnest location especially on the Y axis (red circle)

Table 2.2 Comparison between PLK and PMD

		PLK	PMD
Nature		Central or paracentral ectasia	Peripheral ectasia
Age of presentation		Early teens	20–40
Slitlamp and Scheimpflug image		Central or paracentral thinning	Inferior peripheral thinning
Curvature map		Butterfly	Butterfly
Elevation maps	Cone	Central or paracentral cone	Central, paracentral, or inferior peripheral cone
	Kissing birds	Present occasionally	Present in early and moderate cases
Thickness map	"Bell" sign	Absent	Present in moderate and advanced cases
	Thinnest location	May be displaced	Usually largely displaced
Keratoconus curve diagram		Deviated	Deviated and usually inverted in advanced cases

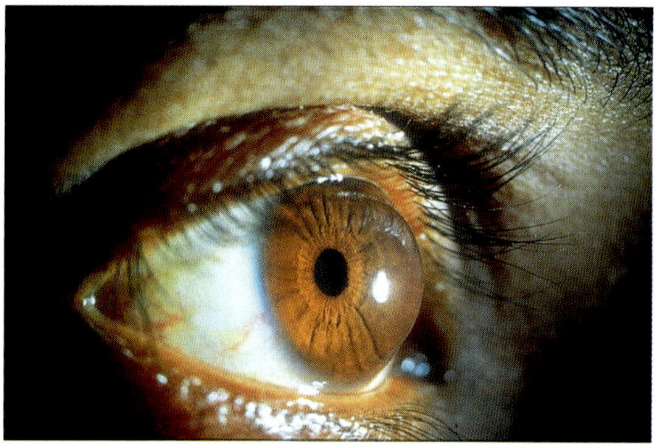

Fig. 2.59 Keratoglobus. A generalized bulging and thinning of the cornea

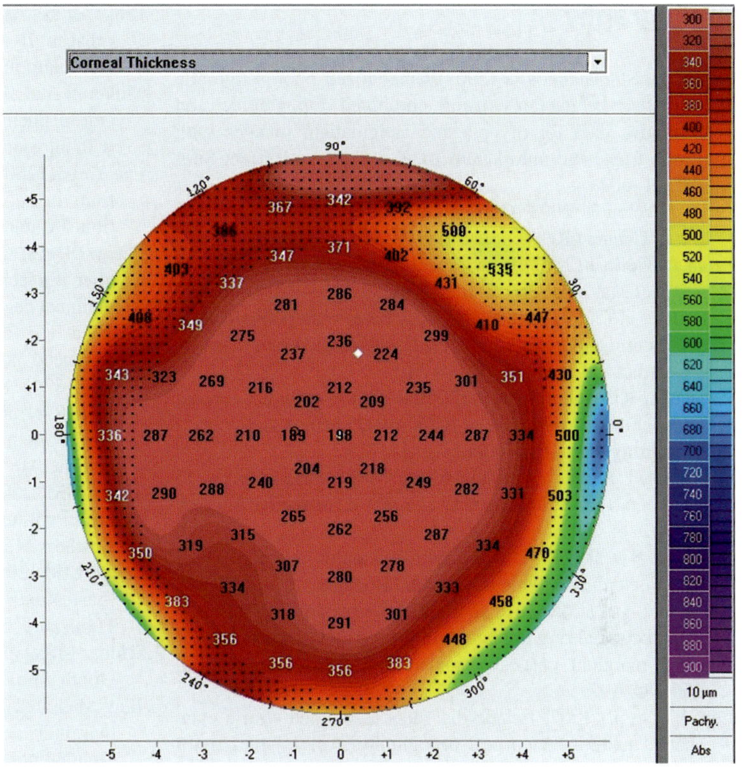

Fig. 2.60 The corneal thickness map in keratoglobus. Note the generalized thinning including the limbal part of the cornea, which differentiates between keratoglobus and the globus morphological pattern of keratoconus

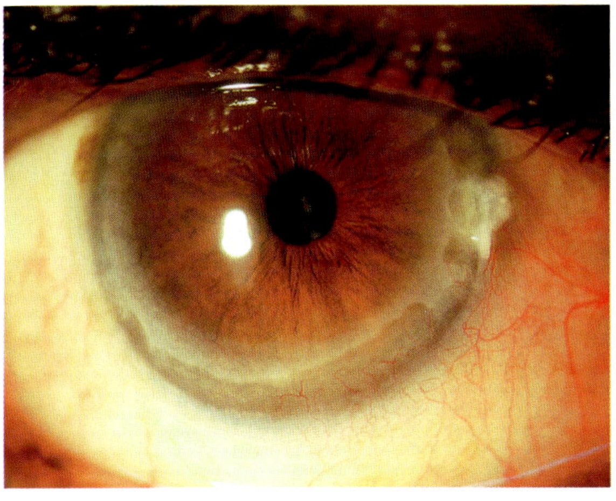

Fig. 2.61 Terrien marginal degeneration. Note the lipid deposition

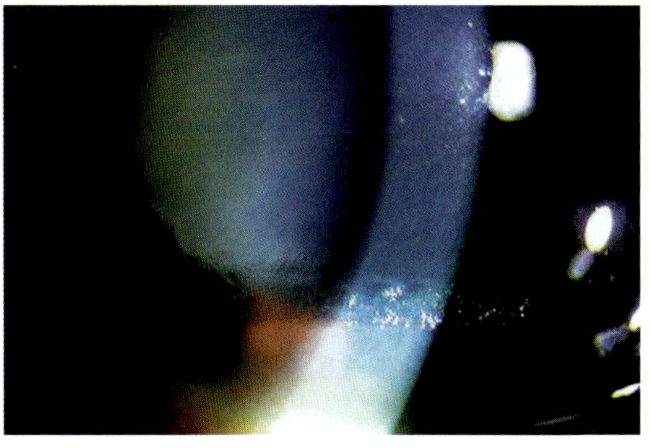

Fig. 2.62 Furrow degeneration

Bibliography

Alpins N, Stamatelatos G (2007) Customized photoastigmatic refractive keratectomy using combined topographic and refractive data for myopia and astigmatism in eyes with forme fruste and mild keratoconus. J Cataract Refract Surg 33:591–602

Colin J, Velou S (2003) Current surgical options for keratoconus. J Cataract Refract Surg 29:379–386

Ertan A, Colin J (2007) Intracorneal rings for keratoconus and keratectasia. J Cataract Refract Surg 33:1303–1314

Fogla R et al (2003) Keratectasia in 2 cases with pellucid marginal corneal degeneration after laser in situ keratomileusis. J Cataract Refract Surg 29:788–791

Gruenauer-Kloevekorn C et al (2006) Pellucid marginal corneal degeneration: evaluation of the corneal surface and contact lens fitting. Br J Ophthalmol 90:318–323

Holladay JT (2008). Detecting forme fruste keratoconus with the Pentacam. Supplement to cataract & refractive surgery today Feb: 11,12

Karimian F et al (2008) Topographic evaluation of relatives of patients with keratoconus. Cornea 27:874–878

Kubaloglu A et al (2010) A single 210-degree arc length intrastromal corneal ring implantation for the management of pellucid marginal corneal degeneration. Am J Ophthalmol 150:185–192

Lee WW et al (2007) Ectatic disorders associated with a claw shaped pattern on corneal topography. Am J Ophthalmol 144:154–156

Lim L et al (2007) Evaluation of keratoconus in asians: role of orbscan II and tomey TMS-2 corneal topography. Am J Ophthalmol 143:390–400

Mularoni A et al (2005) Conservative treatment of early and moderate pellucid marginal degeneration. A new refractive approach with intracorneal rings. Ophthalmology 112:660–666

Oie Y et al (2008) Characteristics of ocular higher-order aberrations in patients with pellucid marginal corneal degeneration. J Cataract Refract Surg 34:1928–1934

Piñero DP et al (2009) Refractive and corneal aberrometric changes after intracorneal ring implantation in corneas with pellucid marginal degeneration. Ophthalmology 116:1656–1664

Rasheed K, Rabinowitz YS (2000) Surgical treatment of advanced pellucid marginal degeneration. Ophthalmology 107:1836–1840

Santo MR et al (1999) Corneal topography in asymptomatic family members of a patient with pellucid marginal degeneration. Am J Ophthalmol 127:205–207

Sinjab MM (2009) Corneal topography in clinical practice (pentacam system): basics and clinical interpretation. Jaypee Brothers Medical Publishers, New Delhi

Sinjab MM (2010) Step by step reading pentacam topography (basics and case study series). Jaypee-Highlights Medical Publishers, New Delhi

Sridhar MS et al (2004) Pellucid marginal corneal degeneration. Ophthalmology 111:1102–1107

Tang M et al (2005) Characteristics of keratoconus and pellucid marginal degeneration in mean curvature maps. Am J Ophthalmol 140:993–1001

3 Management of Keratoconus

3.1 Introduction

Management of KC has advanced during the last few years and still in progress. As there are new modalities of treatment, it is better to say that there are traditional modalities and modern modalities of treatment rather than saying old and new. That is because the old modalities such as spectacle correction, contact lenses, penetrating keratoplasty (PKP), and conductive keratoplasty is still used although the demand upon the last two modalities has been decreased by the modern alternatives. In this chapter, there will be a high concentration on the main two modern modalities of treatment: the intracorneal rings (ICRs) and the corneal collagen cross-linking (CxL). These treatment modalities are relatively new and caution should be taken when taking the decision to use them and the surgeon should be aware of their indications, contraindications, conditions, and complications, hence the aim of this book.

3.2 Management Modalities

KC treatment modalities can be divided into interventional and noninterventional.

3.2.1 Noninterventional Managements

Noninterventional managements include spectacle correction and the very advanced technology of contact lenses.

3.2.1.1 Spectacle Correction

In very early cases of KC, spectacles can suffice to correct for the regular astigmatism and the very low amounts of irregular astigmatism. But in moderate cases, spectacles may still be the best choice when the case is stable and the refractive error, and quality and quantity of vision are reasonable.

3.2.1.2 Contact Lenses

As the condition progresses, spectacles may no longer provide the patient with a satisfactory degree of visual acuity. Once the cylindrical power increases beyond 4.0 dpt, visual intolerance may occur at which time contact lenses are needed. Contact lenses provide a regular refracting surface over the cone by means of tear fluid filling the gap between the irregular corneal surface and the smooth regular inner surface of the lens, thereby creating the effect of a smoother cornea.

Traditionally, contact lenses for KC have been the "hard" or rigid gas-permeable variety, although manufacturers have also produced specialized "soft" or hydrophilic lenses. A soft lens has a tendency to conform to the conical shape of the cornea, thus diminishing its effect. To counter this, hybrid lenses have been developed which are hard in the center and encompassed by a soft skirt. Soft or hybrid lenses do not however prove effective for every patient. Recently, newer soft lenses developed for KC have had successes to a good extent.

Some patients also find good vision correction and comfort with a "piggyback" lens combination, in which RGP lenses are worn over soft lenses, both providing a

M.M. Sinjab, *Quick Guide to the Management of Keratoconus*,
DOI 10.1007/978-3-642-21840-8_3, © Springer-Verlag Berlin Heidelberg 2012

degree of vision correction. One form of piggyback lens makes use of a soft lens with a countersunk central area to accept the rigid lens. Fitting a piggyback lens combination requires experience on the part of the lens fitter, and tolerance on the part of the keratoconic patient.

However, advances in both lens designs and materials have greatly increased the proportion of KC patients who can be fitted with contact lenses. The following types of contact lenses are used:

(a) Standard, large diameter (9.7), RGP.
(b) Aspherical lenses for moderate nipple cones.
(c) Small steep lenses for moderate-to-severe nipple cones.
(d) Specially designed lenses for steep oval and globus cones when standard spherical lenses have failed.
(e) Gas-permeable preformed scleral lenses can be tried in extremely distorted corneas. These lenses cover a greater proportion of the surface of the eye and hence can offer improved stability and comfort. They also vault over the cornea and so minimize any trauma being placed on it. The larger size of the lenses may make them unappealing or awkward to use for some people at first; however, their easier handling can find favor with patients after they have had some practice with using them. Traditionally, Scleral Lenses have been offered in KC cases so advanced that a transplant is the only option, but increasingly they are being successfully used for lower grades of KC where there are problems with corneal contact lens intolerance

In addition to the therapeutic use of contact lenses, they play a very important role in the diagnostic procedure in KC management; when there is no significant difference between uncorrected visual acuity (UCVA) and best spectacle-corrected visual acuity (BSCVA), for example: UCVA = 0.2 and BSCVA = 0.3, two causes should be put in mind: either amblyopia or high order aberrations (HOAs). To distinguish between these two causes, an RGP lens is used and the best corrected visual acuity is measured over the lens. When amblyopia is the reason, no significant improvement will be found. Trial of RGP gives us an impression of the expected visual outcome and visual prognosis when interventional procedures are needed.

3.2.2 Interventional Procedures

3.2.2.1 Conductive Keratoplasty (CK)

It is using heat to alter the curvature of the cornea. It was first used to treat hyperopia. CK uses a low-energy radiofrequency current to heat the peripheral cornea. This results in shrinkage of the peripheral stromal collagen, and therefore flattens the peripheral cornea, and steepens the central cornea.

In KC, CK is applied on the flat axis to steepen this axis and to decrease astigmatism (Fig. 3.1). It can be applied either symmetrically or asymmetrically according to corneal irregular astigmatism.

CK is generally only a temporary measure, because re-steepening usually ensue, therefore it can be combined with CxL to stabilize the results. On the other hand, the results are not always predictable because there are many factors playing a role in this field, the most important of which is the widely variable tissue response to thermal treatment. In other words, this procedure can be considered of historical interest.

3.2.2.2 Penetrating Keratoplasty

Between 10% and 25% of cases of KC progress to the point where visual rehabilitation is no longer possible, especially in those who present at a young age (younger than 20) and with keratometry measurements > 60 dpt and/or corneal thickness < 400 μ at the thinnest location.

In the past, such patients have had only one realistic surgical option: a full thickness corneal transplant or penetrating keratoplasty. KC is one of the most common indications for penetrating keratoplasty accounting for around 15–25% of such surgeries.

As the cornea is avascular, the donor and host do not have to be tissue matched and eye banks – after checking for communicable diseases and tissue quality – can provide suitable tissue within a few days or weeks. Following surgery, visual recovery typically takes several weeks/months, with full stabilization often taking up to a year after which time the sutures can be removed.

Corneal transplantation in KC is considered relatively low risk, in terms of graft rejection and other postoperative complications, as these eyes do not typically exhibit corneal neovascularization and other ocular pathologies. Despite these facts, there are reported complications such as allograft rejection, iatrogenic astigmatism, significant endothelial cell loss (especially

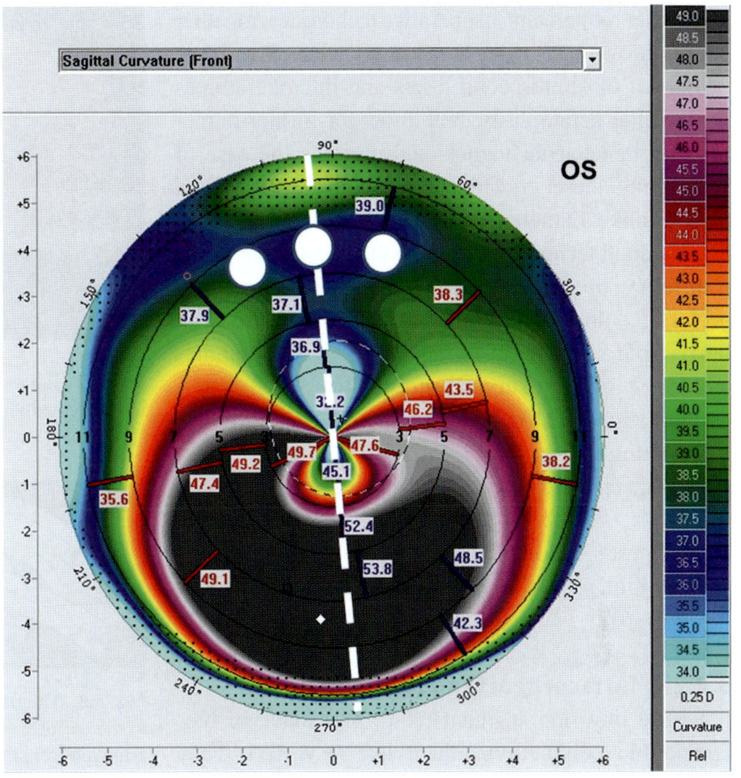

Fig. 3.1 Thermokeratoplasty. It is applied on the flat axis (*white line* and *white spots*) to steepen it and decrease astigmatism

when the life expectancy is long), side effects caused by long-term use of topical corticosteroids (e.g., secondary glaucoma and cataract), and recurrence of KC on the graft itself. Clear grafts are obtained in over 95% of cases but optical outcomes may be unsatisfactory because of the iatrogenic astigmatism and anisometropia. Between 30% and 50% of grafted eyes still require contact lens correction for best acuity or further keratorefractive surgical procedures such as astigmatic keratotomies, or in more recent years, topography-guided excimer laser procedures.

Recently, penetrating keratoplasty is indicated in patients with advanced progressive disease with significant corneal scarring.

3.2.2.3 Lamellar Keratoplasty (DALK)

In KC, the corneal endothelium is generally intact and healthy, even after many cases of acute hydrops. While corneal stromal rejection episodes can occur, it is known that with time, host keratocytes migrate into and replace donor cells and that most rejection episodes (especially after 12 months) are invariably endothelial in origin.

It is for these reasons that there has been a trend over recent years to perform lamellar (partial thickness), rather than full thickness, penetrating techniques. Such procedures offer replacement of the diseased (stromal) part of the keratoconic cornea, while leaving the healthy non-diseased endothelial cells relatively intact. This negates the risk of endothelial rejection and theoretically improves the postoperative mechanical stability of the cornea, with less chance of wound dehiscence and possibly less induction of iatrogenic astigmatism.

Lamellar keratoplasty has been shown to result in less endothelial cell loss, less intraocular pressure problems than full thickness techniques, a reduction in rejection episodes, and, in some cases, a reduction of induced astigmatism.

However, while some series have achieved comparable visual outcomes, others have demonstrated that in terms of BSCVA of 10/10 or better, penetrating techniques slightly outperform deep lamellar procedures and that while endothelial rejection is negated, stromal rejection very rarely can occur.

Further refinements in operative techniques, together with improvements in technologies, such as the implementation of femtosecond lasers and microkeratomes for lamellar keratoplasty, will allow for further refinement of lamellar techniques and improve the ease of performing these procedures for both surgeons and patients alike. Lamellar keratoplasty, with the advanced femtosecond technology, may be the first choice in the near future, providing an effective, technically easy-to-perform, outpatient, local anesthetic procedure with fairly rapid visual recovery and good visual outcomes and long-term graft survival and stability.

Indications of DALK regarding KC:

- Anterior corneal scars
- Advanced disease with stress lines and clear cornea
- K-max > 65 dpt
- Thinnest location < 350 μ
- Very high refractive error (sphere > −6 and/or cylinder > −6)

3.2.2.4 Intracorneal Rings (ICRs)

ICRs are tiny ring segments (Fig. 3.2) made of biocompatible polymethylmethacrylate (PMMA). They are inserted into the cornea to regularize its surface and achieve some refractive correction. Intracorneal ring segment implantation is a safe and reversible procedure that does not affect the central visual axis of the cornea. It is considered as an alternative aiming at delaying the need for corneal grafting procedures in KC patients. However, long-term stability remains the concern of many studies.

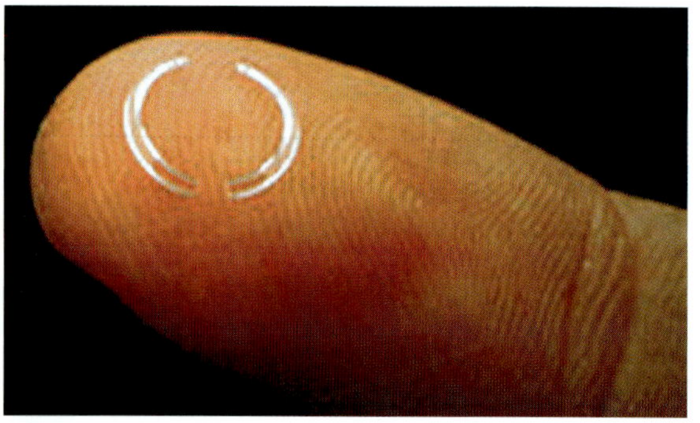

Fig. 3.2 Intracorneal rings: tiny segments made of biocompatible polymethylmethacrylate (PMMA)

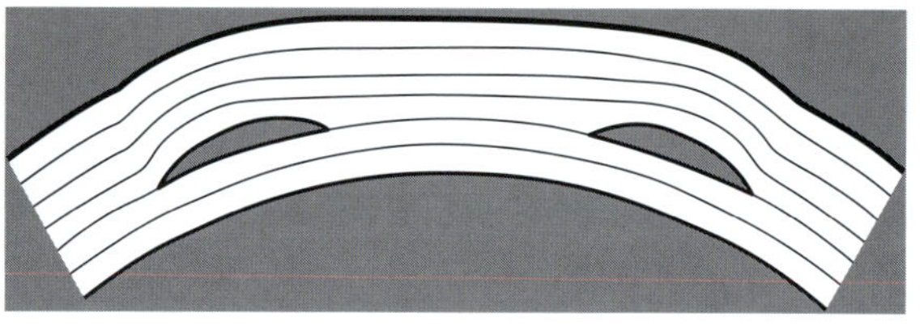

Fig. 3.3 The Barraquer thickness law. When a material is added to the periphery of the cornea or an equal amount of material is removed from the central area, a flattening effect is achieved. In contrast, when a material is added to the center or removed from the corneal periphery, the surface curvature is steepened

Mechanism of Actions

In general, ICRs act by an arc-shortening effect, flatten the center of the cornea, and provide a biomechanical support for the thin ectatic cornea. The changes in corneal structure induced by the rings can be roughly predicted by the Barraquer thickness law; that is, when a material is added to the periphery of the cornea or an equal amount of material is removed from the central area, a flattening effect is achieved (Fig. 3.3). In contrast, when a material is added to the center or removed from the corneal periphery, the surface curvature is steepened. The corrective result varies according to the thickness and the diameter of the segment (Fig. 3.4).

Every segment has a double effect (Fig. 3.5): a, a flattening effect along the virtual line (cd) connecting the two ends of the segment, and b, a steepening effect perpendicular to the line (cd) achieved by the skew action of the ring established by the difference between the plane of the segment and the plane of the cornea at the insertion area (Fig. 3.6a, b). Therefore, each segment flattens the axis that is parallel to line (cd) and steepens the perpendicular axis. For this reason, the segments are implanted on the steep axis. The flattening action of the arc is greater when the arc is longer (e.g., 160° arcs are stronger than 120° arcs), and vice versa, the perpendicular steepening action is greater when the arc is smaller (e.g., 90° arcs are stronger than 120° arcs). On the other hand, the overall flattening of the central cornea is greater with thicker segments (e.g., 300 μ arcs are stronger than 150 μ arcs).

The location of the ring has also an important role; the closer the segment to the center of the cornea, the stronger the skewing effect will be (i.e., astigmatic correction), and the farer the segment from the center of the cornea, the better the flattening effect will be (i.e., myopic correction). Therefore, segments implanted on the 5 mm circle (like Ferrara and Keraring) have better effect on astigmatism, and those implanted on the 7 mm (such as INTACS) have better effect on myopia. Since getting closer to the center of the cornea carries

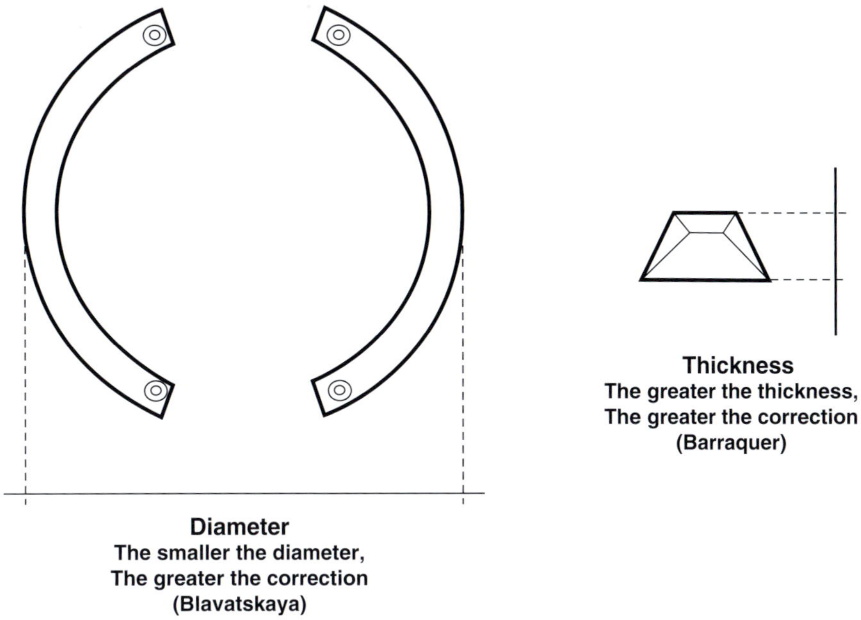

Fig. 3.4 Principle of action of intra corneal rings. The corrective result varies according to the thickness and the diameter of the segment. The greater the thickness, the greater the correction (Barraquer principle). The smaller the diameter, the greater the correction (Blavatskaya principle)

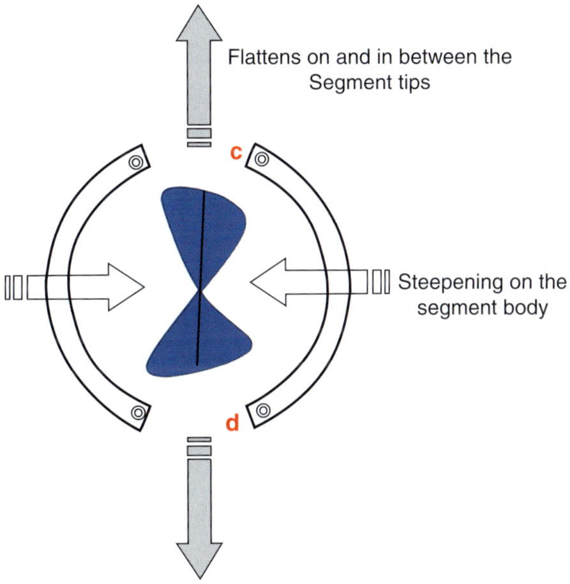

Fig. 3.5 Mechanism of action of intracorneal rings. Every segment has two effects: a flattening effect on the virtual line (*cd*) connecting between the two tips of the segment; thus the segment is implanted on the steep axis, and a steepening effect on the flat axis achieved by the skew action of the segment

the problem of night glare, new designs of the segments were developed to be implanted on the 6 mm circle, such as Kera6 and INTACS SK. In general, by using the 6 mm segments, less night glare (if any) is encountered, and better effect on both myopia and astigmatism is achieved.

In summary, if a case requires correcting myopia more than astigmatism, longer and thicker arcs are needed and vice versa. However, each company has its own nomogram and guidelines to choose the segments. The surgeon thereafter may modify the nomogram according to his/her accumulative experience.

Most of the effect of the ICRs is noticed on the anterior surface of the cornea and to less extent on the posterior surface as shown in Figs. 3.7–3.13. Figure 3.7 represents the change in the sagittal curvature map of the anterior corneal surface where the left column is the preoperative map, the middle column is the postoperative map and the right map is the difference (change) map. In the same way, Fig. 3.8 represents changes in the anterior tangential curvature map, Fig. 3.9 is for the posterior sagittal map, Fig. 3.10 is for the posterior tangential map, Fig. 3.11 is for the anterior elevation map, Fig. 3.12 is for the posterior elevation map and finally, Fig. 3.13 is for the keratometric power deviation map. The latter – very briefly – reflects the changes that happen on the posterior corneal surface. When reviewing all these figures, it is clear that improvements mainly occur on the anterior corneal surface.

Conditions to Use ICRs

The term (conditions) is preferred rather than indications, because the indication here is clearly KC, but

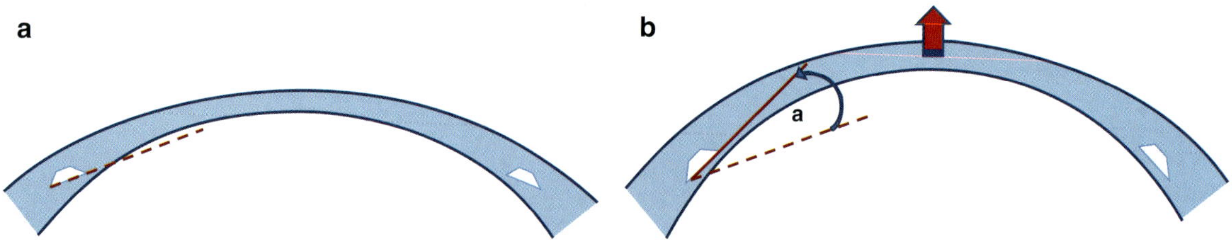

Fig. 3.6 (**a**) and (**b**) The skew action of the segment. (**a**) The position of the segment when implanted, (**b**) the final position of the segment after the skew; i.e., taking angle $\hat{a}$

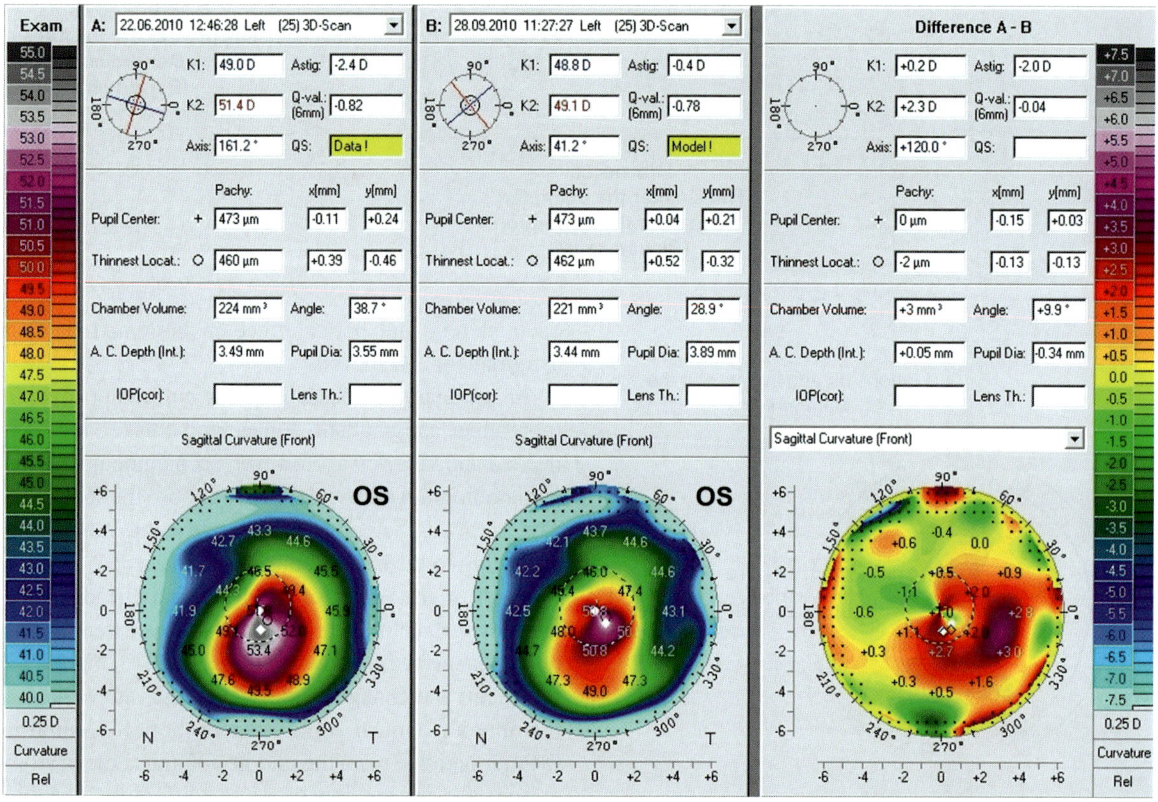

Fig. 3.7 Corneal response to intracorneal rings implantation. Changes on the *anterior sagittal* curvature map. The right column reflects these changes. Look at the central part, there is a *significant* change

there are guidelines to follow and limits to stop at when deciding to use ICRs.

Guidelines

- Corneal thickness > 350 µ at the thinnest location
- Maximal K-reading < 60 dpt
- Refractive error (S.E) < −6 dpt
- Clear cornea with no central scars or stress lines

The expert surgeons may go beyond these guidelines in selected cases.

Factors for Poor Visual Outcome

1. Preoperative Km > 55 dpt
2. Preoperative pachymetry at thinnest location 350–400 µ
3. Paracentral opacities

Contraindications

- High visual expectations.
- Uncontrolled autoimmune, collagen vascular, and immunodeficiency diseases because of high incidence

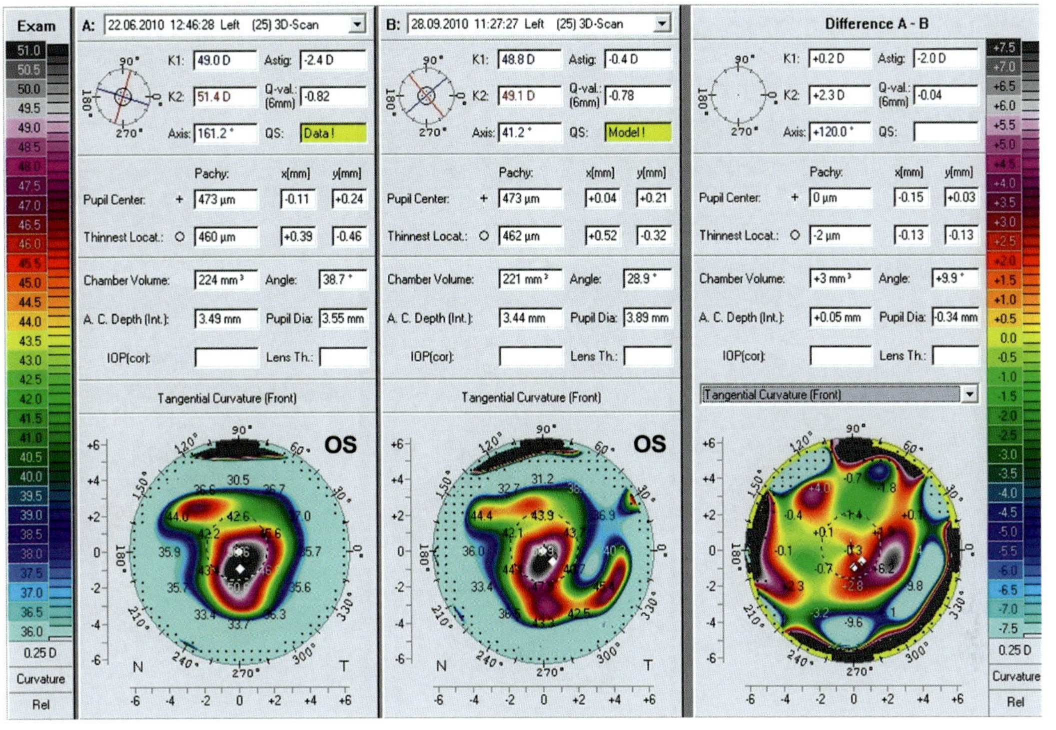

Fig. 3.8 Corneal response to intracorneal rings implantation. Changes on the *anterior tangential* curvature map. The right column reflects these changes. Look at the central part, there is a *significant* change

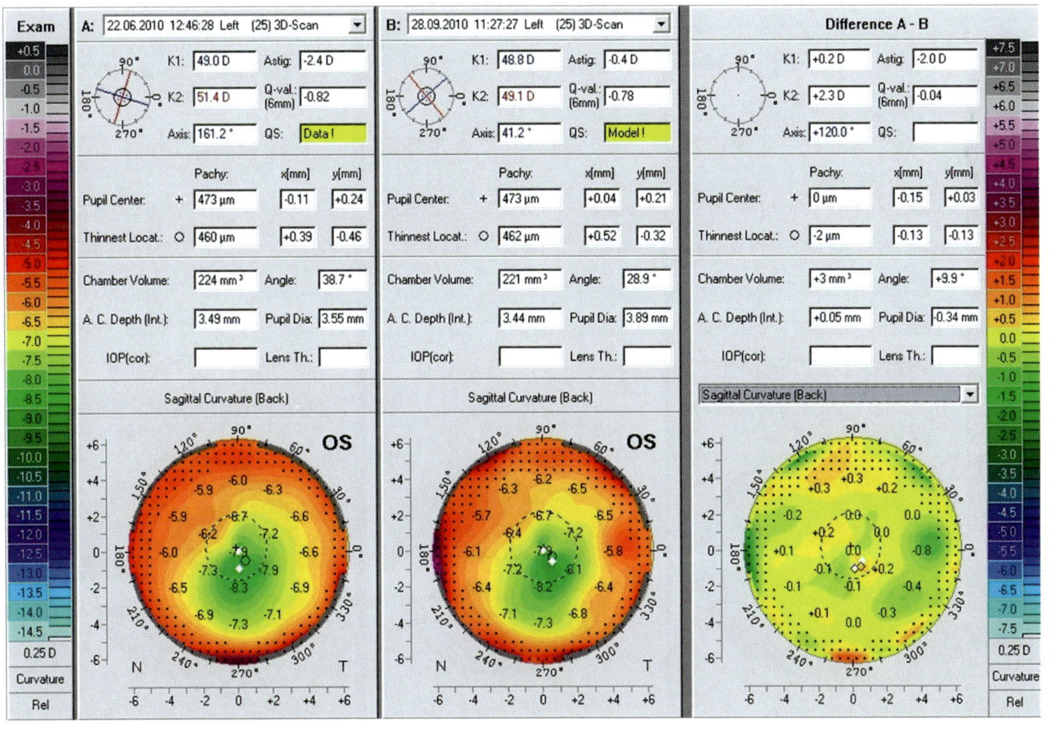

Fig. 3.9 Corneal response to intracorneal rings implantation. Changes on the *posterior sagittal* curvature map. The right column reflects these changes. Look at the central part, there is an *insignificant* change

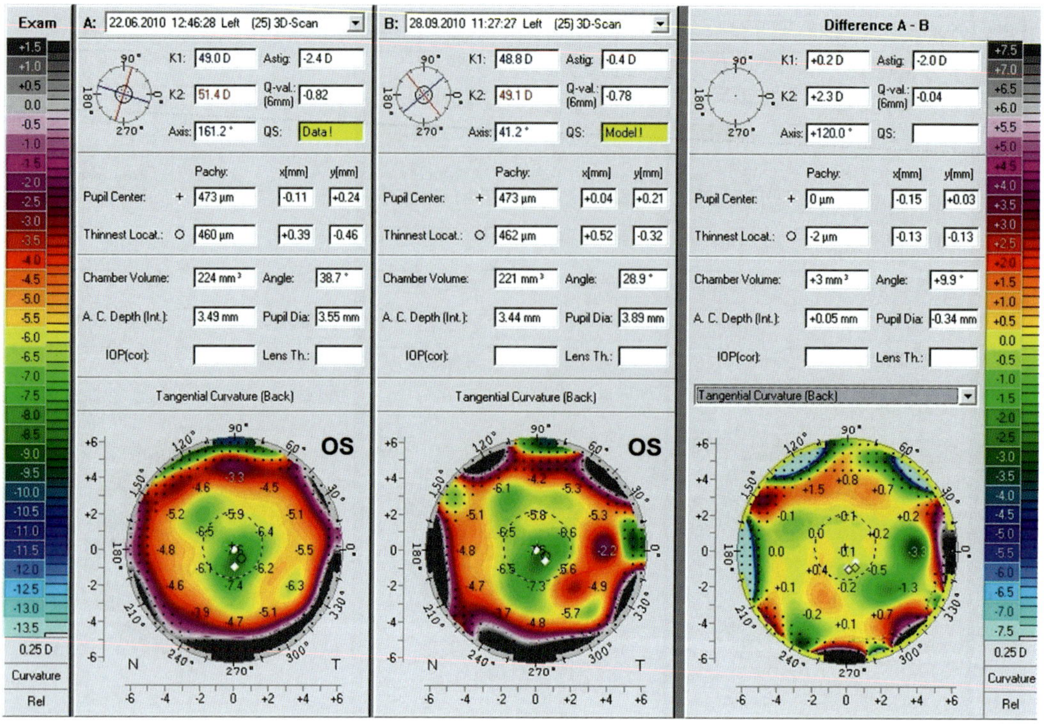

Fig. 3.10 Corneal response to intracorneal rings implantation. Changes on the *posterior tangential* curvature map. The right column reflects these changes. Look at the central part, there is an *insignificant* change

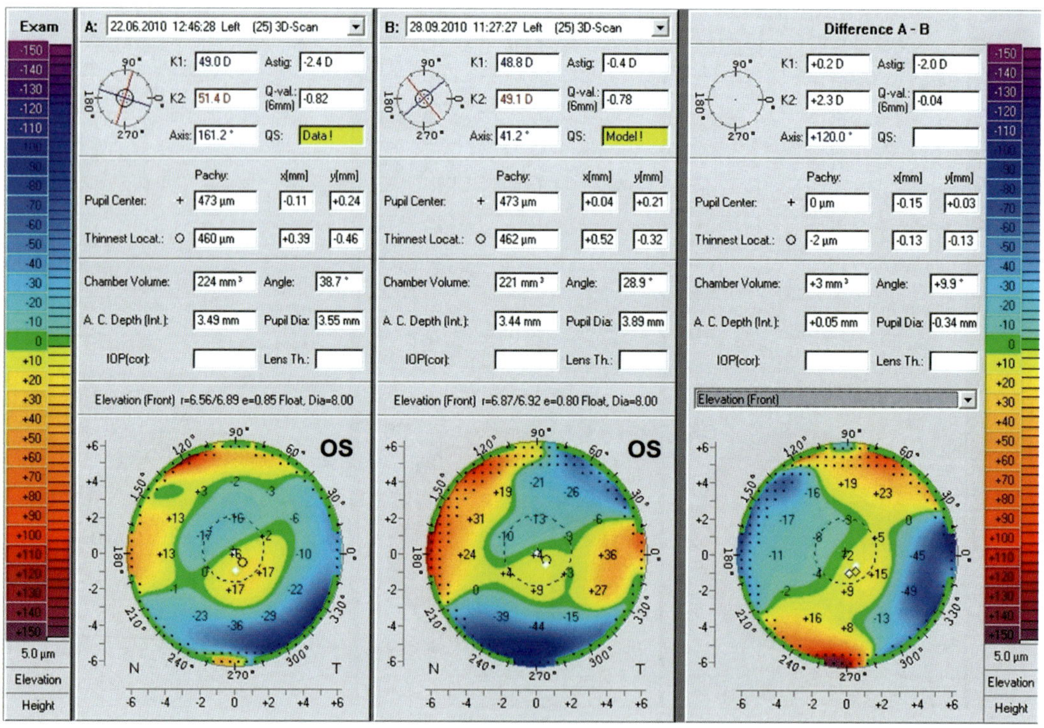

Fig. 3.11 Corneal response to intracorneal rings implantation. Changes on the *anterior elevation map*. The right column reflects these changes. Look at the central part, there is a *significant* change

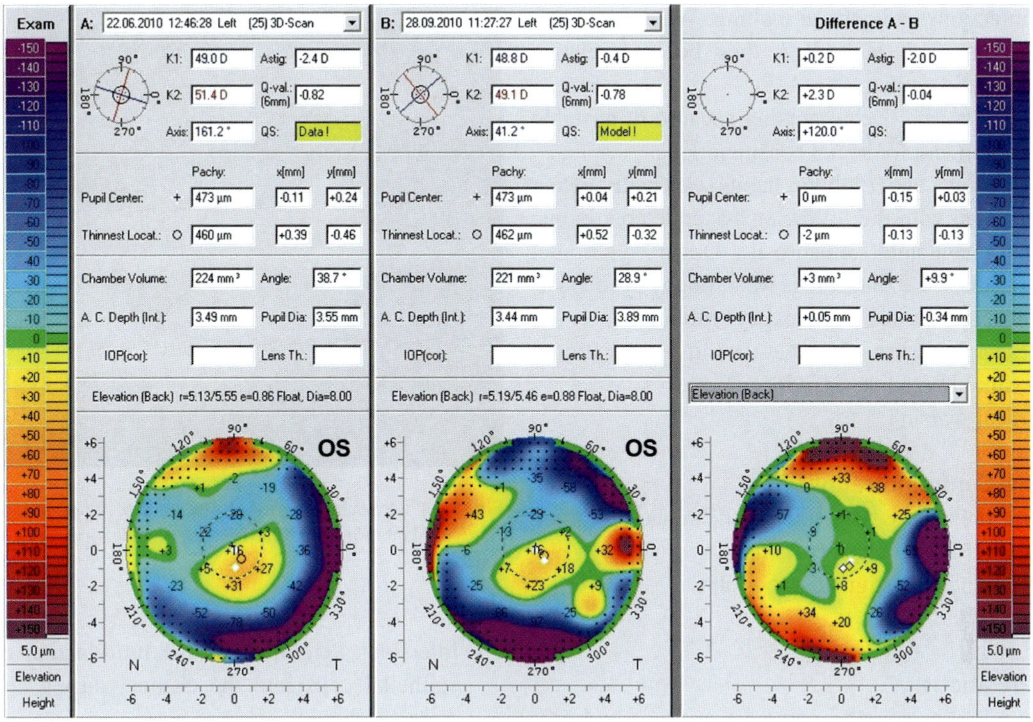

Fig. 3.12 Corneal response to intracorneal rings implantation. Changes on the *posterior elevation map*. The right column reflects these changes. Look at the central part, there is an *insignificant* change

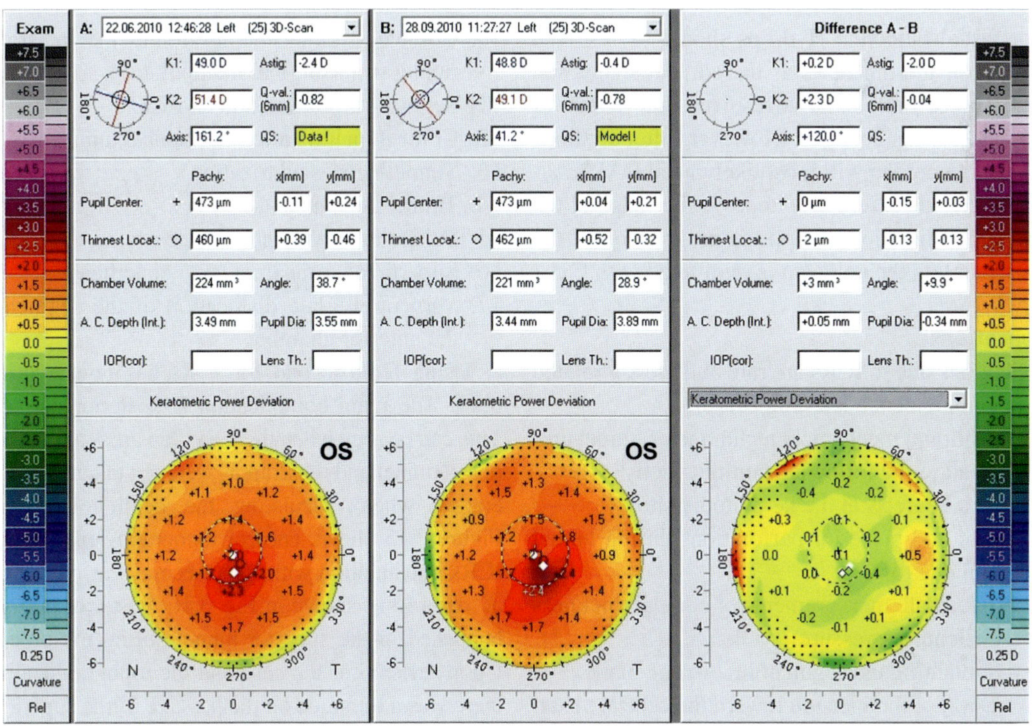

Fig. 3.13 Corneal response to intracorneal rings implantation. Changes on the *keratometric power deviation (KPD) map*. The right column reflects these changes. Look at the central part, there is an *insignificant* change. The KPD very briefly reflects the changes that happen on the posterior corneal surface

of infections and corneal melting. When these diseases are well controlled, they become relative contraindications.

- Pregnancy and during nursing because of unstable refraction and for social considerations.
- Continuous eye rubbing habits especially when associated with the following systemic conditions: Leber congenital amaurosis, Down syndrome, atopic disease, contact lens wear, floppy eyelid syndrome, and nervous habitual eye rubbing.
- Corneal thickness <350 μ at the thinnest location.
- Maximal K-reading >65 dpt.
- Corneal scarring.

Relative Contraindications

- Corneal thickness 350–400 μ at the thinnest location
- Maximal K-readings 60–65 dpt
- Topographical astigmatism>–6dpt
- Stress lines

Considerations

- Central or paracentral corneal scaring or hydrops: In patients with large (>4 mm) dense scars that completely obstruct the papillary area, ICRs are unlikely to be effective. Reticular scaring (Fig. 3.14) does not preclude ICRs but maybe responsible for poor visual outcome. Hydrops should be resolved before considering ICRs as the corneal shape will change once the edema is resolved and degree of corneal scaring emerges. However, after hydrops cornea, the cornea will most likely need DALK.
- Progressive disease: ICRs improve the shape of the cornea but they do not stop the progression of the disease unless the collagen is reinforced with CxL.

Complications

Complications due to ICRs are rare and mostly related to the beginning of the learning curve.

The traditional mechanical technique of tunnel creation can lead to the following complications:

1. Epithelial defects at the keratotomy site
2. Anterior and posterior perforations during tunnel creation due to:
   (a) Inaccurate measurements of corneal thickness
   (b) Inadequate pressure
   (c) Implanting the segment in a wrong plane
3. Extension of the incision toward the central visual axis or toward the limbus
4. Shallow placement and/or uneven placement of the segments

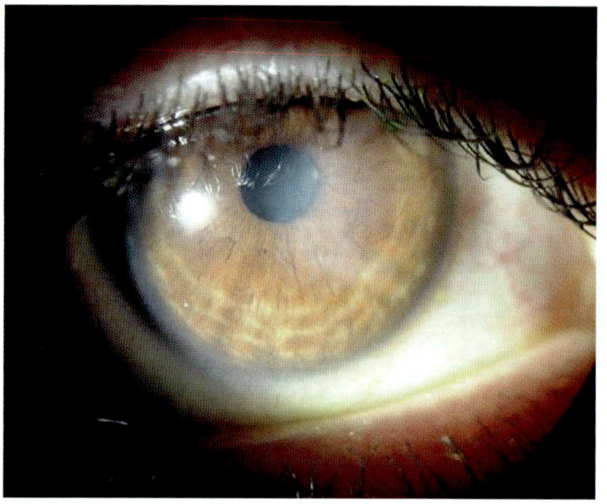

Fig. 3.14 Reticular scarring. It does not preclude intracorneal ring implantation but maybe responsible for poor visual outcome

5. Infectious keratitis with the introduction of the epithelial cells into the channel during channel dissection
6. Asymmetric placement
7. Persisting incisional gaping
8. Decentration
9. Stromal thinning
10. Corneal stromal edema around the incision and tunnel from surgical manipulation
11. Segment migration and extrusion
12. Corneal melting after mechanical tunnel dissection
13. Tunnel neovascularization
14. Tunnel deposits
15. Subconjunctival hemorrhage
16. Superficial corneal incision opacification
17. Very rarely, late dislocation of the segment into the anterior chamber

Using femtosecond for ICRs has fewer complications. The main complication is posterior perforation. This can be seen when there are thin areas along the proposed tunnel and those areas were not taken into consideration when calculating the depth of dissection. Figure 3.15 shows corneal topography of a KC case. ICRs implantation with femtosecond was planned to be at axis 140 as shown in Fig. 3.16. Posterior perforation happened in the superior tunnel during the procedure. Upon revision of the case and the topographical maps, there was a thin area on the passage of the superior tunnel; this area was thinner than the 80% of the depth at the sight of incision. Figure 3.17 shows cone location on the tangential map. Figure 3.18 shows the thickness map.

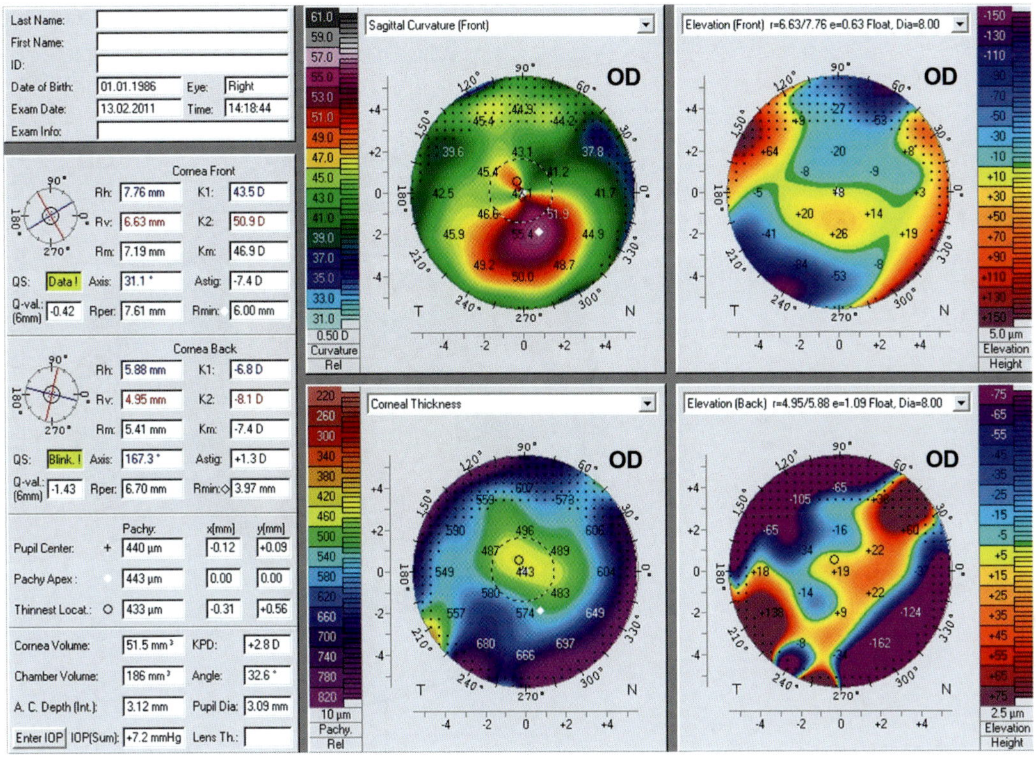

Fig. 3.15 A case of keratoconus. Intracorneal ring implantation was planned to be performed using the femtosecond

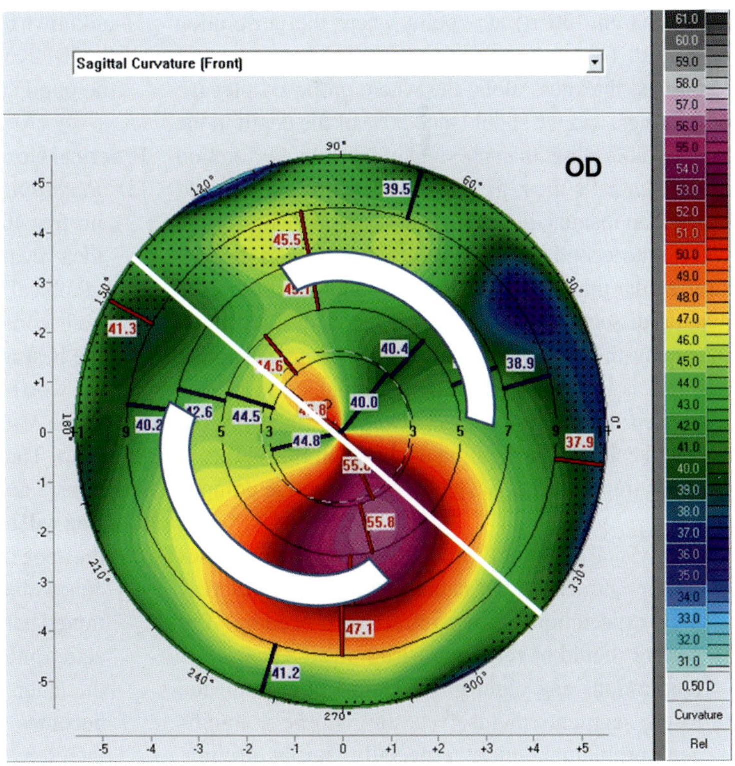

Fig. 3.16 Two tunnels were made using the femtosecond

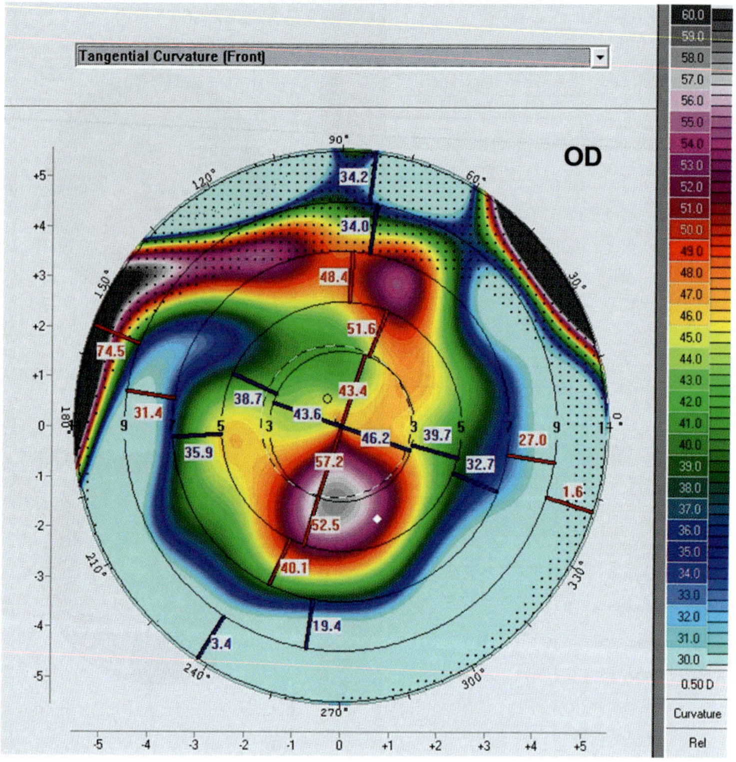

Fig. 3.17 Cone location on the anterior tangential map

Note the thin area on the passage of the superior tunnel, the yellow discussion triangle shows the very small safety margin (30 μ) at a point where the perforation happened. This case shows that we should pay attention to corneal thickness along the whole proposed passage of the rings, and we should take 80% of the depth in the thinnest area rather than the sight of incision. Perforation in such cases is most likely to occur with femtosecond rather than manual dissection. That is because dissection with femtosecond takes one level that may pass through an irregular thin area and thus perforation occurs, while manual dissection takes a layer rather than a level and maintains this layer throughout the passage. Another example is a PMD, if the ring is implanted in a level calculated depending on the thickness at incision; the case will end with perforation as shown in Fig. 3.19.

ICRs implantation has also two refractive complications:

- Poor visual outcome: Although uncommon, it causes disappointment to the patient who always has very high expectations in any refractive procedure. The patient should be told such a truth in advance.
- Aberrations and night glare: Halos may occur due to the segments themselves, this will be a significant problem at night especially during driving. Such a problem can be expected when the pupil diameter is>7 mm in dim light. This problem usually diminishes gradually after 6 months for unknown reason and rarely persists. Using Alphagan 0.15% eye drops (brimonidine titrate) to constrict the pupil at nighttime is an option.

Practical Notes in Using the Rings

(a) *Regarding topographical patterns*: After reviewing his first 400 cases of ICRs, the author could build an idea regarding the relationship between the topographical pattern and postoperative improvement in both corneal topography and BSCVA. In general, the best results can be obtained with pattern 1 and the worst results are with pattern 6, while in pattern 7, the results are unpredictable (author's classification). There may be an explanation for this. In patterns 5 and 6, which are PMD or PLK, the inferior ring will be implanted in a position that goes through the apex of the cone (Fig. 3.20a–c). The apex of the cone is the weakest part in the cornea, and as mentioned before, the ring acts in two directions, but its action must come from out of the cone to change the latter. When the ring goes through the cone, it becomes inside the supposed field of action and, therefore, composes a barrier against the desired change. On the other hand, caution should be taken

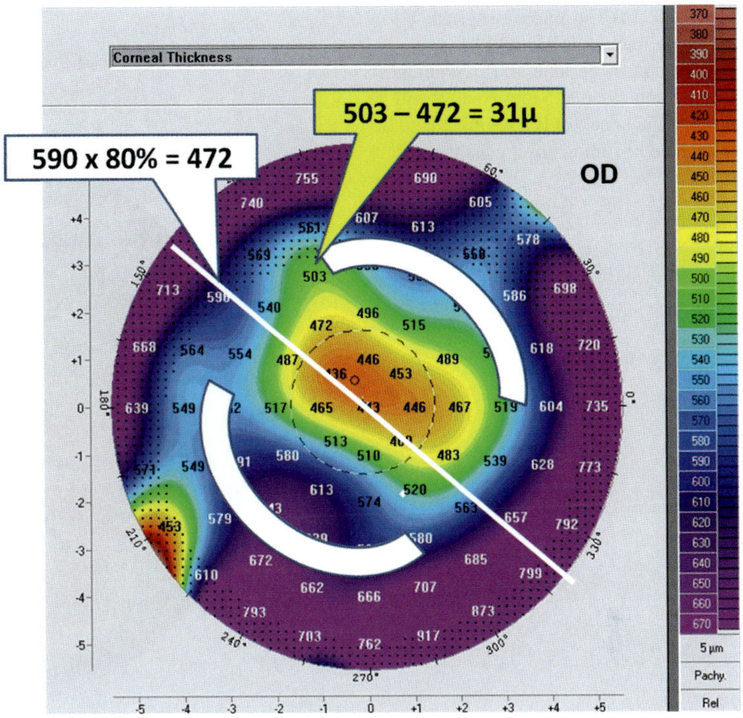

Fig. 3.18 Corneal thickness map demonstrates a thin area on the passage of the superior tunnel, note the 31 μ safety margin, which is insufficient to supply an intact passage

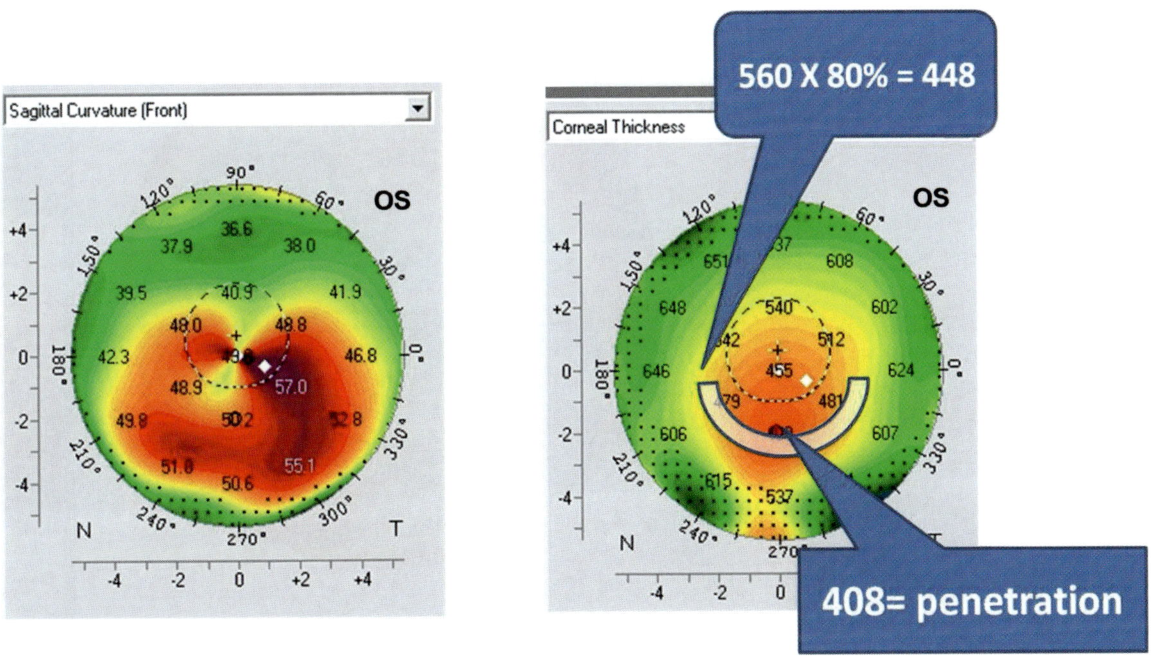

Fig. 3.19 PMD case. If a ring is implanted in the inferior cornea, there will be an intrusion of the ring into the anterior chamber. Note that the level of implantation will be shallower than the 80% of the entrance

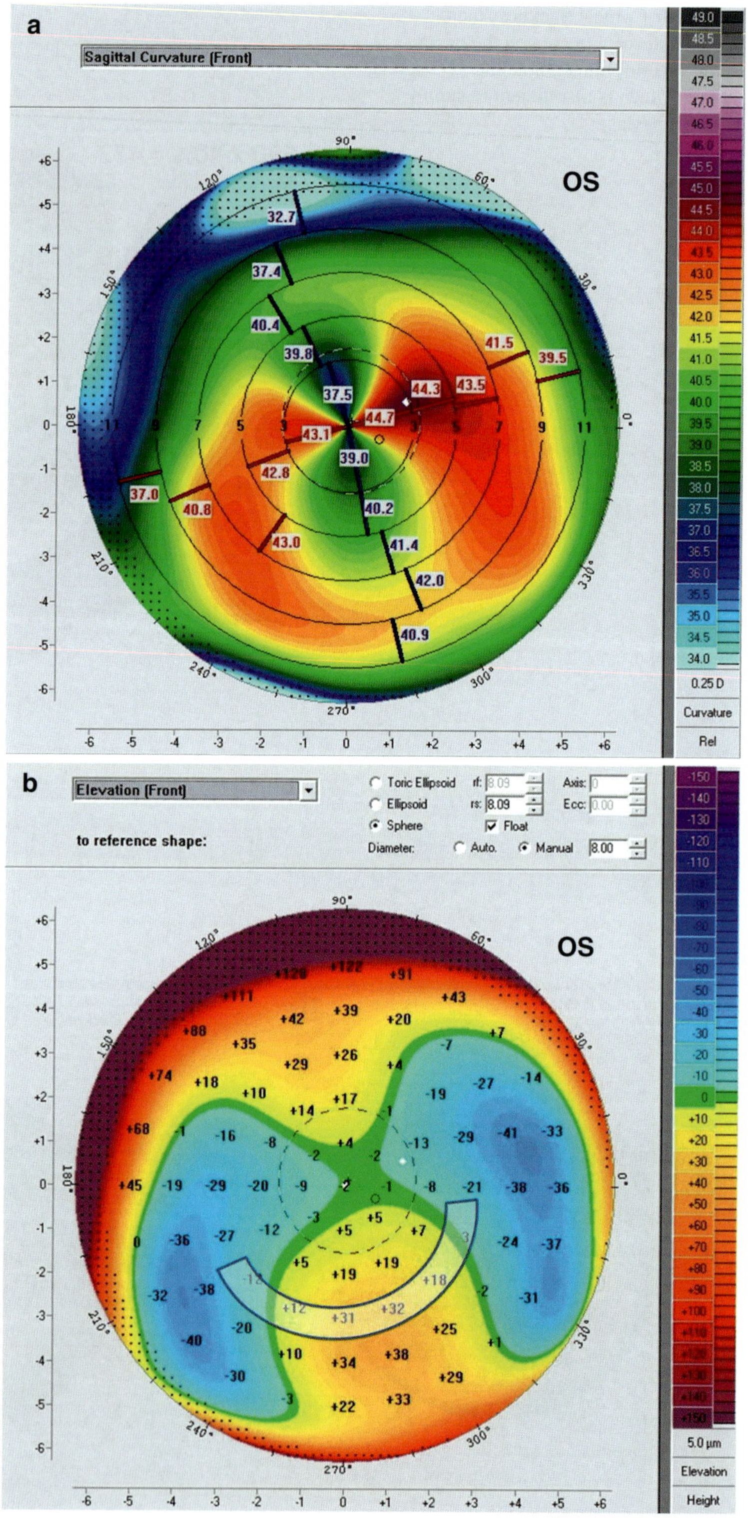

Fig. 3.20 (**a**) The anterior sagittal curvature map in PMD and PLK. (**b**) The cone is peripheral. If a segment is to be implanted at 5 mm zone, it will go through the cone. (**c**) If a segment is to be implanted at 7 mm, still it goes through the cone

Fig. 3.20 (continued)

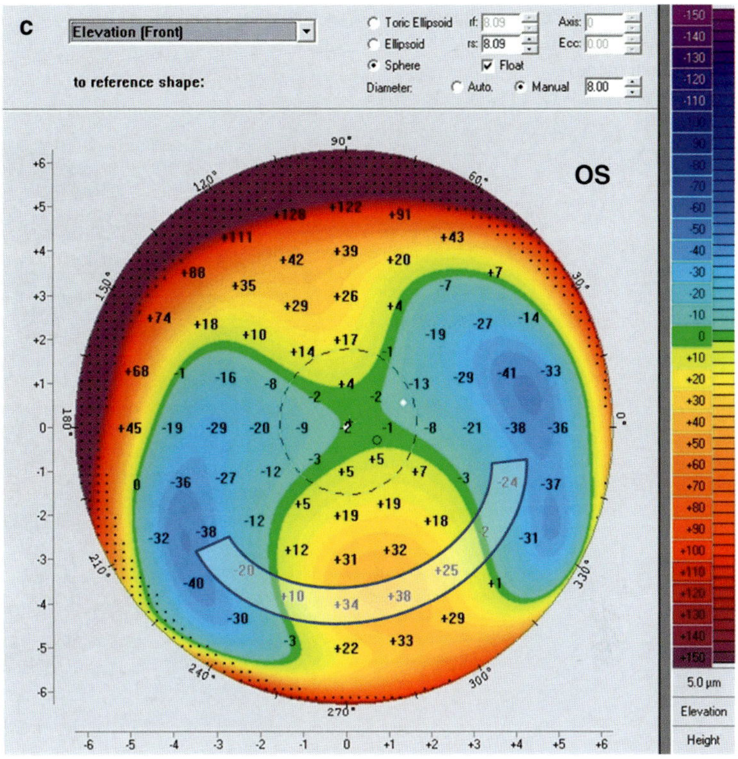

in this situation; the thinnest location may happen on the passage of the ring (particularly in PMD as mentioned before) leading to the risk of penetration. In such a case, it is strongly recommended to put the ring on the 7-mm zone to avoid the apex of the cone in order to achieve the desired effect and to avoid the thin area, but in advanced cases of PMD when the cone is very inferior, even those rings that are implanted at 7 mm zone may not be helpful as shown in Fig. 3.20c.

(b) *Regarding morphology of KC*: Nipple and oval patterns are more prone to respond to treatment, whereas globus cone may not. This is logical because the larger the cone the bigger the process that is needed to make a change. On the other hand, nipple and oval cones are usually found at the beginning of the disease where more elastic tissue is still available. The same can be applied to corneal thickness and K-readings. The thinner the cornea, the less the available elastic tissue and the less the response will be. Similarly, the higher the K-readings, the more advanced the disease and the less the response will be.

(c) *Regarding cone location*: When the cone is central (Fig. 3.21), usually two symmetric rings are needed. When the cone is not central (Fig. 3.22), either one ring or two asymmetric rings are needed. On the other hand, cone location is important for the choosing the zone of implantation and to avoid penetration as mentioned previously.

(d) *Regarding the refractive error*: The fact that ICRs are mainly to regularize corneal surface should be kept in mind. This will be achieved when irregular corneal astigmatism is minimized or at least inverted into regular astigmatism to improve the quality of vision. For this reason, correction of the spherical component of the refractive error is not the main goal. That is because the spherical component may be due to the cone itself or it might be of axial or refractive origin (such as nuclear sclerosis). A hyperopic component is sometimes found in the refractive error in KC. This is usually due to low K-readings in the center of the cornea which is found with peripheral cones and with PMD (see Fig. 3.20a and note the very low K-readings in the green area and in the very center of the cornea). Since the spherical component is not the main issue, the patient should never be told that this procedure is a refractive procedure that corrects his/her refractive error completely.

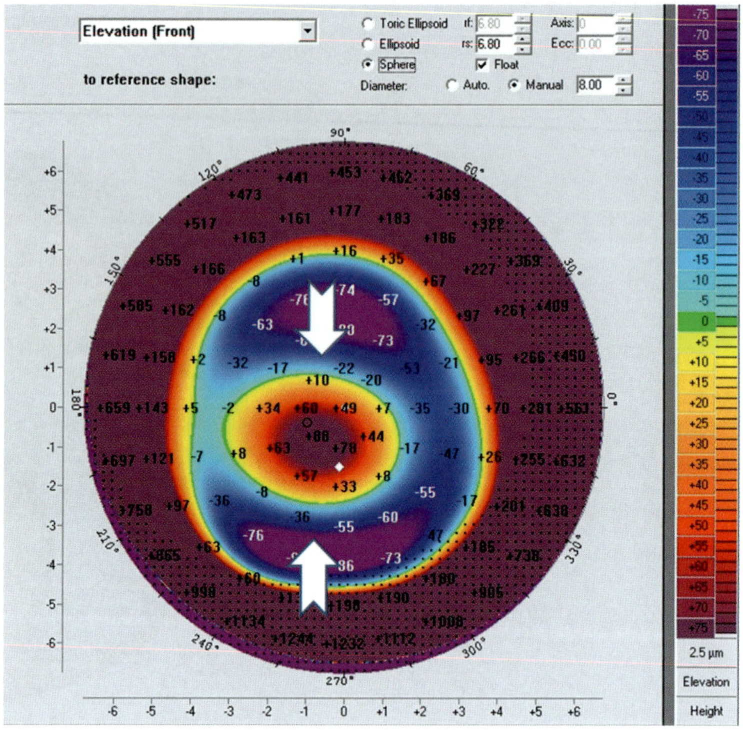

Fig. 3.21 A central cone as it appears on the anterior elevation map (BFTE float mode)

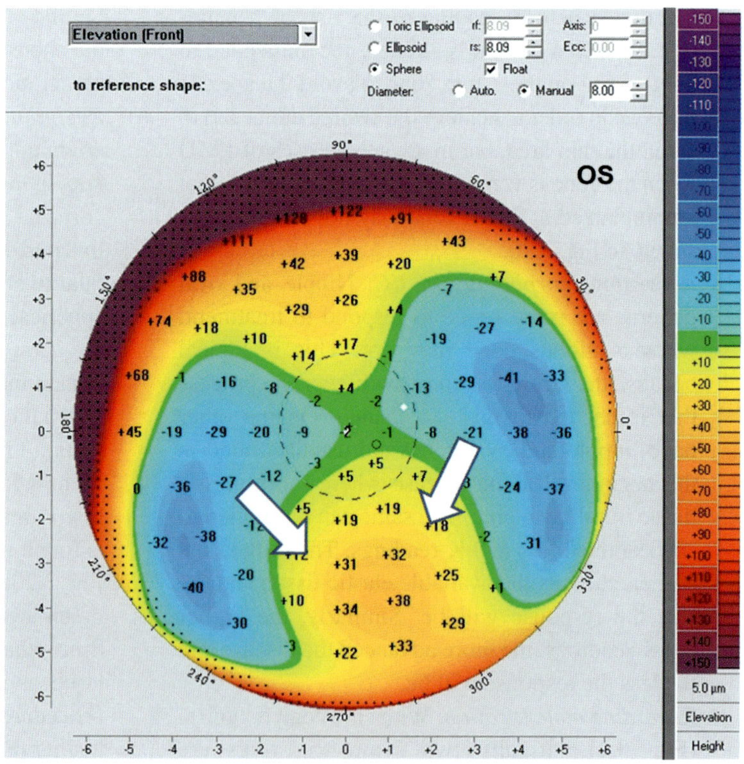

Fig. 3.22 A peripheral cone as it appears on the anterior elevation map (BFTE float mode); the white arrows point at the location of the cone

(e) *Regarding visual acuity*: As mentioned above, this procedure aims at improving the quality of vision, and to some extent correcting visual acuity. Comparing BSCVA with UCVA of the patient is very important because it gives an idea about the severity of the problem and the prognosis of the visual outcome. As an example, a patient with KC with UCVA=0.3 and BSCVA=0.4, this means one of two things: First, the patient is suffering from severe HOAs, second, the patient has a kind of tortional amblyopia! To distinguish between these two causes, it is very useful to check visual acuity with RGB contact lenses; the lens – with the tear film – composes a smooth surface in front of the cornea and, therefore, visual acuity will highly improve when the cause is HOAs. ICRs are useful – to some extent – when HAOs are the problem and they are not useful when the tortional amblyopia is. In general, severely impaired visual acuity bears unpredictable prognosis.

(f) *Regarding using contact lenses after ICR implantation*: One of the benefits of ICRs is making contact lenses tolerable. The ICRs regularize the cornea and, therefore, toric contact lenses (or specially designed soft lenses) can be used to correct the residual astigmatism and sphere.

3.2.2.5 Corneal Collagen Cross-Linking

Introduction

Riboflavin/ultraviolet A (UVA) – induced collagen cross-linking of the cornea (CxL) is a novel approach that aims at increasing the mechanical and biochemical stability of the stromal tissue. Its goal is to slow down or arrest KC progression to delay or avoid recourse to keratoplasty. The purpose of this treatment is to create additional chemical bonds inside the corneal stroma by means of photopolymerization in the anterior two thirds of the stroma, while minimizing exposure to the surrounding structure of the eye. Figure 3.23 demonstrates the main goal of CxL, which is to increase corneal stiffness and to achieve corneal stability. Figure 3.24 shows that in KC, there is lack of inter-collagen fiber bonding, which will increase after CxL as shown in Fig. 3.25. Very briefly, after topical anesthesia is applied and the epithelium removed, the cornea is rinsed with riboflavin 0.1% solution and exposed to UV light at a wavelength of 370 nm and irradiance of 3 mW/cm^2 for 30 min (Fig. 3.26).

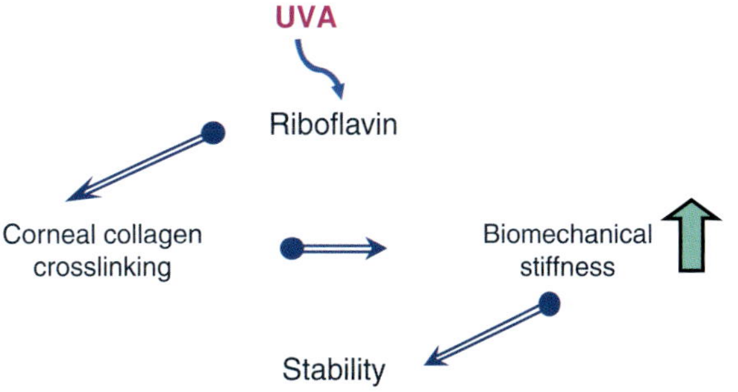

Fig. 3.23 Corneal cross-linking. The aim of this procedure is to increase corneal stiffness and achieve corneal stability

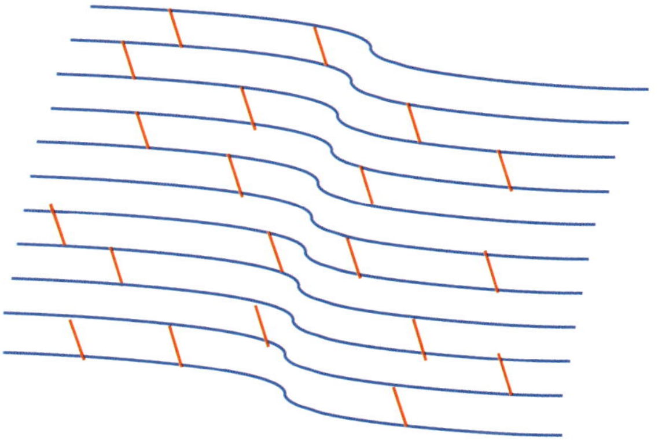

Fig. 3.24 Inter-collagen fiber bonding. In keratoconus, there is a deficiency in the bonds

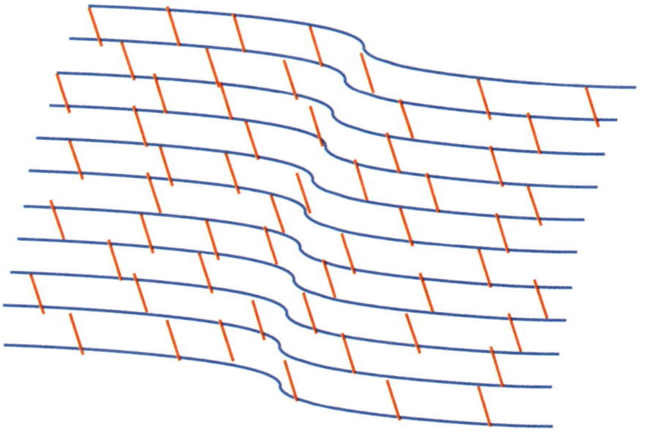

Fig. 3.25 Inter-collagen fiber bonding. Corneal cross-linking increases the number of bonds

Indications

(a) Documented progression of KC in the preoperative months. Progression parameters include at least one of the followings (during 1 year of follow-up):
   - Change of K-max by > 1 dpt
   - Thinning of the cornea by > 30 μ
   - Increase of topographical astigmatism by > 1 dpt

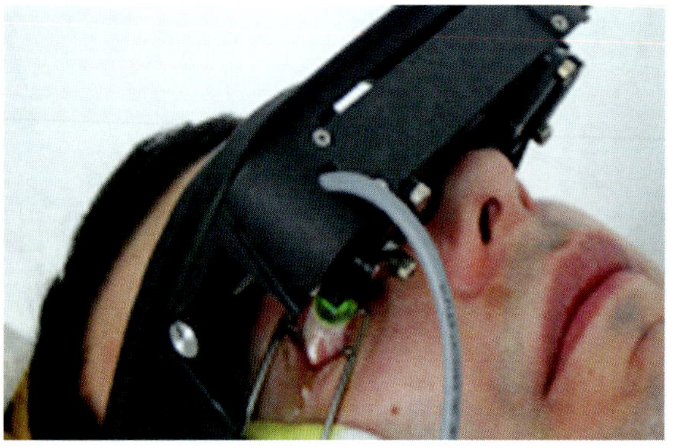

Fig. 3.26 One of corneal cross-linking machines

(b) KC with age under 20 years old
(c) PMD
(d) To stabilize or to prepare the cornea with KC before PRK
(e) Forme fruste KC before PRK
(f) Corneal ectasia after refractive surgery
(g) Corneal deformation after radial keratectomy

There are non-refractive indications for CxL mentioned by some researchers such as bollous keratopathy and infectious keratitis. This book focuses on refractive indications which are KC, PLK, FFKC, PMD, and post lasik ectasia.

Conditions

Upon decision, the following questions mount:
(a) Is the cornea suitable for CxL? i.e., clear cornea and corneal thickness at the thinnest location is > 400 μ.
(b) Are there any risk factors that might lead to unpleasant healing responses?
(c) What does the patient expect from the procedure (visual expectation)?
(d) Is the aim of CxL to stop the progression or to prepare the cornea for PRK or for both?

The importance of such questions will be highlighted in the case study chapter.

Contraindications

The answers to the above questions compose part of the contraindications for CxL. Contraindications include:
(a) Corneal thickness < 400 μ at thinnest location because of danger of damaging the endothelium. Figure 3.27 shows the safety margin of the procedure.
(b) K-max > 60 dpt.
(c) High visual expectations.
(d) Corneal epithelial healing disorders.
(e) Previous herpes keratitis.
(f) Corneal melting disorders (rheumatoid…).
(g) Pregnancy.
(h) Continuous eye rubbing habits especially when associated with the following systemic conditions: Leber congenital amaurosis, Down syndrome, atopic disease, contact lens wear, floppy eyelid syndrome, and nervous habitual eye rubbing.
(i) Corneal scaring.

Expected Changes After CxL

CxL starts acting immediately during the operation. Apart from the biochemical bonding, CxL affects two main aspects of the cornea, the curvature and the thickness. Collagen fibers not only bond to each other, but also they shrink. As a result, the cone will be displaced toward the center of the cornea, which by itself becomes more regular. These changes lead to an increase of K-readings almost by 2.0–2.5 dpt, an increase of minus spherical component of the refractive error by 2.0–2.5 dpt. Figure 3.28 is a comparison between topographical parameters of pre-CxL and 1.5 months post-CxL, where A is the post-op (left column) and B is the pre-op (right column). Yellow arrows point at anterior corneal astigmatism; note its increase at 1.5 months. Red arrows point at the steep K-readings, note the increase. Blue arrows point at corneal thickness at the thinnest location, note the decrease. These changes are also visible on the anterior sagittal and tangential curvature maps and also on the anterior elevation map as shown in Figs. 3.29–3.31. However, the changes in K-readings and the spherical refractive error are usually temporary; they may last for 3 or 4 months after the operation and then diminish gradually and may be followed by a reduction of K-max. On the other hand, CxL causes a reduction of central corneal thickness by 30–50 μ as shown in Figs. 3.28 and 3.32. This may be explained by corneal dehydration induced by the intensive exposure to UV light during the treatment. This thinning of the cornea is usually temporary and the cornea retains its original preoperative thickness within about 1 year. Nevertheless, from a topographical point of view, changes in the cornea mainly happen on the anterior surface rather than the posterior surface. Figures 3.33 and 3.34 show the changes that happened in the anterior surface, whereas Figs. 3.35 and 3.36 show the changes that happened in the posterior surface, it is very clear that the anterior surface is the main field for

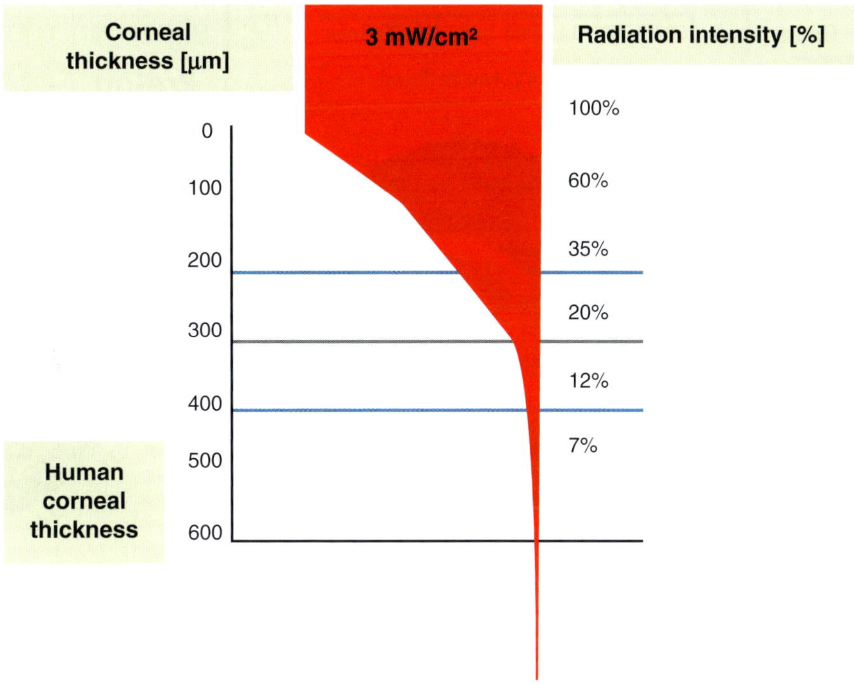

Fig. 3.27 Safety margin of corneal cross-linking. When UV light penetrates a saturated stroma with riboflavin, it will be absorbed and a small safe amount will reach the endothelium

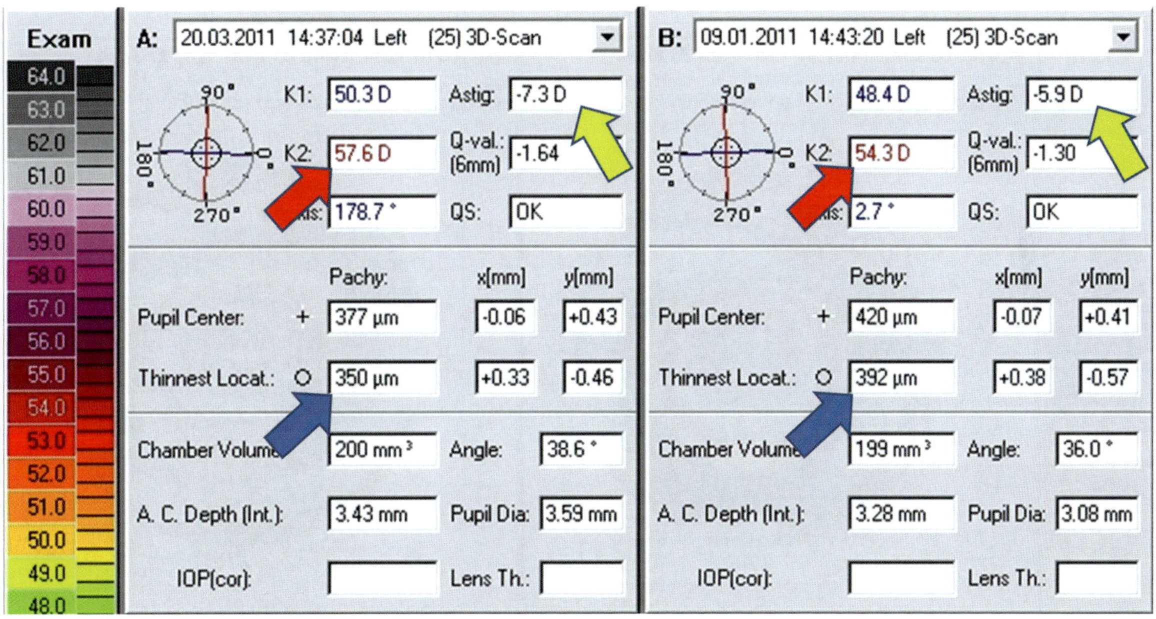

Fig. 3.28 (**a**) comparison between topographical parameters before CxL and 1.5 months after CxL, where A is the post-op map (*left* column) and (**b**) is the pre-op map (*right* column). *Yellow* arrows point at anterior corneal astigmatism; note its increase at 1.5 months. *Red* arrows point at the steep K-readings, note the increase. *Blue* arrows point at corneal thickness at the thinnest location, note the decrease

changes. Finally, mainly the anterior two thirds of the cornea are affected by CxL, this can be seen by the anterior OCT. Figure 3.37 is an anterior OCT of a cross-linked cornea, notice the demarcation line between the anterior two thirds and the posterior third of the stroma. This demarcation line is due to the difference between the (hyper-reflective) cross-linked tissue and the residual posterior less-crossed-linked tissue.

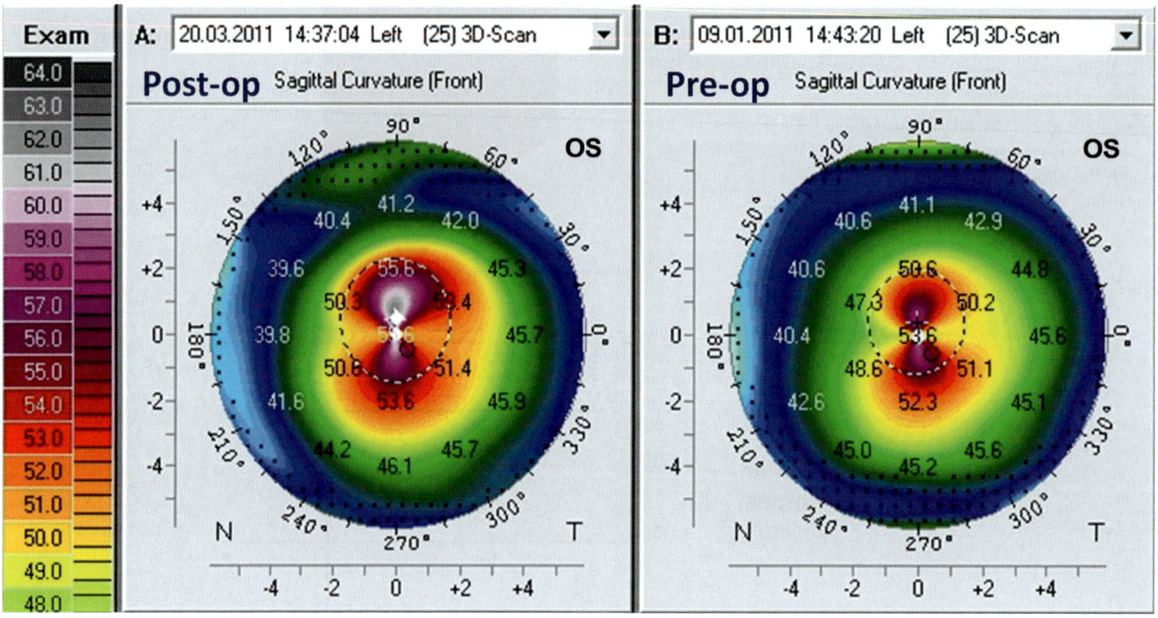

Fig. 3.29 Changes on the anterior sagittal curvature map after CxL; same case of figure 3.28; notice the increase in K-readings in the first 3 months after the procedure

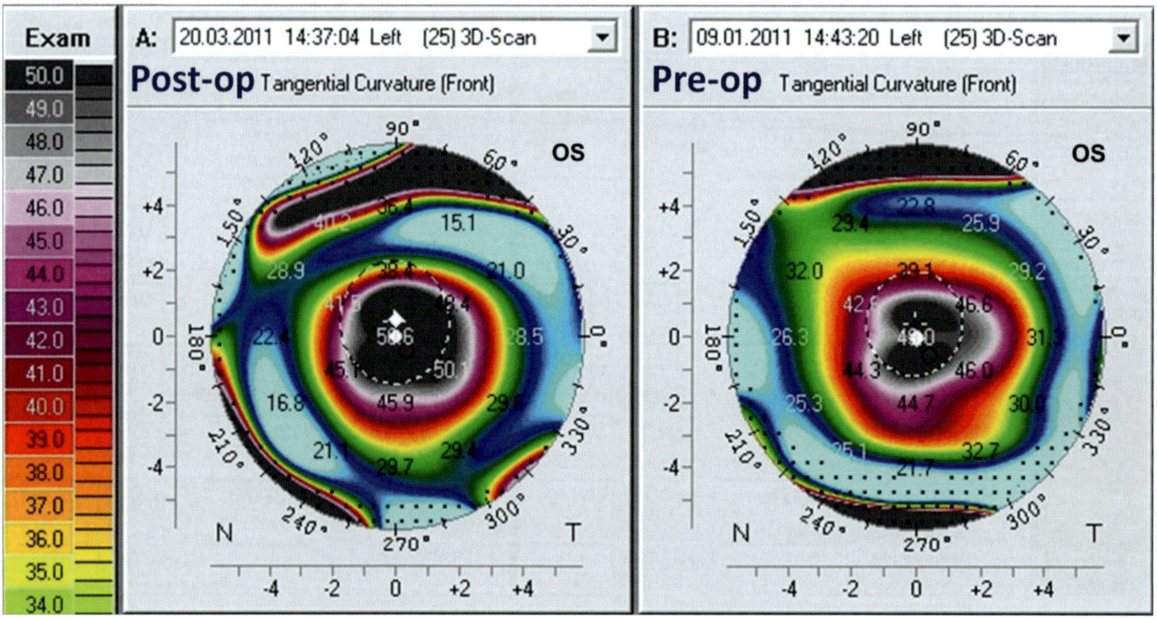

Fig. 3.30 Changes on the anterior tangential curvature map after CxL; same case of figure 3.28; the increase in K-readings is more obvious here than in the sagital curvature map

Typical Final Clinical Outcomes

(a) Reduction of K-max by 1.0–2.0 dpt
(b) Stability that is statistically proven over 48 months
(c) 1–2 line gain in BSCVA
(d) Low-tomoderate haze up to 6 months post surgery

CxL for PRK

When CxL is indicated to prepare the keratoconic cornea for PRK, there are important considerations and guidelines to be followed:

As mentioned above, CxL affects corneal thickness. Shrinkage of about 30–50 μ will follow the procedure;

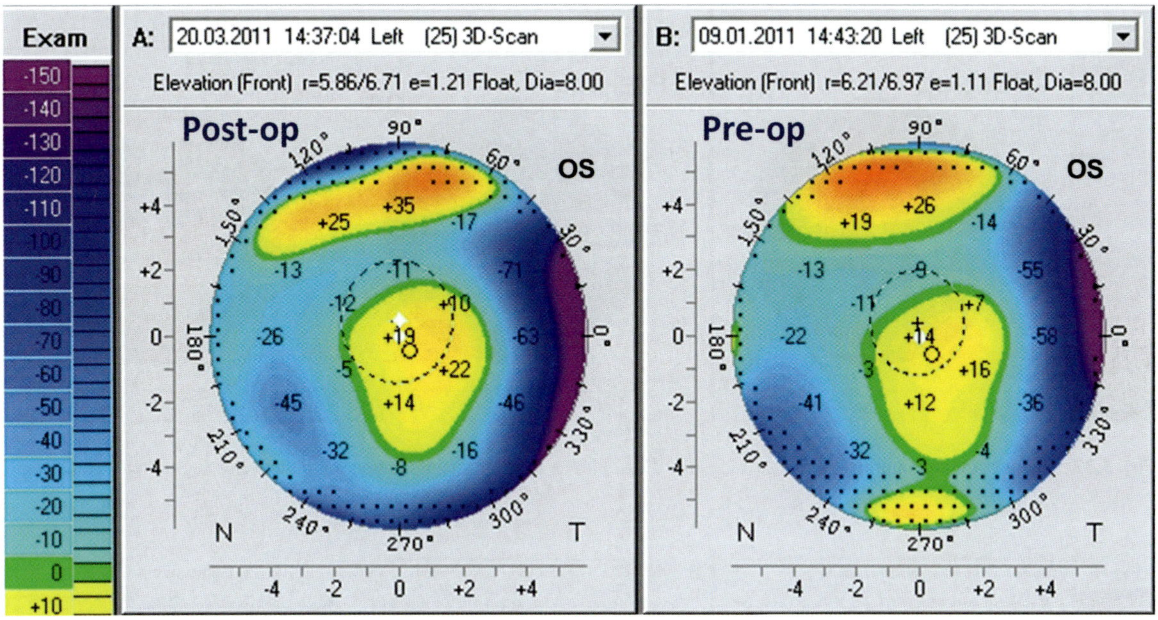

Fig. 3.31 Changes on the anterior elevation map after CxL; same case of figure 3.28; notice the increase in anterior elevations

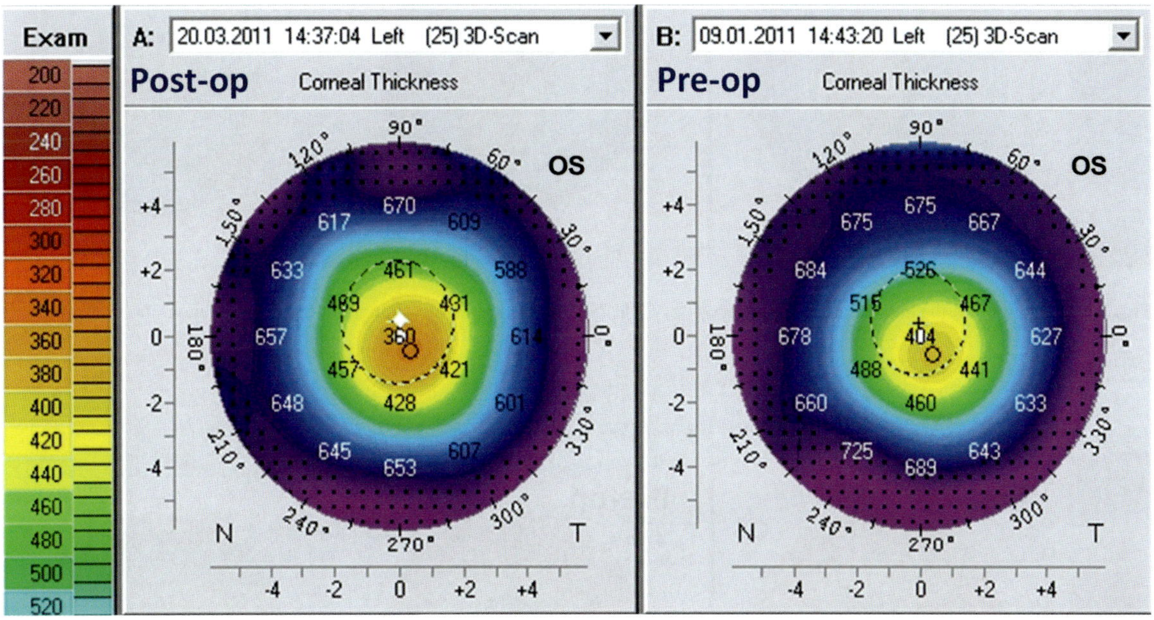

Fig. 3.32 Changes on the thickness map after CxL; same case of figure 3.28; notice the decrease in thickness which is usually temporary

thereafter, the cornea retains its previous thickness almost 1 year after the procedure.

There are two conditions when doing topography-guided (TG) PRK on a cross-linked cornea:

- The maximal ablation depth must not exceed 40–50 μ. Exceeding this ablation depth weakens the structure of the cornea which is already weak.
- The proposed residual corneal thickness after the procedure should not be less than 400 u including the epithelium for the same reason above.
- It is very important to know that more tissue is ablated during the TG PRK (compared with the standard treatment), that is because the procedure has a dual role: regularizing the corneal surface and

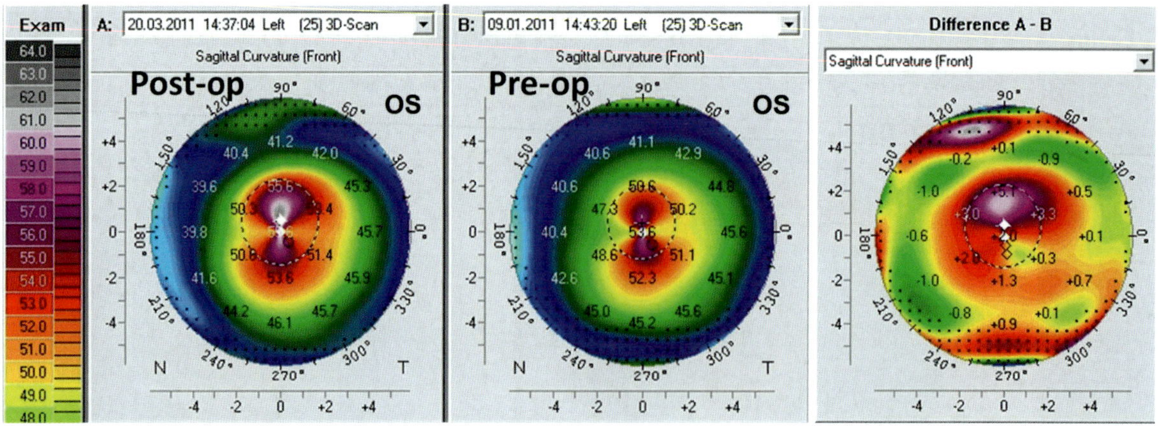

Fig. 3.33 Changes on the anterior corneal surface after CxL. Notice the significant change on the anterior sagittal curvature map

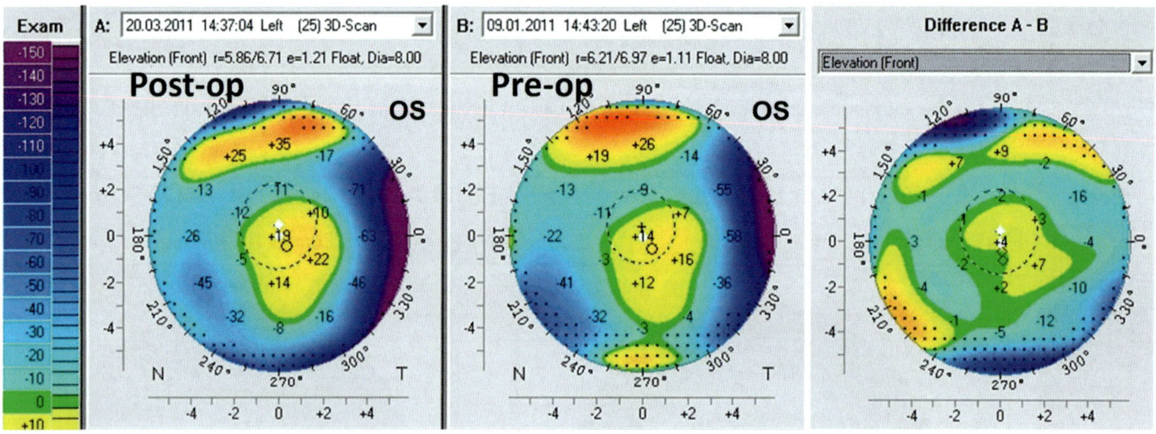

Fig. 3.34 Changes on the anterior corneal surface after CxL. Notice the significant change on the anterior elevation map

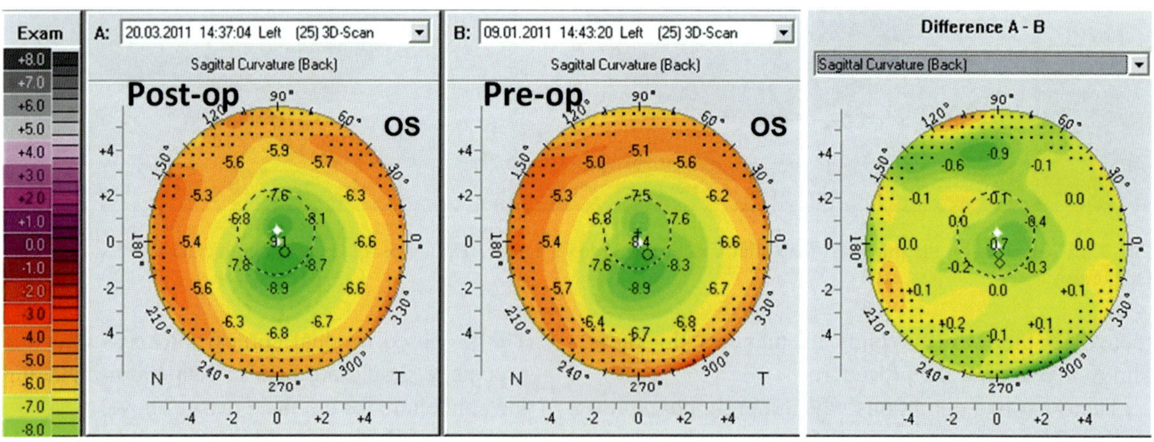

Fig. 3.35 Changes on the posterior corneal surface after CxL. Notice the insignificant change on the posterior sagital curvature map

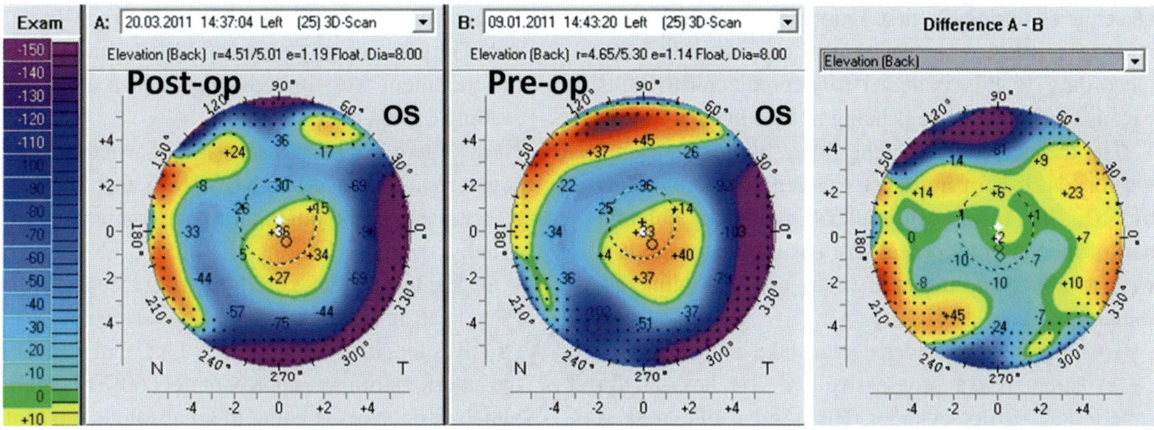

Fig. 3.36 Changes on the posterior corneal surface after CxL. Note the insignificant change on the posterior elevation map

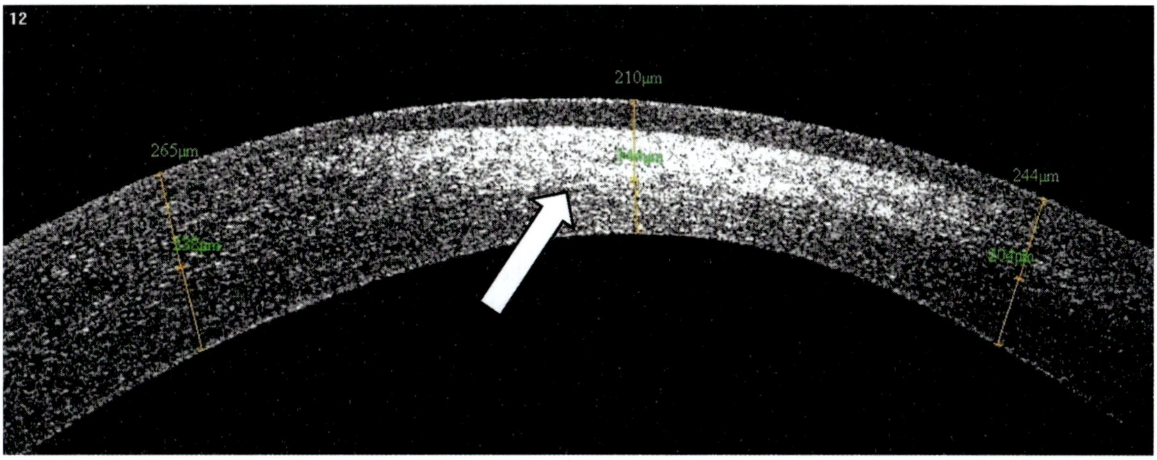

Fig. 3.37 Anterior OCT showing the demarcation line after CxL. The hyper-reflective anterior area represents the cross-linked tissue; it composes nearly two thirds of corneal thickness in the central area of the cornea, while it composes nearly half thickness at periphery. The cross-linked tissue acts as a barrier in the front cornea preventing the bulging-out posterior mechanical forces. The white arrow points at the level of the demarcation line

correcting the refractive error, this means that with the allowed 40–50 u of ablation, less than −4.0 dpt can be treated.

When adding the refractive error correction to the TG PRK profile, astigmatism has the priority over the spherical component because the former is the main issue in KC. As an example, suppose that the TG PRK profile will ablate 25 μ, and the patient has a refractive error of −3.0 dpt sphere and −2.0 dpt cylinder. Including the astigmatism within the profile will drain the allowed maximal ablation depth (50 μ), which means that the spherical component will not be corrected. This is of course better than including the spherical component and leaving the astigmatism.

There are two controversies regarding PRK and CxL:

1. The first, doing CxL first followed by TG PRK after at least 6 months.
2. The second, doing both procedures in the same session. Even this issue has two techniques: Some surgeons prefer to do TG PRK first followed by CxL immediately, and others prefer to do the opposite.

The thesis behind the first idea (6 months apart) is: When the cornea is cross-linked, there will be biomechanical changes in the anterior two thirds of the cornea. These changes begin immediately after CxL and continue over 48 months, but 90% of the changes will be achieved during the first 6 months. Therefore, combining TG PRK with CxL in the same session leads (according to this opinion) to unpredictable results because unstable tissue is being treated in such a case.

The thesis behind the other idea (both in the same session) is: It is of nonsense to strengthen the cornea by CxL, then re-weaken it after 6 months by ablating part of the anterior corneal stiff tissue. Therefore, it is wise to ablate the diseased tissue and cross-link the remaining tissue.

To apply the above ideas, let us take an example:

A patient has a progressive KC. He has −3 dpt sphere and −3 dpt cylinder. His corneal thickness is 490 μ at the thinnest location. Suppose that CxL with TG PRK are planned. Although the patient has 90 μ above the 400 μ, still we should be limited to the allowed 40 μ of ablation depth. The TG PRK may correct the irregularity of the corneal surface using the 40 μ and one may try adding −3 D cylinder to the correction profile if the maximal depth of the profile does not exceed the 40 μ. A smaller optical zone can be chosen to increase the ability to treat the astigmatism, e.g., 6 mm instead of 6.5 mm.

Complications

Complications of CxL are rarely encountered. They include:

(a) Herpetic keratitis with iritis even in patients with no history of herpetic disease, and in cases with an ocular herpes history, systemic anti-herpes therapy is clearly indicated.
(b) Induction of diffuse lamellar keratitis after CxL in a patient with post LASIK ectasia. Using topical steroids should precede CxL in cases of iatrogenic keratoectasia.
(c) Loss in BSCVA of 2 or more Snellen lines after 6 months to 1 year postoperatively. A refractive surgical procedure is considered safe if this complication rate is lower than 5%. Risk factors for visual loss after CxL seem to be (1) age over 35 years and (2) a BSCVA of 20/25 or better. From a strategic viewpoint, it may be that the earlier CxL is performed, the better for the patient.
(d) Failures (failures to stop the progression or failures to achieve the demarcation line): Although failures are not considered complications, they may have an impact on the complication rate. In one study, the only identified risk factor for failure was a K-max reading greater than 58.00 dpt. The efficacy of CxL would likely increase if the treatment was limited to eyes with a K-max reading of less than 58.00 dpt.
(e) Haze: There has been discussion of whether haze is a normal finding after CxL and whether the haze affects vision. Although haze occurs after CxL, it usually decreases during the first postoperative year. The haze after CxL differs from the haze after PRK in stromal depth. Whereas haze after PRK is strictly subepithelial, haze after CxL extends into the anterior stroma to approximately 60% of depth, which is on average equal to an absolute depth of 300 nm. The nature of this haze is unclear but may be due to loss of keratocytes or to dehydration.
(f) Corneal melting: It is a rare complication reported following CxL treatment. Frequent instillation of topical anesthetic agents during the procedure, NSAIDs instillation, and Acanthamoeba infection were suggested to lead to the activation of multiple noxious mechanisms that finally causes ulceration and corneal melting. Therefore, it is recommended to avoid NSAIDs and contact lenses during the healing process of the epithelium when performing CxL. If prescribed, the patient should be informed of the risk of wearing a contact lens and instructed in its correct use. The risk of bacterial keratitis during the healing process of the epithelium may be greatly reduced with the use of proper prophylactic antibiotic agents, but prophylactic coverage with topical antiamebic and antifungal drugs is not considered. The role of keratocyte apoptosis must be investigated. The patient must be informed of the safety and possible side effects of the therapy. Stressing the importance of avoiding exposure to fresh water while wearing contact lenses is fundamental.
(g) Very rare cases of microbial keratitis with Acanthamoeba and pseudomonas were reported.

3.2.2.6 Intraocular Refractive Lenses

Intraocular refractive lenses (IORLs) or phakic IOLs are lenses used to correct high refractive errors. There are two types regarding the location of implantation: posterior chamber (PC) IORLs and anterior chamber IORLs. There are two types of the latter: angle-supported (AS) lenses and iris-supported (IS) lenses.

Indications

This procedure can be a single or an additive procedure in KC patients; the following are suggestions for treatment:

- When the case is stable and there is high refractive error (>−6 dpt S.E) and BSCVA is reasonable, it can be a single procedure.
- When the case is stable and there is high refractive error (>−6 dpt S.E) and BSCVA is unreasonable because of high corneal irregularities, it can be an additive procedure in combination with ICRs.
- When the case is unstable and there is high refractive error (>−6 dpt S.E) and BSCVA is reasonable, it can be an additive procedure in combination with CXL.
- When the case is unstable and there is high refractive error (>−6 dpt S.E) and BSCVA is unreasonable, it can be an additive procedure in combination with ICRs and CXL.

Table 3.1 summarizes the above guidelines. The above guidelines are general and other guidelines should be considered such as corneal thickness, K-readings, etc.

Conditions

(a) The anterior chamber depth (ACD) measured from the endothelium must be at least 2.8 mm.
(b) Stable refraction.

Contraindications

(a) ACD <2.8
(b) Myopia other than axial
(c) Evidence of nuclear sclerosis or developing cataract
(d) History of uveitis
(e) Presence of anterior or posterior synechiae
(f) Corneal dystrophy
(g) Glaucoma or IOP higher than 20 mmHg
(h) Any other pathology in the anterior segment
(i) Personal or family history of retinal detachment
(j) Diabetes mellitus

Some of the above contraindications depend on the discretion of the surgeon and the needs of the patients.

Relative contraindications include the following:

(a) The patient should not rub the eye. Patients who cannot follow these instructions should not be implanted with a phakic IOL.
(b) The smallest available posterior chamber phakic lens is of 11-mm total diameter. The total diameter of the lens is calculated by adding 0.5 mm to the white-to-white limbal diameter. The minimum white-to-white diameter should be 11 mm. Any degree of microcornea from this size is a contraindication. In the case of an iris claw lens, it is possible to have customized, smaller lenses. While the normal phakic lens is 8.5 mm wide, the iris claw lens may be made as small as 6 mm, thus greatly extending its application.

Table 3.1 Guidelines for managing KC with IORLs

Stability	S.E	BSCVA	Management
Stable	>−6	Reasonable	IORLs
Stable	>−6	Reasonable	ICRs+IORLs
Unstable	>−6	Unreasonable	CxL+ICRs
Unstable	>−6	Unreasonable	CxL+ICRs+IORLs

Considerations

Ophthalmic Examination

All patients should undergo a complete ophthalmic examination:

(a) Manifest and cycloplegic refraction
(b) Uncorrected visual acuity
(c) Spectacle and/or contact lens corrected visual acuity
(d) Slit lamp examination of the anterior segment and ocular adnexa
(e) IOP
(f) Pupil size measurement under scotopic conditions
(g) Corneal endothelial cell count with specular endothelial microscopy
(h) Biometry to calculate axial length of the eyeball and the anterior chamber
(i) White-to-white corneal diameter measurement, if contemplating angle-supported or posterior chamber implants
(j) Videokeratography and keratometry
(k) Fundus examination by indirect ophthalmoscopy
(l) Anatomical imaging by anterior OCT or UBM.

Basic Concepts

When planning for an IORL implant, the surgeon should answer the following questions:

(a) What is the minimum age at which the lens is to be implanted?
(b) What is the minimum or the maximum refractive error to be treated?

(c) What should be the lowest limit for anterior chamber depth?
(d) What is the lowest corneal diameter at which lens implantation will be refused?
(e) How accurate is the white-to-white diameter on the basis of which the length of an implant lens is to be derived?
(f) What is the smallest size of the lens available?
(g) How can the risk of complications be minimized? What are those complications? What are the chances of occurrence?

Complications

In general, early complications are related to the design of the lens and the meticulous details of the surgery. Late postoperative complications are related to the interaction of the IORL and the intimate ocular tissues during the lifetime of the patient. After surgery, the implanted eyes should be monitored at least yearly, and for those with PC IORLs, monitoring should include UBM.

(a) Angle-supported IORLs:

The angle-supported (AS) IORL has two features; it lies completely in front of the pupil, and it is supported by the delicate tissues of the angle of the anterior chamber. Successful AS-IORLs should have some properties (defined by Charles Kelman) that should:

- Not put pressure on the angle
- Not move in the anterior chamber
- Not flex against the peripheral endothelium
- Not rub against the iris
- Not cause damage to the natural lens on insertion
- Not require an incision of more than 1.5–2 mm
- Not be difficult to insert
- Not be difficult to remove
- Not be difficult to exchange

Additionally, anatomical imaging (by anterior OCT or UBM) is important for correct AS-IORLs sizing:

- Correct measurement of angle-to-angle distance for IORL diameter.
- Sufficient clearance with the endothelium (more than 1.5 mm).
- Sufficient clearance with the crystalline lens (more than 700 μm).
  1. Intraoperative complications:
     - Hemorrhage may occur due to trauma to ciliary body or iridectomy
     - Ocular hypotony
     - Damage to the natural crystalline lens, endothelium, or iris
  2. Postoperative complications:
     - Ocular hypertension
     - Acute uveitis
     - Decentration, displacement, or rotation of the IORL causing reduced vision, prism effect, glare, or diplopia
     - Endophthalmitis
     - Injury to endothelium when lens is undersized and hence rotates and moves Anterior-Posteriorly
     - Corneal edema
     - Residual refractive error
     - Tenderness due to press upon the ciliary body especially if the lens has been placed vertically
     - Low-grade UGH syndrome
     - Cystoid macular edema
     - Oval pupil or distorted pupil

(b) Iris-supported IORLs:

1. Intraoperative complications:
   - Off-center fixation
   - Iris prolapse
   - Endothelial touch
   - Hemorrhage due to pull on the iris root, and during peripheral iridectomy
   - Crystalline lens injury due to clumsy efforts at iris enclavation
2. Postoperative complications:
   - Ocular hypertension
   - Early dislocation due to inadequate fixation.
   - Late dislocation due to trauma, or to iris atrophy within the lens claw
   - Early or late anterior uveitis
   - Corneal decompensation due to forcible rubbing. Corneal decompensation may occur if a dislocated phakic lens is not corrected or explanted well in time.
   - Endophthalmitis
   - Cystoid macular edema
   - Reduced vision, glare, halos, or diplopia
   - Residual refractive error

In general, most complications encountered with IS-IORLs are surgeon related, and can be avoided with good selection of candidates and perfect surgery.

In the selection of the candidates, special attention should be paid the anterior chamber depth and to iris shape. Patients with shallow anterior chamber and/or convex iris should be excluded.

During surgery, the key points to have perfect surgery are avoiding trauma and putting sufficient amount of iris tissue grasped by the haptics.

(c) Posterior chamber IORLs:

1. Intraoperative complications: Most intraoperative complications are rare and almost always related to human errors. The most important complication is trauma to the crystalline lens, which may or may not manifest later.
2. Early postoperative complications:
   - Pupillary block glaucoma due to the blockage of previous laser iridotomies or viscoelastic material residue in the posterior chamber. It shows itself within the first 24–48 h.
   - Loss of BSCVA
   - Overcorrection and under correction.
   - Quality of vision disturbances
   - Inflammation
   - Endophthalmitis
3. Late postoperative complications:
   - Iatrogenic anterior subcapsular cataract may develop because of contact with the natural crystalline lens. Many patients develop cataract within 2 years. This complication is size related; a small IORL has greater chances of having direct contact with the crystalline lens. Sizing should not be based on external anatomy or white-to-white distance which correlates poorly with the internal anatomy; thus, sizing should be done by UBM and then calculated by accomplished software.
   - Uveitis may occur in acute or chronic form.
   - Pigment dispersion may be seen on the artificial lens or the natural lens.
   - Late glaucoma may occur because of crowding of the angle and pigment deposits in the angle.
   - In some cases, the pupil may become partially dilated and not responding to the usual miotics.
   - Corneal decompensation.
   - Vitreoretinal complications such as progressive posterior retinal atrophy, spontaneous or neovascular macular hemorrhage, and rhegmatogenous retinal detachment.
   - Zonular damage, decentration, anterior and posterior dislocation.

3.2.3 Combination Between Treatment Modalities

It is not unusual that a KC case can be (or needs to be) treated with more than one treatment modality as shown in many studies. For example, a progressive case with high refractive error and good BSCVA can be treated by CxL to stabilize the cornea and IORLs to correct the high refractive error. A second example, a progressive moderate KC with moderate refractive error can be treated either by CxL and contact lenses if the patient is tolerant, or by CxL and spectacles, or by CxL and ICRs. A third example, a stable case of moderate KC with very high refractive error but with good BSCVA can be treated by ICRs then by IORLs in a second stage. In other words, combination between treatment modalities gives the opportunity to correct as much as possible corneal irregularity and refractive error, but with the least number of procedures.

3.3 Management Parameters

3.3.1 Introduction

Before starting discussion of management parameters, there are general considerations regarding full evaluation of the patient:

- Using RGP lenses must be stopped for at least 2 weeks before evaluation of any KC case to achieve a correct measurement of the corneal shape.
- Anecdotally reported refractive changes do not serve as a basis for decision making.
- Measurements previously performed in other clinics cannot be a basis for a treatment decision but can give an idea of the progression of the disease.
- Corneal topography should be done with Scheimpflug imaging and it will be more accurate when combined with Placido imaging system.
- Progression of the ectasia can only be determined by follow-ups.
- Family history should be considered.

3.3.2 Management Parameters

Taking the right decision in treating KC is not a simple process; it depends on important parameters. Patient's age, sex, and environment should be considered and it is important to know whether the disease has stopped progression or not. There are also important parameters related to the cornea itself such as corneal thickness at the thinnest location, maximal K-readings, corneal transparency, and the existence of stress lines. Patient's refractive error, UCVA and BSVA with and without the pin hole test (± PH) are also important factors affecting the decision.

3.3.2.1 Age

Patient's age is important for three reasons:

The younger the patient, the higher the possibility that the disease to be progressive.

The younger the patient, the more elastic the cornea and the more response to treatment the cornea shows.

CxL has higher ratio of complications in patients older than 35 years old.

3.3.2.2 Sex

Patient's sex is important for the following reasons:

(a) KC is prone to progress in females more than in males because of estrogen, especially during pregnancy and with taking anti-pregnancy estrogenic tablets. Therefore, it is recommended to think of CxL in females when they are in the productive age even in stable cases (when other parameters are suitable) to prevent deterioration of the case during pregnancy.
(b) It has been found in one study that there was a ratio of pre-cross-linked pregnant women who have lost the effect of CxL after pregnancy and they should be re-cross-linked.
(c) Both CxL and ICRs are contraindicated during pregnancy because of changes in corneal structure and because of social considerations.

3.3.2.3 Environment

One of the proposed factors for KC is environment; the incidence of the disease increases in dry and cold areas, especially in mountain populations. May be the high inter-marriage percentage in such relatively socially closed areas may exaggerate the problem, this is particularly seen in the Middle East, where cases are found to be more aggressive and in younger ages.

3.3.2.4 Progression

As mentioned previously, progression is defined as an increase in K-max by more than 1 dpt or corneal thinning at the thinnest location by more than 30 μ or an increase of topographical astigmatism by more than 1 dpt within 1 year of follow-up. It happens during the young age, usually till mid 20s and rarely after 30, hence the need for close follow-ups of patient's young brothers and sisters who may develop the disease, and also the need to stop the progression of the patient's disease as soon as possible.

3.3.2.5 Corneal Thickness

Thickness of the diseased cornea is important for the following reasons:

The thinner the cornea the higher the alert for advanced disease.

It is contraindicated to cross-link corneas thinner than 400 μ at the thinnest location.

It is not useful and not reasonable to implant ICRs in corneas thinner than 350 μ at the thinnest location.

The response of the cornea to ICRs decreases when the cornea is thin (<400 μ) or thick (>550 μ). The cause in both cases is the low percentage of collagen fibers, which are responsible for corneal elasticity, and the high percentage of viscous matrix, which is responsible for corneal viscosity. The high viscosity and the low elasticity lessen the corneal response needed by the ICRs to do their job.

3.3.2.6 K-max

It is well known that with high K-readings (>58 dpt), the response to ICRs decreases and the complications after CxL increase.

3.3.2.7 Refractive Errors and the Visual Acuity

Refractive error should be determined by both manifest spectacle refraction and cycloplegic refraction. Measuring uncorrected visual acuity (UCVA) and best spectacle-corrected visual acuity (BSCVA) with and without the pin hole test (±PH) is essential. The effect of refractive error, UCVA, and BSCVA was discussed previously, but in general, the followings are recommendations:

When sphere is ≤ -3 dpt and cylinder is ≤ -3 dpt, think of CxL and PRK.

When sphere is −3–6 dpt and cylinder is −3–6 dpt, think of ICRs.

When sphere is ≥ -6 dpt and/or cylinder is ≥ -6 dpt, think of IORLs or DALK.

3.3.2.8 Corneal Transparency and Stress Lines

When the cornea is not transparent due to central scaring or hydrops cornea, PKP and DALK are the main choices that should be discussed with the patient.

On the other hand, clear cornea with stress lines is an indicator of an advanced disease where the following are usually found: K-max > 60 dpt, high refractive error (S.E > −6 dpt), and corneal thickness < 350 μ. In such cases, DALK is usually indicated. In the author's experience with such cases, still other parameters can be considered such as the refractive error, UCVA, and BSCVA of the patient and there might be other choices such as ICRs with or without IORLs unless the disease is progressive.

3.3.2.9 PMD

Beside the previously mentioned two points (thinnest location and field of action), there is an important point regarding PKP and DALK. A number of surgical procedures have been performed to provide visual rehabilitation.

Standard-sized penetrating keratoplasty may produce poor results because the inferior edge of the transplant has to be sutured to an abnormally thin cornea, causing a high degree of post keratoplasty astigmatism in the short- and long-term periods. Continued thinning of the host cornea in the inferior aspect produces a situation similar to the situation that indicated surgery.

Large-diameter grafts have been tried to remove as much of the affected cornea as possible, with good success. However, because of the proximity to the limbus and its blood vessels, these grafts may be prone to rejection.

Regular-sized grafts that are deliberately decentered in the inferior aspect also work poorly. The degree of astigmatism is large because of decentered graft, and the incidence of rejection is high because of the proximity to the limbus.

Thermokeratoplasty and epikeratophakia are of only historical interest because the results obtained with these techniques are extremely poor.

Excision of a crescent wedge of corneal tissue from the inferior cornea, followed by tight suturing, has been reported to reduce the corneal ectasia.

The procedure is usually well tolerated; however, the effect is typically short lived, and thinning and ectasia recur.

In addition, this procedure may be hazardous in inexperienced hands. Several instances of wound dehiscence and resultant flat anterior chambers with its attendant problems have been reported with attempts of this procedure.

Crescent lamellar keratoplasty, in which a crescent transplant is performed to reinforce the area of thinning, has been described, but it may result in a high degree of astigmatism that necessitates subsequent central penetrating keratoplasty.

Currently, the combination of peripheral lamellar crescent keratoplasty, followed by a central penetrating keratoplasty after a few months, is a favored surgical treatment.

The lamellar transplant restores normal thickness to the inferior cornea and enables good edge-to-edge apposition at the time of penetrating keratoplasty, reducing the possibility of high post keratoplasty astigmatism.

Furthermore, the central graft that is now sutured to normal-thickness host tissue can be treated with videokeratography-guided selective removal of sutures and astigmatic keratotomy in the usual way to reduce any residual astigmatism.

Performing two keratoplasty procedures at different times necessitates the use of two separate corneas. By performing the two procedures in the same sitting, tissue from the same donor may be used, potentially reducing the antigenic load.

Because a central graft almost always is needed, performing both procedures at the same time significantly decreases the time needed to attain best corrected acuity. This consideration is important, as patients are often young and in the active and working phase of their lives.

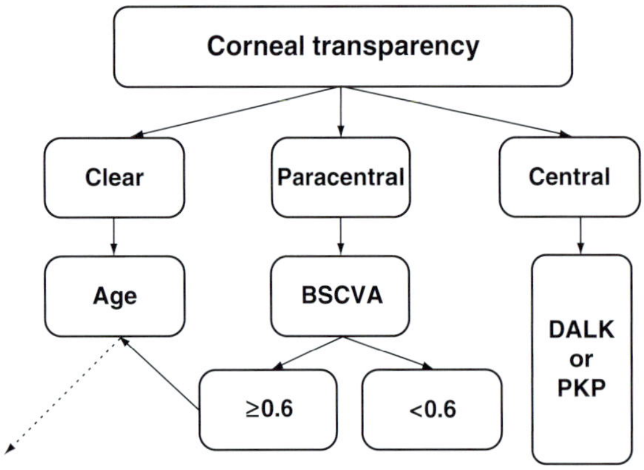

Fig. 3.38 Corneal transparency. There are three probabilities: (1) the cornea is clear, go through age; (2) a paracentral scar, see the BSCVA, if the latter is ≥0.6, go through age, otherwise do DALK or PKP depending on the level of the scar; (3) a central scar, do DALK or PKP depending on the level of the scar

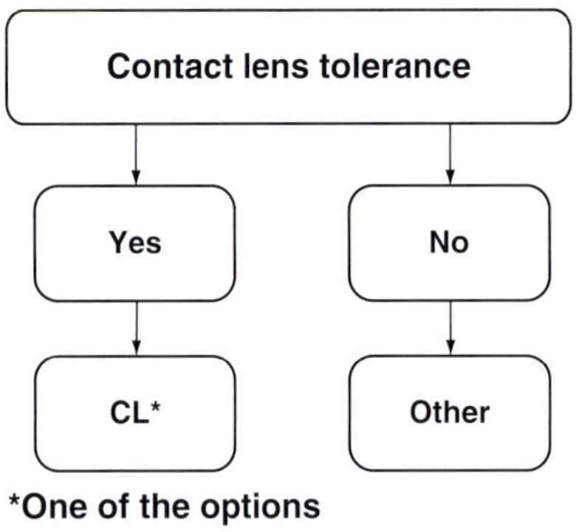

Fig. 3.39 Contact lens tolerance. If the patient is tolerant, CLs are one of the options; otherwise think of other modalities

3.4 The Systematic Plan for Managing Keratoconus

The author's systematic approach depends on determination of the following factors in the same following order:

1. Corneal transparency and stress lines
2. Age
3. Progression
4. Contact lens tolerance
5. Refractive error
6. UCVA and BSCVA with and without pinhole test. Best corrected visual acuity over gas-permeable contact lens should be tried if possible.
7. K-max

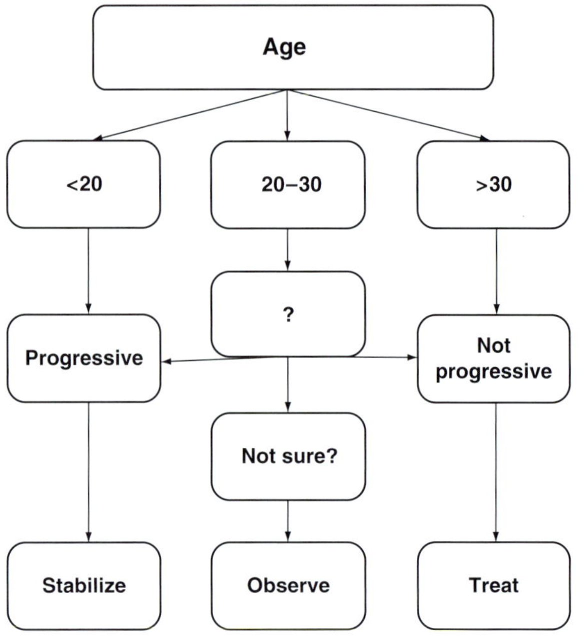

Fig. 3.40 Age. If the patient is younger than 20 years old, the disease should be considered as progressive and should be stabilized; if the patient is older than 30 years old, the disease can be considered as not progressive and can be treated; if the patient's age is 20–30-years old, the disease should be monitored

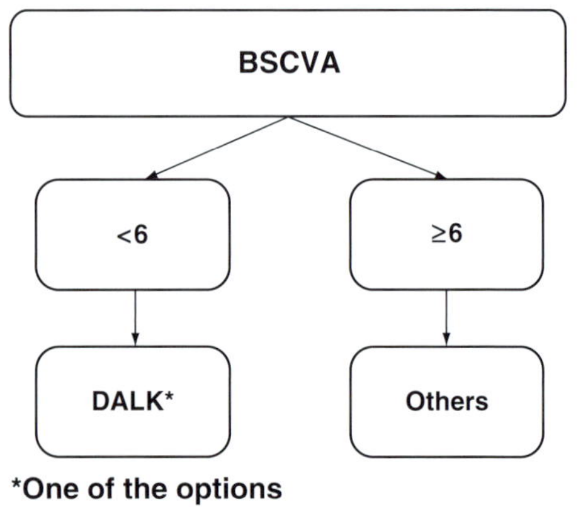

Fig. 3.41 BSCVA. Six over ten is the cutoff point

8. Corneal thickness
9. Sex

Figures from 3.38–3.45 illustrate management suggestion charts according to the mentioned factors. Figures from 3.46–3.49 summarize management suggestions and the main factors.

Table 3.2 is suggested as a checklist.

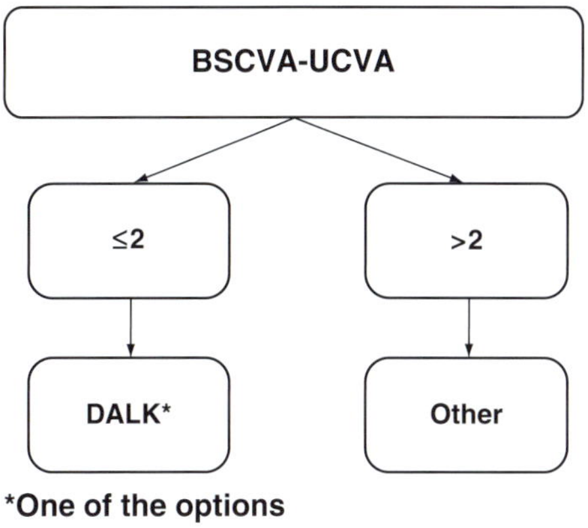

Fig. 3.42 Difference between BSCVA and UCVA. The cutoff point is two Snellen lines. This gives an impression about prognosis

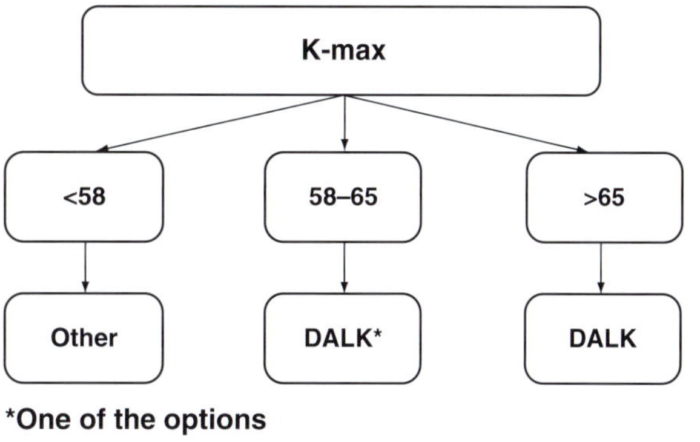

Fig. 3.44 Maximal K-readings. When K-max is >65 dpt, DALK should be performed, but it becomes an option when K-max is 58–65 dpt. When K-max is <58 dpt, options other than DALK are considered

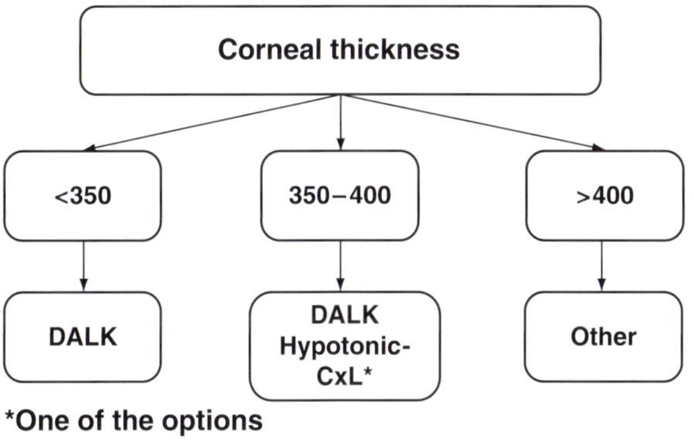

Fig. 3.43 Corneal thickness at the thinnest location. When corneal thickness is <350 μ, DALK will be a medical indication rather than a refractive indication since the cornea becomes very weak and tears in Descemets layer may happen leading to hydrops cornea. When corneal thickness is 350–400 μ, DALK or Hypotonic CxL is one of the options. When corneal thickness is >400 μ, options other than DALK are considered

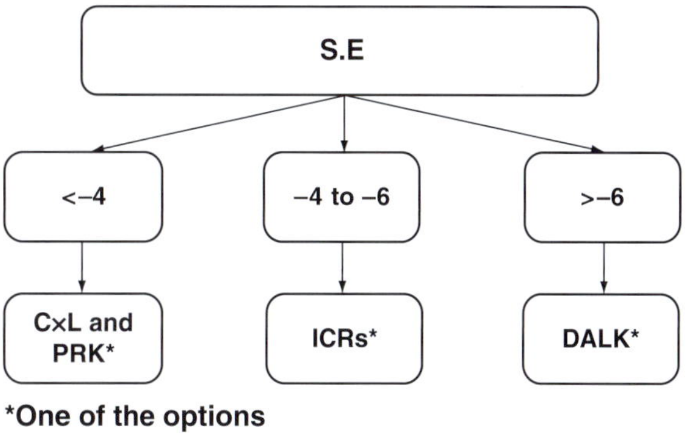

Fig. 3.45 Spherical equivalent (*SE*). When the SE is <–4 dpt, CxL with TG PRK can be performed since this refractive error can be corrected within the allowed 50 μ of ablation. When the SE is –4 to –6 dpt, ICRs implantation is one of the options. When the SE is >–6 dpt, DALK will be one of the options

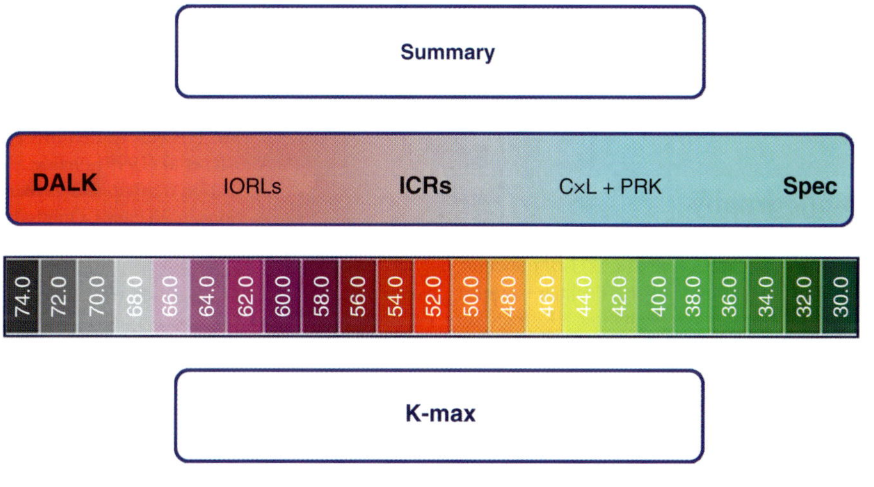

Fig. 3.46 Range of management modalities according to K-max. The higher the K-max, the closer the approach will be toward DALK. The lower the K-max, the closer the approach will be toward conservative treatments such spectacles

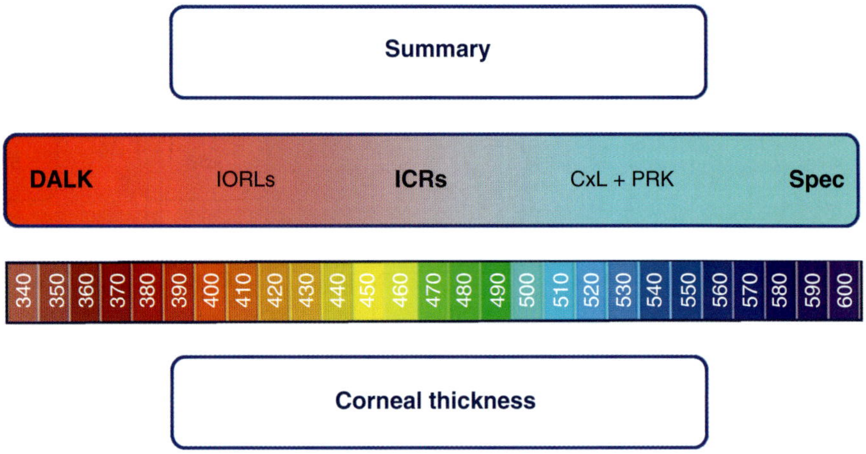

Fig. 3.47 Range of management modalities according to corneal thickness. The lower the thickness, the closer the approach will be toward DALK. The higher the thickness, the closer the approach will be toward conservative treatments such spectacles

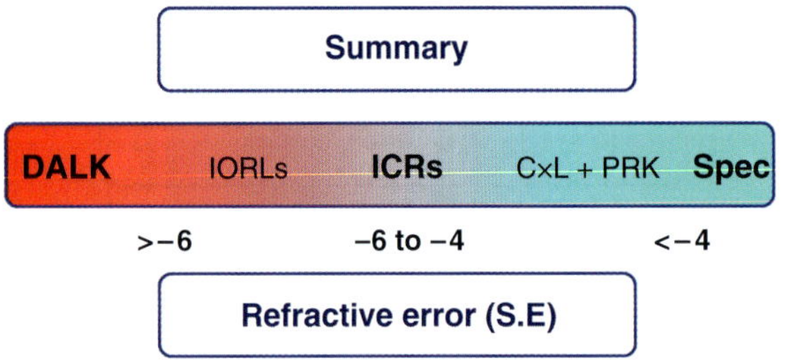

Fig. 3.48 Range of management modalities according to refractive error. The higher the S.E, the closer the approach will be toward DALK. The lower the S.E, the closer the approach will be toward conservative treatments such spectacles

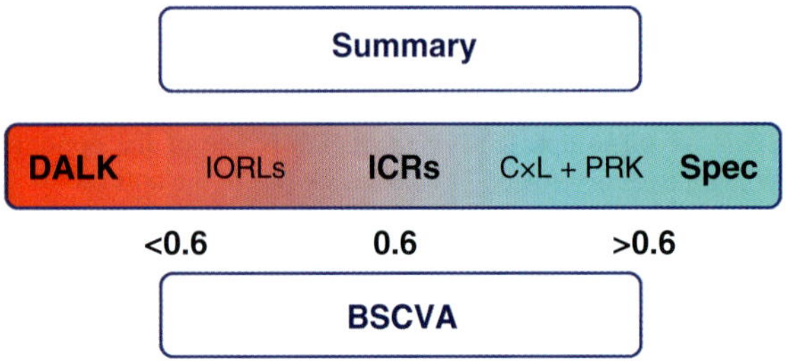

Fig. 3.49 Range of management modalities according to BSCVA. The worse the BSCVA, the closer the approach will be toward DALK. The better the BSCVA, the closer the approach will be toward conservative treatments such spectacles

Table 3.2 A suggested table for patient's data and the related management (s)

Factors	Patient data	Suggested treatment
Transparency and stress lines		
Age		
Progression		
CL tolerance		
Refractive error (S.E)		
BSCVA vs. UCVA		
K-max		
Corneal thickness @ thinnest location		
Sex		
Management summary		

Bibliography

Aguilar-Valenzuela L et al (2003) Intraocular pressure in myopic patients after Worst-Fechner anterior chamber phakic intraocular lens implantation. J Refract Surg 19(2):131–136

Alessandro M et al (2005) Conservative treatment of early an moderate pellucid marginal degeneration: a new refractive approach with intracorneal rings. Ophthalmology 112: 660–666

Alfonso FJ et al (2011) Intrastromal corneal ring segments and posterior chamber phakic intraocular lens implantation for keratoconus correction. J Cataract Refract Surg 37:706–713

Alio JL, Azar DT (2008) Management of complications in refractive surgery. Springer, Heidelberg

Alio JL, De La Hoz F and Ismail MM (1993). Subclinical inflammatory reaction induced by phakic anterior chamber lenses for the correction of high myopia: ocular lenses for the correction of high myopia. Avaliable at http://www.tandf.co.uk/swets.asp. In: Ocular immunology and inflammation, Vol 1. Swets & Zeitlinger 219–223.

Alio JL et al (1999) Phakic anterior chamber lenses for the correction o myopia: a 7-year cumulative analysis of complications in 26 cases. Ophthalmology 106(3):458–466

Alio JL et al (2006a) Analysis of results related to good and bad outcomes of intacs implantation for keratoconus correction. J Cataract Refract Surg 32:756–761

Alio JL et al (2006b) Intracorneal ring segments for keratoconus correction: long-term follow-up. J Cataract Refract Surg 32:978–985

Allemann N et al (2000) Myopic angle-supported intraocular lenses: two-year follow-up. Ophthalmology 107(8):1549–1554

Ardjomand N et al (2002) Pupillary block after phakic anterior chamber intraocular lens implantation. J Cataract Refract Surg 28(6):1080–1081

Arne JL, Lesueur LC (2000) Phakic posterior chamber lenses for high myopia: functional and anatomical outcomes. J Cataract Refract Surg 26(3):369–374

Arriola-Villalobos P (2009) Intrastromal corneal ring segment implantation for high astigmatism after penetrating keratoplasty. J Cataract Refract Surg 35:1878–1884

Asano-Kato N et al (2005) Experience with the Artisan phakic intraocular lens in Asian eyes. J Cataract Refract Surg 31(5):910–915

Assetto V et al (1996) Collamer intraocular contact lens to correct high myopia. J Cataract Refract Surg 22(5):551–556

Assil KK (2008). The ARTISAN myopia lens: interim results of the US FDA clinical study. Available at http://emedicine.medscape.com/article/1221908-overview. Accessed Dec 2008.

Benedetti S et al (2005) Correction of myopia of 7 to 24 diopters with the Artisan phakic intraocular lens: two-year follow-up. J Refract Surg 21(2):116–126

Caroline P et al. (2006). Etiology, diagnosis, and management of keratoconus: new thoughts and new understandings. Pacific University College of Optometry. Retrieved on 26 March 2006.

Colin J (2006) European clinical evaluation: use of intacs for the treatment of keratoconus. J Cataract Refract Surg 32:747–755

Colin J, Velou S (2003) Current surgical options for keratoconus. J Cataract Refract Surg 29:379–386

Colin CK et al (2007) Effect of inferior-segment intacs with and without C3-R on keratoconus. J Cataract Refract Surg 33:75–80

Consuelo F et al (2010) Causes of intrastromal corneal ring segment explantation: clinicopathologic correlation analysis. J Cataract Refract Surg 36:970–977

Coskunseven E et al (2009) Effect of treatment sequence in combined intrastromal corneal rings and corneal collagen crosslinking for keratoconus. J Cataract Refract Surg 35(12):2084–2091

Dejaco-Ruhswurm I et al (2002) Long-term endothelial changes in phakic eyes with posterior chamber intraocular lenses. J Cataract Refract Surg 28(9):1589–1593

Ertan A (2009) Early and severe keratoconus treatment options: do intacs intracorneal rings ensure optimal outcomes? Ophthalmol Times Eur 5(2): 2–4

Ertan A, Bahadir MJ (2006) Intrastromal ring segment insertion using a femtosecondlaser to correct pellucid marginal corneal degeneration. J Cataract Refract Surg 32(10): 1710–1716

Ertan A, Colin J (2007) Intracorneal rings for keratoconus and keratectasia. J Cataract Refract Surg 33:1303–1314

Espandar L, Meyer J (2010) Keratoconus: overview and update on treatment. Middle East Afr J Ophthalmol 17(1):15–20

Fechner PU (1990) Intraocular lenses for the correction of myopia in phakic eyes: short-term success and long-term caution. Refract Corneal Surg 6(4):242–244

Fechner PU (1999) Cataract formation with a phakic IOL. J Cataract Refract Surg 25(4):461–462

Fechner PU, Wichmann W (1993) Correction of myopia by implantation of minus optic (Worst iris claw) lenses into the anterior chamber of phakic eyes. Eur J Implant Refract Surg 5:55–59

Fechner PU et al (1989) The correction of myopia by lens implantation into phakic eyes. Am J Ophthalmol 107(6):659–663

Fechner PU et al (1991) Correction of myopia by implantation of a concave Worst-iris claw lens into phakic eyes. Refract Corneal Surg 7(4):286–298

Fechner PU et al (1996) Posterior chamber myopia lenses in phakic eyes. J Cataract Refract Surg 22(2):178–182

Frederik Raiskup-Wolf et al (2008) Collagen crosslinking with riboflavin and ultraviolet-A light in keratoconus: long-term results. J Cataract Refract Surg 34:796–801

Fyodorov SN et al (1993) Clinical and functional follow-up of minus IOL implantation in high grade myopia. Oftalmochirurgia 2:12–17

Ghajarnia M et al (2008) Descemet detachment after femtosecond-laser-assisted placement of intrastromal ring segments in pellucid marginal degeneration. J Cataract Refract Surg 34(12):2174–2176

Gonvers M et al (2001) Implantable contact lens for moderate to high myopia: short-term follow-up of 2 models. J Cataract Refract Surg 27(3):380–388

Greenstein SA et al (2010) Natural history of corneal haze after collagen crosslinking for keratoconus and corneal ectasia: Scheimpflug and biomicroscopic analysis. J Cataract Refract Surg 36:2105–2114

Greenstein SA et al (2011) Corneal thickness changes after corneal collagen crosslinking for keratoconus and corneal ectasia: one-year results. J Cataract Refract Surg 37(4): 691–700

Grewal DS et al (2009) Corneal collagen crosslinking using riboflavin and ultraviolet-A light for keratoconus one-year analysis using Scheimpflu imaging. J Cataract Refract Surg 35:425–432

He X et al (2010) Measurement of corneal changes after collagen crosslinking using a noninvasive ultrasound system. J Cataract Refract Surg 36(7):1207–1212

Hersh PS et al (2011) Corneal collagen crosslinking for keratoconus and corneal ectasia: one-year results. J Cataract Refract Surg 37(1):149–160

Jankov Ii MR et al (2010) Corneal collagen cross-linking. Middle East Afr J Ophthalmol 17(1):21–27

Javadi MA et al (2004) Lamellar crescentic resection for pellucid marginal corneal degeneration. J Refract Surg 20(2): 162–165

Javadi MA et al (2005) Outcomes of penetrating keratoplasty in keratoconus. Cornea 24(8):941–946

Jimenez-Alfaro I et al (2001) Safety of posterior chamber phakic intraocular lenses for the correction of high myopia: anterior segment changes after posterior chamber phakic intraocular lens implantation. Ophthalmology 108(1):90–99

Kamburoglu G et al (2007) Implantation of Artisan toric phakic intraocular lens following intacs in a patient with keratoconus. J Cataract Refract Surg 33:528–530

Kashani AA (1996) Phakic posterior chamber intraocular lenses for the correction of high myopia. J Refract Surg 12(4): 454–456

Kohlhaas M et al (2006) Biomechanical evidence of the distribution of cross-links in corneas treated with riboflavin and ultraviolet A light. J Cataract Refract Surg 2:279–283

Koller T et al (2009) Complication and failure rates after corneal crosslinking. J Cataract Refract Surg 35:1358–1362

Kolli S, Aslanides IM (2010) Safety and efficacy of collagen crosslinking for the treatment of keratoconus. Expert Opin Drug Saf 9(6):949–957

Krumeich JH, Duncker G (2006) Intrastromal corneal ring in penetrating keratoplasty: evidence-based update 4 years after implantation. J Cataract Refract Surg 32:993–998

Kubaloglu A et al (2010) Comparison of mechanical and femtosecond laser tunnel creation for intrastromal corneal ring segment implantation in keratoconus prospective randomized clinical trial. J Cataract Refract Surg 36:1556–1561

Kymionis GD (2011) Corneal collagen cross linking - PLUS. Open Ophthalmol J 5:10

Kymionis DG et al (2004) Intacs for early pellucid marginal degeneration. J Cataract Refract Surg 30(1):230–233

Kymionis DG et al (2007) Herpetic keratitis with iritis after corneal crosslinking with riboflavin and ultraviolet A for keratoconus. J Cataract Refract Surg 33:1982–1984

Kymionis GD et al (2009a) Intraoperative pachymetric measurements during corneal collagen cross-linking with riboflavin and ultraviolet A irradiation. Ophthalmology 116(12): 2336–2339

Kymionis GD et al (2009b) Management of pellucid marginal corneal degeneration with simultaneous customized photorefractive keratectomy and collagen crosslinking. J Cataract Refract Surg 35(7):1298–1301

Kymionis GD et al (2010) Photorefractive keratectomy followed by same-day corneal collagen crosslinking after intrastromal corneal ring segment implantation for pellucid marginal degeneration. J Cataract Refract Surg 36(10):1783–1785

Labiris G et al (2011) Corneal melting after collagen crosslinking for keratoconus: a case report. J Med Case Reports 5(1):152

Landesz M et al (2001) Iris-claw phakic intraocular lens for high myopia. J Refract Surg 17(6):634–640

Malecaze FJ et al (2002) A randomized paired eye comparison of two techniques for treating moderately high myopia: LASIK and artisan phakic lens. Ophthalmology 109(9): 1622–1630

Maloney RK et al (2002) Artisan phakic intraocular lens for myopia: short-term results of a prospective, multicenter study. Ophthalmology 109(9):1631–1641

McCall AS et al (2010) Mechanisms of corneal tissue crosslinking in response to treatment with topical riboflavin and long-wavelength ultraviolet radiation (UVA). Invest Ophthalmol Vis Sci 51(1):129–138

Meek MK et al (2005) Changes in collagen orientation and distribution in keratoconus corneas. Invest Ophthalmol & Vis Sci Vol. 46, No. 6

Menezo JL et al (1996) Iris-fixated Worst claw versus sulcus-fixated posterior chamber lenses in the absence of capsular support. J Cataract Refract Surg 22(10):1476–1484

Menezo JL et al (1998) Endothelial study of iris-claw phakic lens: four year follow-up. J Cataract Refract Surg 24(8): 1039–1049

Menezo JL et al (2004) Phakic intraocular lenses to correct high myopia: Adatomed, Staar, and Artisan. J Cataract Refract Surg 30(1):33–44

Navas A, Suarez R (2009) One-year follow-up of toric intraocular lens implantation in forme fruste keratoconus. J Cataract Refract Surg 35:2024–2027

Nuzzi G, Cantù C (2002) Vitreous hemorrhage following phakic anterior chamber intraocular lens implantation in severe myopia. Eur J Ophthalmol 12(1):69–72

Park S et al (2010) Late dislocation of intrastromal corneal ring segment into the anterior chamber. J Cataract Refract Surg 36:2003–2005

Perez-Santonja JJ et al (2009a) Microbial keratitis after corneal collagen corneal crosslinking and bandage contact lens use. J Cataract Refract Surg 35:788–791

Perez-Santonja JJ et al (2009b) Microbial keratitis after corneal collagen crosslinking. J Cataract Refract Surg 35:1138–1140

Pérez-Santonja JJ et al (1996a) Chronic subclinical inflammation in phakic eyes with intraocular lenses to correct myopia. J Cataract Refract Surg 22(2):183–187

Pérez-Santonja JJ et al (1996b) Endothelial changes in phakic eyes with anterior chamber intraocular lenses to correct high myopia. J Cataract Refract Surg 22(8):1017–1022

Pérez-Santonja JJ et al (2000) Surgical correction of severe myopia with a angle-supported phakic intraocular lens. J Cataract Refract Surg 26(9):1288–1302

Pérez-Torregrosa VT et al (1995) Digital system measurement of decentration of Worst-Fechner iris claw myopia intraocular lens. J Refract Surg 11(1):26–30

Pokroy R, Levinger S (2006) Intacs adjustment surgery for keratoconus. J Cataract Refract Surg 32:986–992

Raiskup F and Spoerl E (2011) Corneal cross-linking with hypoosmolar riboflavin solution in thin keratoconic corneas. Am J Ophthalmol (article in press: published online in 28 April 2011)

Rama P et al (2009) Acanthamoeba keratitis with perforation after corneal crosslinking and bandage contact lens use. J Cataract Refract Surg 35:788–791

Rasheed K, Rabinowitz YS (1997) Results of combined lamellar and penetrating keratoplasty for pellucid marginal degeneration. Ophthalmol Suppl; Oct: 191

Rodriguez AL et al (2007) Penetrating keratoplasty versus intrastromal corneal ring segments to correct bilateral corneal ectasia: preliminary study. J Cataract Refract Surg 33:488–496

Rodriguez LA et al (2009) Treatment of six cases of advanced ectasia after LASIK with 6-mm intacs SK. J Refract Surg 25:1116–1119

Rodriguez-Prats J et al (2003) Intracorneal rings for the correction o pellucid marginal degeneration. J Cataract Refract Surg 29:1421–1424

Rosen E, Gore C (1998) Staar Collamer posterior chamber phakic intraocular lens to correct myopia and hyperopia. J Cataract Refract Surg 24(5):596–606

Rubinstein MP, Sud S (1999) The use of hybrid lenses in management of the irregular cornea. Cont Lens Anterior Eye 22(3):87–90

Ruiz-Moreno JM et al (2003) Choroidal neovascularization in phakic eyes with anterior chamber intraocular lenses to correct high myopia. J Cataract Refract Surg 29(2):270–274

Sansanayudh W et al (2010) Intrastromal corneal ring segment SK implantation for moderate to severe keratoconus. J Cataract Refract Surg 36:110–113

Schanzlin DJ et al (1983) Crescentic lamellar keratoplasty for pellucid marginal degeneration. Am J Ophthalmol 96(2): 253–254

Schirmbeck T et al (2005) Efficacy and low cost in keratoconus treatment with rigid gas-permeable contact lens. Arq Bras Oftalmol 68(2):219–222

Senthil S, Reddy KP (2006) A retrospective analysis of the first Indian experience on Artisan phakic intraocular lens. Indian J Ophthalmol 54(4):251–255

Sharma N et al (2010) Pseudomonas keratitis after collagen crosslinking for keratoconus: case report and review of literature. J Catarac Refract Surg 36:517–520

Spoerl E et al (2004a) Increased resistance of crosslinked cornea against enzymatic digestion. Curr Eye Res 29(1): 35–40

Spoerl E et al (2004b) Thermomechanical behavior of collagen-cross-linked porcine cornea. Ophthalmologica 218(2): 136–140

Spoerl E et al (2011) Corneal cross-linking and safety issues. Open Ophthalmol J 5:14–16

Stulting RD et al (2008) Three-year results of Artisan/Verisyse phakic intraocular lens implantation: results of the United States Food And Drug Administration clinical trial. Ophthalmology 115(3):464–472

Verma A (2008) Phakic IOL myopia. Available at http://emedicine.medscape.com/article/1221908-overview.

Vinciguerra P et al (2009) Intraoperative and postoperative effects of corneal collagen cross-linking on progressive keratoconus. Arch Ophthalmol 127(10):1258–1265

Wachler BSB (2008) Modern management of keratoconus. Jaypee Brothers medical Publishers, New Delhi: 75–228

Weissman BA, Yeung KK (2006) Keratoconus. eMedicine: keratoconus. Available at http://en.wikipedia.org/wiki/Keratoconus. Accessed 12 Feb 2006

Yeung K et al (1995) Clinical experience with piggyback contact lens systems on keratoconic eyes. J Am Optom Assoc 66(9):539–543

4 Case Study

Introduction

Studying any case of KC consists of three steps

Step 1: Analyzing Step

This step consists of

1. Analyzing patient's data including history, clinical examination, and corneal topography. Analyzing corneal topography consists of studying the following maps: the anterior sagittal and tangential curvature maps, the anterior and posterior elevation maps, and the thickness map.
   (i) The anterior sagittal curvature map should be displayed with the distribution of the steep and flat segments on. Studying the anterior sagittal curvature map is essential to determine the topographical *pattern*. Modification of the color scale may be needed in order to clarify the pattern of the cone.
   (ii) The anterior tangential map and the elevation maps in the BFS mode are essential to determine the *shape* and the *location* of the cone.
   (iii) The thickness map is essential for differentiating between PMD and PLK.
2. Krumeich classification is applied to grade the case.

Step 2: Management Suggestion Step

This step consists of

1. Filling the suggested table with patient's data.
2. Filling suggestion(s) for management(s) according to each category alone.
3. Summarizing the most appropriate management(s) at the bottom of the table.

Step 3: Discussion Step

All possibilities of suggested managements will be discussed bearing in mind that the least managements and the least combination between managements should be done.

N.P: Only positive findings will be mentioned in the history taking of the patient.

M.M. Sinjab, *Quick Guide to the Management of Keratoconus*,
DOI 10.1007/978-3-642-21840-8_4, © Springer-Verlag Berlin Heidelberg 2012

4.1 Case 1

A 19-year-old male has a progressive refractive error in both eyes. He is complaining of rapid progression of blurring of vision. He is also intolerant to contact lenses. His manifest refraction (MR) is (Table 4.1.1):

Table 4.1.1 Manifest refraction

Eye	Sphere	Cylinder	Axis	UCVA	BSVCA	BSCVA+PH
OD	−1	−2.5	150	0.6	0.8	0.9
OS	−2.25	−2.25	95	0.5	0.7	0.8

His old correction (3 months ago) is (Table 4.1.2):

Table 4.1.2 Old refraction

Eye	Sphere	Cylinder	Axis
OD	−0.75	−1	140
OS	−1.5	−1.25	135

Slitlamp examination shows clear cornea with no stress lines. Other ocular findings are within normal limits.

Corneal Topography reveals KC in both eyes, more advanced in the left eye.

For educational purposes, the left eye will be studied. Figure 4.1.1 shows corneal topography of the left eye.

4.1.1 Step 1: Analyzing Step

1. The patient is 19 years old, so he is supposed to be in the age of progression.
2. His refractive error is progressing during short periods, this is clear from his complaint and by comparing his old glasses (Table 4.1.2) with his recent MR (Table 4.1.1).
3. The axes of the old glasses, manifest refraction, and topography are different. This means a skew in astigmatism which is usually consistent with KC.

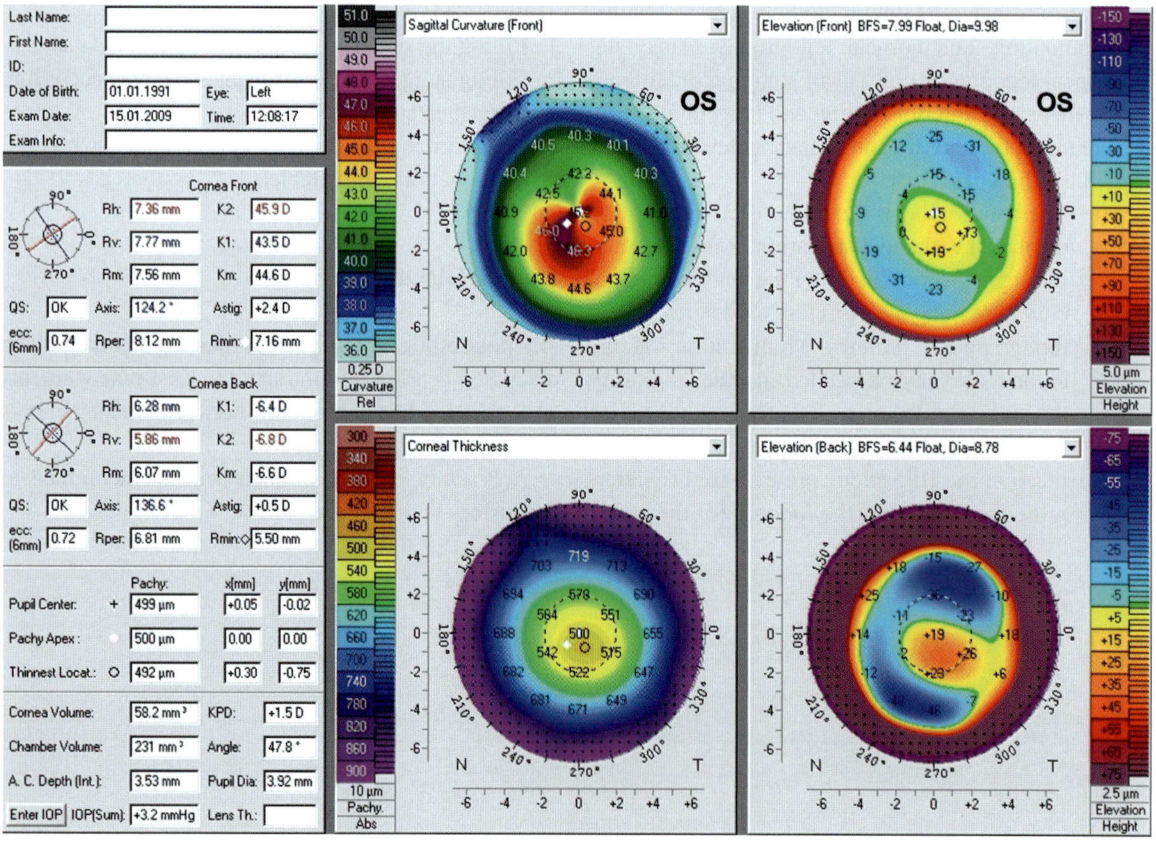

Fig. 4.1.1 Corneal topography of the left eye: mild KC

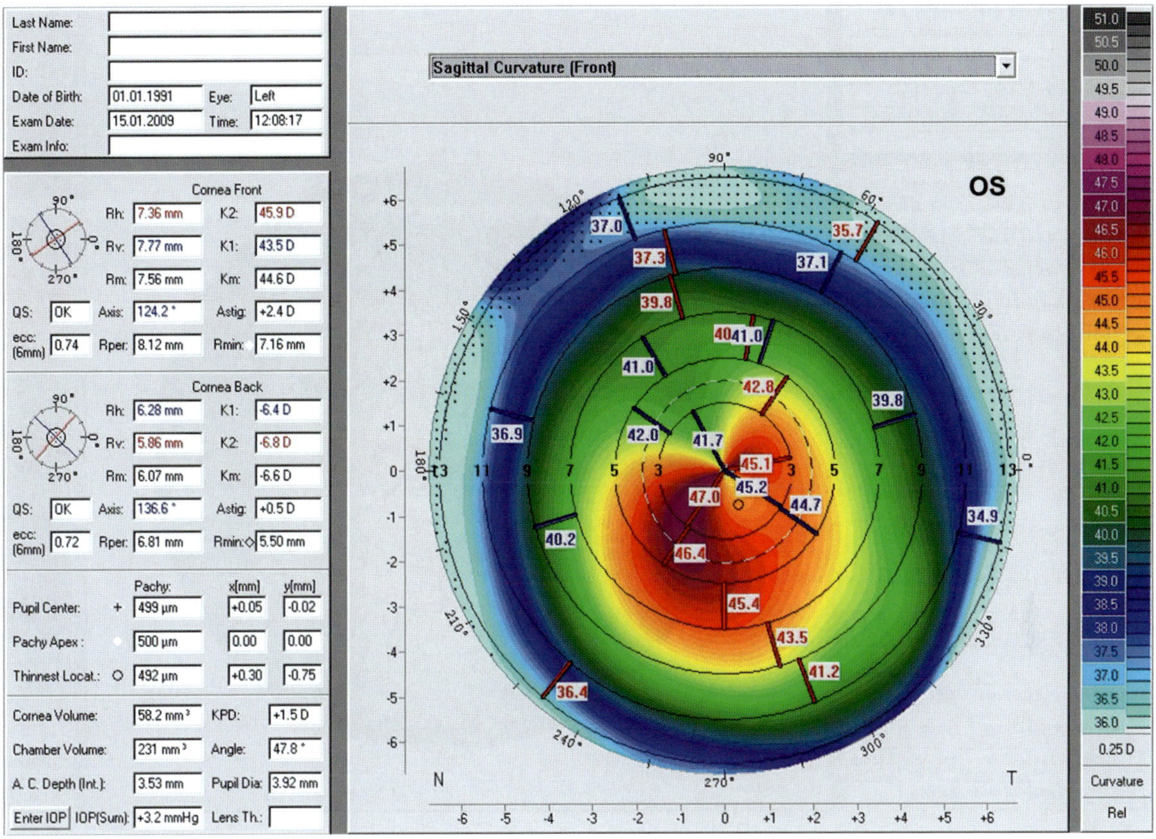

Fig. 4.1.2 Anterior sagittal curvature map. The curvature pattern is AB/SRAX. According to author's classification, it is pattern 2

4. UCVA is primarily good and there is three lines difference between UCVA and BSCVA, this usually carries a good prognosis.
5. Corneal topography of the left eye is taken as an example:
   (a) Figure 4.1.1 shows the main four maps, it is obviously KC.
   (b) Figure 4.1.2 is the anterior sagittal curvature map. The topographical pattern is AB/SRAX; it is AB because the inferior segment of the bow tie is larger than the superior segment and the refractive power of the inferior segment is higher than the superior by more than 1.5 dpt; it is SRAX because of the more than 22° of skew between the axes of the two segments. Since K-readings are not high, the shape of the cone is clear and there is no need for color modification (see Fig. 4.1.3).
6. According to Krumeich classification, this case is grade 1 KC, and according to the author's classification, it is pattern 2.

4.1.2 Step 2: Management Suggestions

Table 4.1.3 summarizes patient data and the corresponding individual suggestion(s) for treatment, and presents a final summary of the best management.

Table 4.1.3 Management suggestions

Factors	Patient data	Suggested treatment
Transparency and stress lines	Transparent with no stress lines	
Age	19	CxL
Progression	Most probably yes	CxL
CL tolerance	No	Other modalities
Refractive error (S.E)	−3.25 dpt	CxL and PRK or ICRs
BSCVA Vs UCVA	3 lines difference	CxL and PRK or ICRs
K-max	47	CxL and PRK
Corneal thickness @ thinnest location	492 µ	CxL and PRK
Sex	Male	
Management summary	CxL with or without PRK	

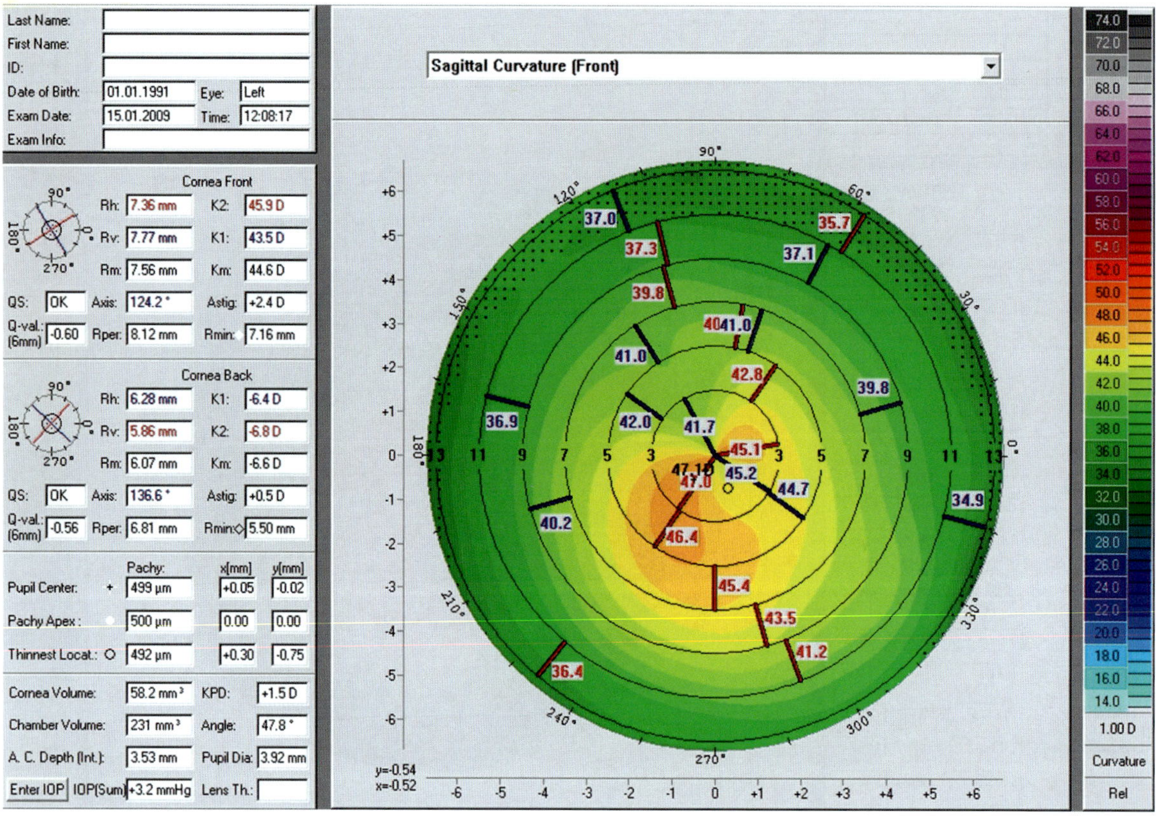

Fig. 4.1.3 Anterior sagittal curvature map after color modification, which is necessary in severe cases to identify the shape of the cone

4.1.3 Step 3: Discussion

1. It is a mild case of KC which does not need aggressive procedures to be managed with.
2. As the case is progressive, the cornea should be cross-linked.
3. As the refractive error is small (< −6 dpt) and the thinnest location is >450 µ, TG PRK is a good choice.

Personally, I do not advise ICRs because of small K-readings and refractive error; using ICRs in such a case carries the possibility of over correction. I do advise CXL with or without TG PRK.

Figure 4.1.4 shows a similar case treated with CxL and TG PRK. A (on the left) is the preoperative curvature map, B (in the middle) is the postoperative curvature map, and C (on the right) is the difference map that shows the correction achieved by the TG PRK. Note the homogenous shape of the cornea after the operation that led to improvement in quality and quantity of vision.

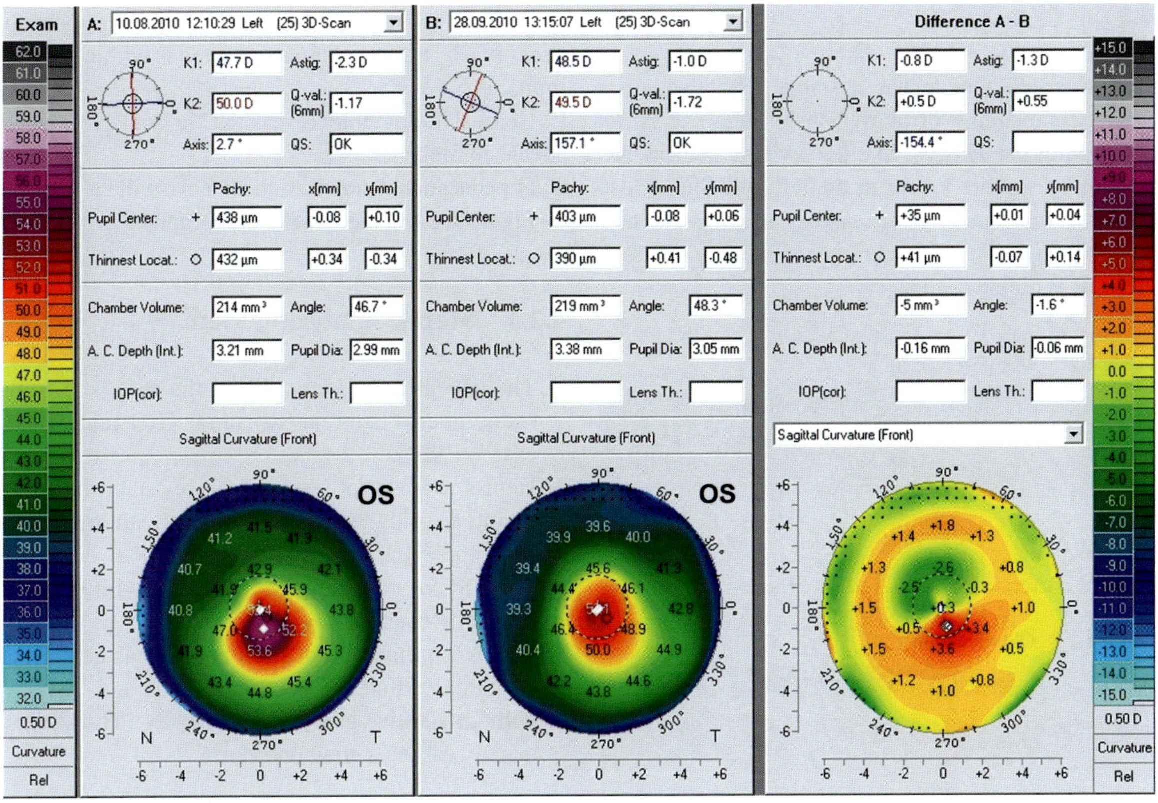

Fig. 4.1.4 A mild KC case treated with CxL and TG PRK. A (on the left) is the pre-op map; B (in the middle) is the post-op map; and C (on the left) is the difference map showing the correction achieved by this procedure

4.2 Case 2

A 41-year-old female has a stable refractive error. She is complaining of blurred vision and she is not happy with her glasses. She knows that she has KC in both eyes, more severe in the left eye. She is also intolerant to contact lenses and is seeking for new solutions.

Her MR is (Table 4.2.1):

Table 4.2.1 Manifest refraction

Eye	Sphere	Cylinder	Axis	UCVA	BSVCA	BSCVA+PH
OD	−3	−2.5	165	0.4	0.5	0.7
OS	−5	−2.5	120	0.05	0.4	0.6

Her old correction (1 year ago) is (Table 4.2.2):

Table 4.2.2 Old refraction

Eye	Sphere	Cylinder	Axis
OD	−2.75	−2.5	155
OS	−5	−3	120

Slitlamp examination shows clear cornea with no stress lines. Other ocular examination is within normal limits.

Corneal Topography reveals KC in both eyes, more advanced in the left eye.

For educational purposes, the left eye will be studied. Figure 4.2.1 is the left eye topography.

4.2.1 Step 1: Analyzing Step

1. The patient is 41 years old, so the case is already stable due to age-related natural CxL (unless the case is PMD).
2. Her refractive error is most probably stable by comparing her old glasses (Table 4.2.2) with her recent MR (Table 4.2.1).
3. The BSCVA cannot reach 10/10 even with PH; this is usually consistent with KC.
4. UCVA is primarily not good but there is an almost four lines difference between UCVA and BSCVA with an additive gain of two lines by PH test, this usually carries a good prognosis.

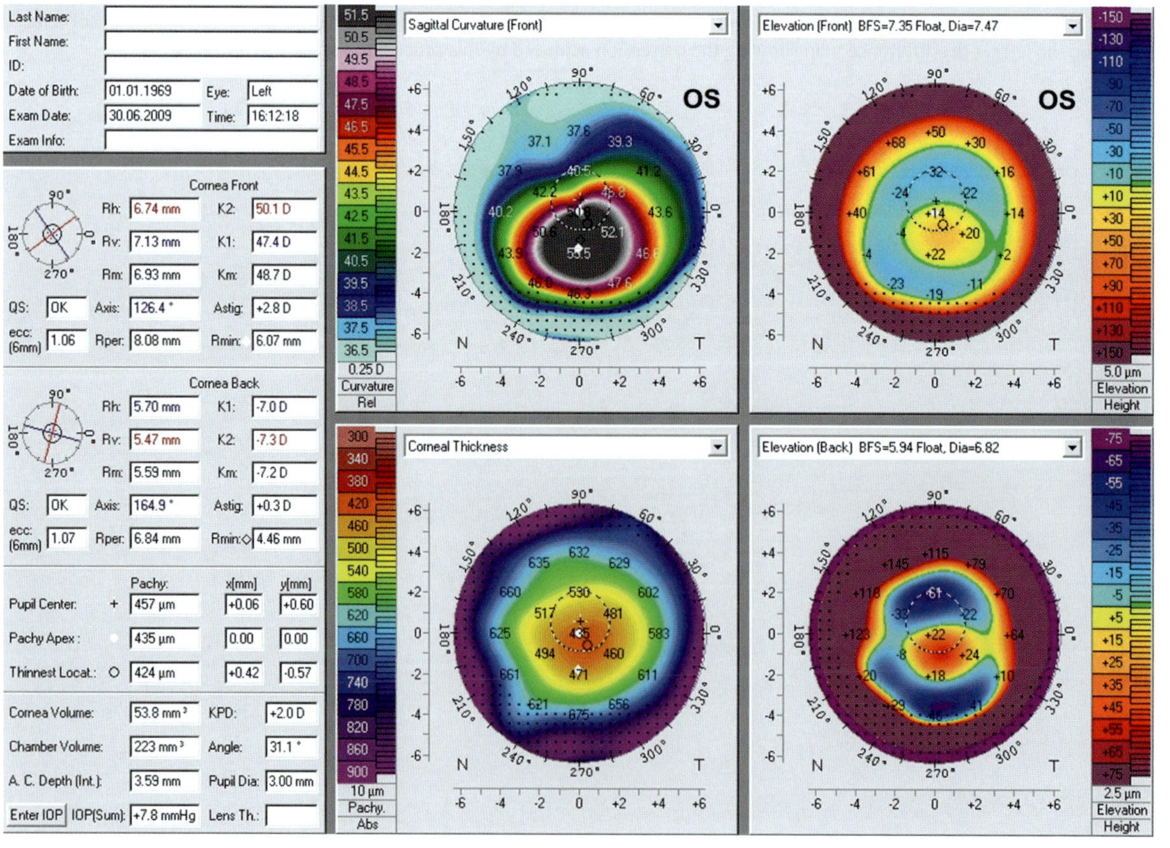

Fig. 4.2.1 Corneal topography of the left eye: moderate KC

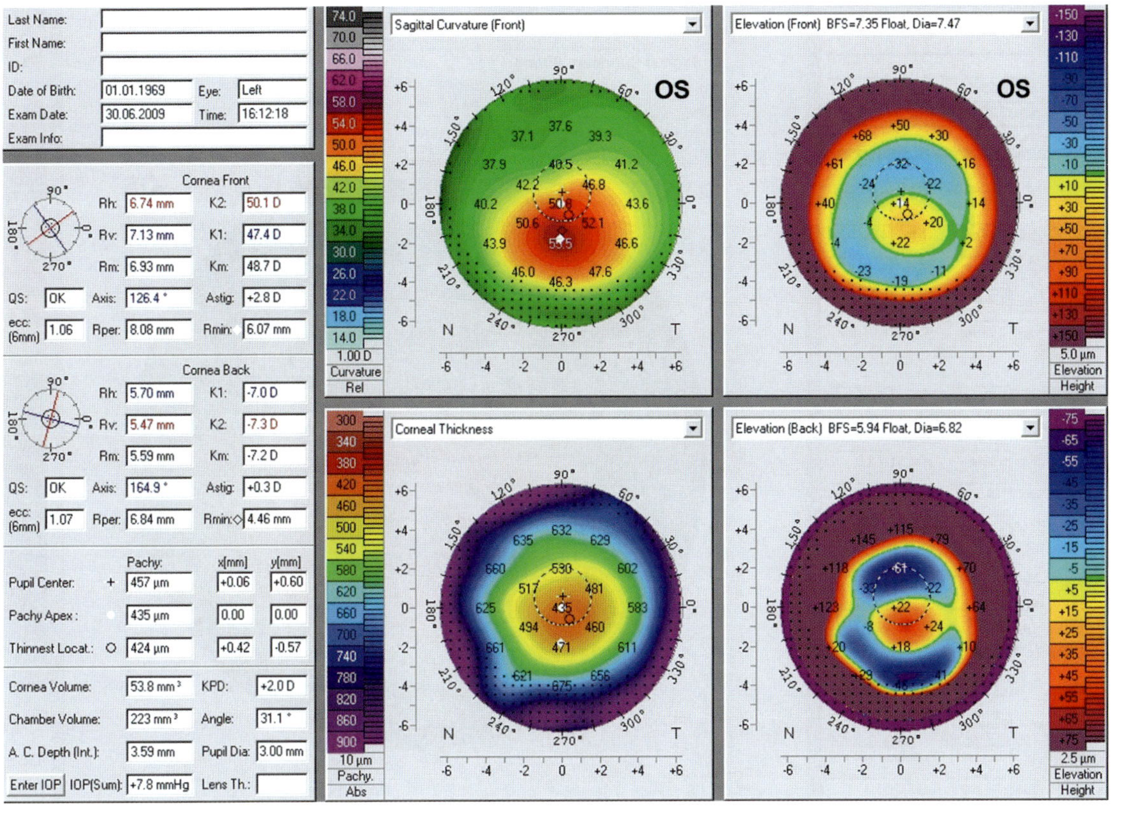

Fig. 4.2.2 Corneal topography of the left eye after color modification to clarify the shape of the cone

5. Corneal topography of the left eye:
   (a) Figure 4.2.1 shows the main four maps.
   (b) Figure 4.2.2 shows the same maps after color modification to clarify the details of the cone.
   (c) Figure 4.2.3 is the anterior sagittal curvature map. The topographical pattern is initially PMD or PLK.
6. According to Krumeich classification, this case is grade 2 KC, and according to the author's classification, it is pattern 5.

4.2.2 Step 2: Management Suggestions

Table 4.2.3 summarizes patient data and the corresponding individual suggestion(s) of treatment, and presents a final summary of the best management.

4.2.3 Step 3: Discussion Step

1. This case seems to be not progressive; thus, CxL is not needed unless the refractive error is to be treated by TG PRK.
2. As the refractive error is not small (> −4 dpt) and the thinnest location is 424 μ, TG PRK is not a good choice.
3. The best choice for this case is inserting ICRs, so let us study the case as a candidate for ICRs.

Figure 4.2.1 shows the main four maps. Choosing the size of the rings and the axis at which they should be inserted relies upon the curvature map. Since the curvature map differs according to misalignment while taking the capture, the surgeon should be sure that this picture is valid and reproducible (please refer to my book: Corneal Topography in Clinical Practice, chapter 15, Jaypee brothers 2009). On the other hand, this curvature map with such color display cannot be reliable; the cone details cannot be identified, so the pictures should be seen after color modification (Fig. 4.2.2).

Figure 4.2.3 shows the single curvature map with the steep and flat axes projected and the color scale changed, the cone details are clearer. In general, the curvature map shows the refractive shape of the cone, and the elevation maps show the anatomical location and height of the cone; therefore, both curvature and elevation maps are important and should be studied carefully. This case is PLK due to two reasons: first,

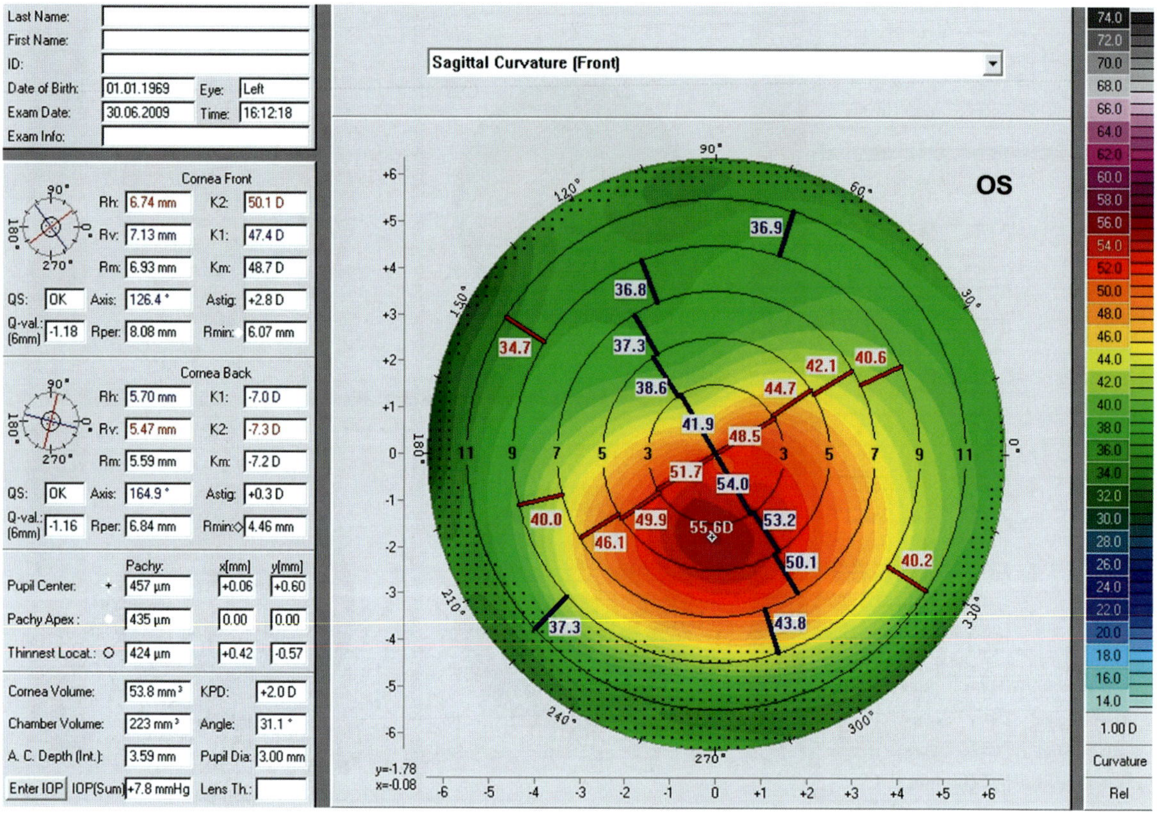

Fig. 4.2.3 The anterior curvature map. The curvature pattern is PMD or PLK. According to author's classification, it is pattern 5

Table 4.2.3 Management suggestions

Factors	Patient data	Suggested treatment
Transparency and stress lines	Transparent with no stress lines	
Age	41	
Progression	No	
CL tolerance	No	Other modalities
Refractive error (S.E)	−6.25 dpt	ICRs
BSCVA Vs UCVA	4 lines difference	CXL and PRK or ICRs
K-max	56	ICRs or CXL and PRK
Corneal thickness at thinnest location	424	ICRs
Sex	Female	
Management summary	ICRs	

the slitlamp view, second, the absence of the bell sign on the thickness map. The cone can be considered as central because it is within the 3-mm central zone; therefore, the cone is not on the site of ICR insertion (Fig. 4.2.4: arrows).

From a practical point of view, this case will be considered as pattern 1 (author's classification) because the apex of the cone is paracentral (see the topographical patterns). Pattern 1 shows the best response when compared with other patterns.

Intracorneal ring implantation was performed in the patient's left eye. Figure 4.2.5 is the 3 months postoperative corneal topography including the main four maps. There has been an improvement in the curvature and the elevation maps. Figure 4.2.6 is the 3 months postoperative anterior sagittal curvature map; and when compared with Fig. 4.2.3, a significant improvement can be seen in the curvature pattern shape, which became more regular, and in K-readings.

Figures 4.2.7 and 4.2.8 are the 6 months postoperative topography. Figure 4.2.9 is the difference map to show the changes that happened during the first 3 months after the operation, the effect of the rings on the anterior corneal surface can be noticed. Figure 4.2.10 is the difference map to show the changes that happened during the second 3 months postoperatively. There were still some improvement but the

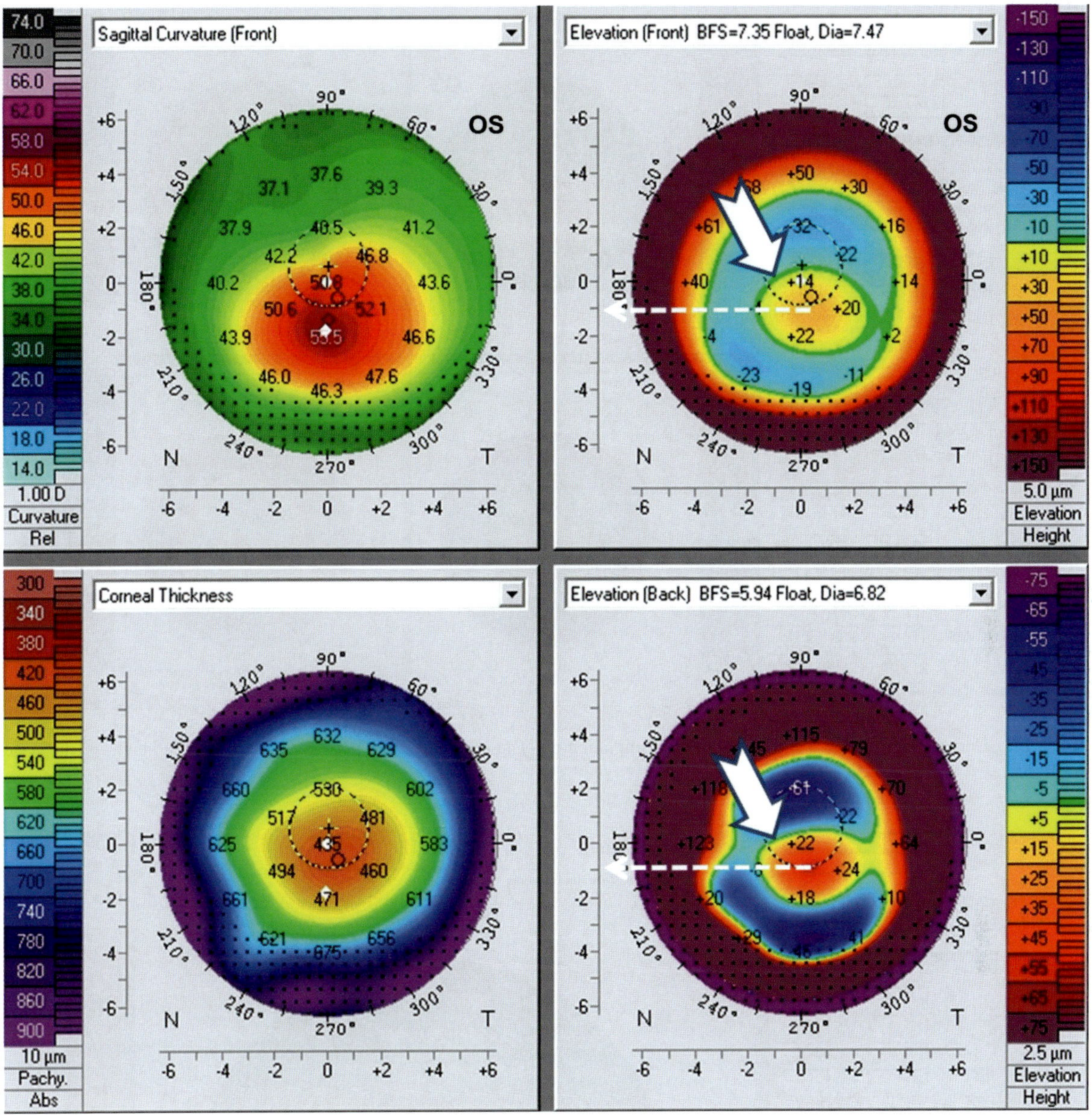

Fig. 4.2.4 Cone location on the elevation maps. The *white arrows* point at the cone. The intermittent *white arrows* point at the location on the scale. The cone can be considered as central because it is within the 3 mm central zone

biggest improvement was during the first 3 months postoperatively.

Figure 4.2.11 is the numerical changes that happened during the first 3 months, and Fig. 4.2.12 is the numerical changes that happened during the second 3 months. Following the changes in the K-readings, the most improvement in K_1 and K_2 was during the first 3 months. It is not uncommon to see also an increase in corneal thickness at the thinnest location (red circles). There was also an improvement in both UCVA and BSCVA as shown in Table 4.2.4.

Table 4.2.4 Postoperative manifest refraction

Eye	Sphere	Cylinder	Axis	UCVA	BSVCA	BSCVA + PH
OS	−1	−0.75	55	0.6	0.9	1.0

In summary, using ICRs in this case was appropriate and the suggested reasons for the good visual outcome are: the cornea was stable, UCVA-BSCVA difference was acceptable, K-max was <58 dpt, corneal thickness was >400 μ, and the refractive error of the patient was reasonable.

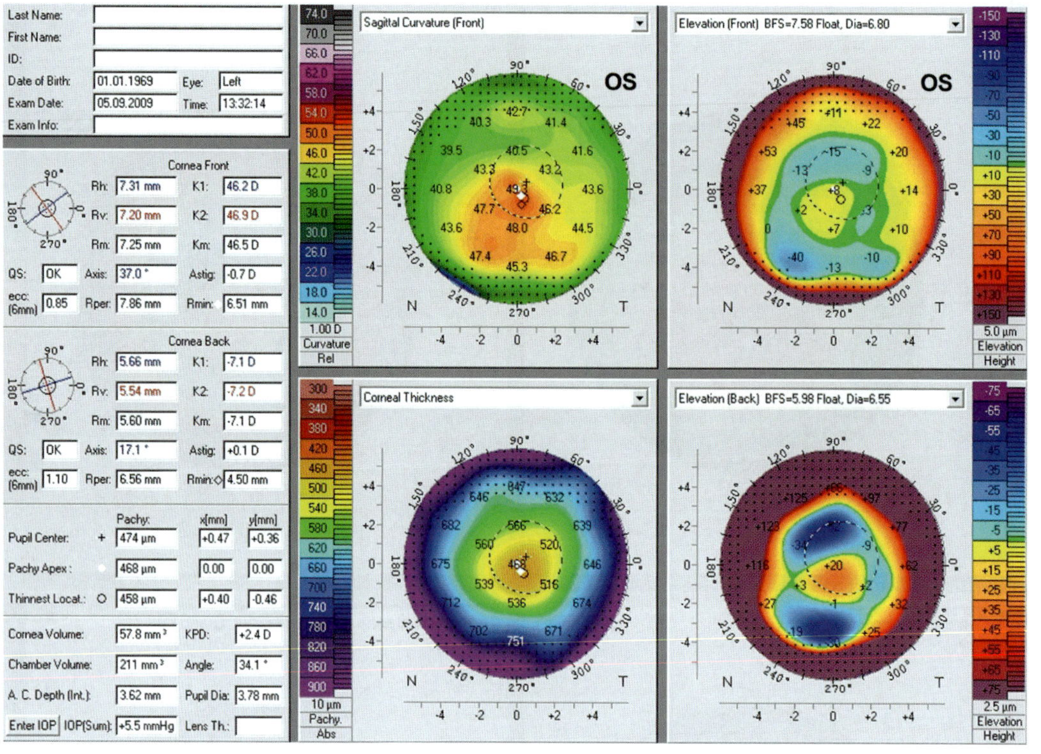

Fig. 4.2.5 Corneal topography 3 months after ICR implantation. The curvature map is more regular and the height of the cone decreased as shown in the elevation maps

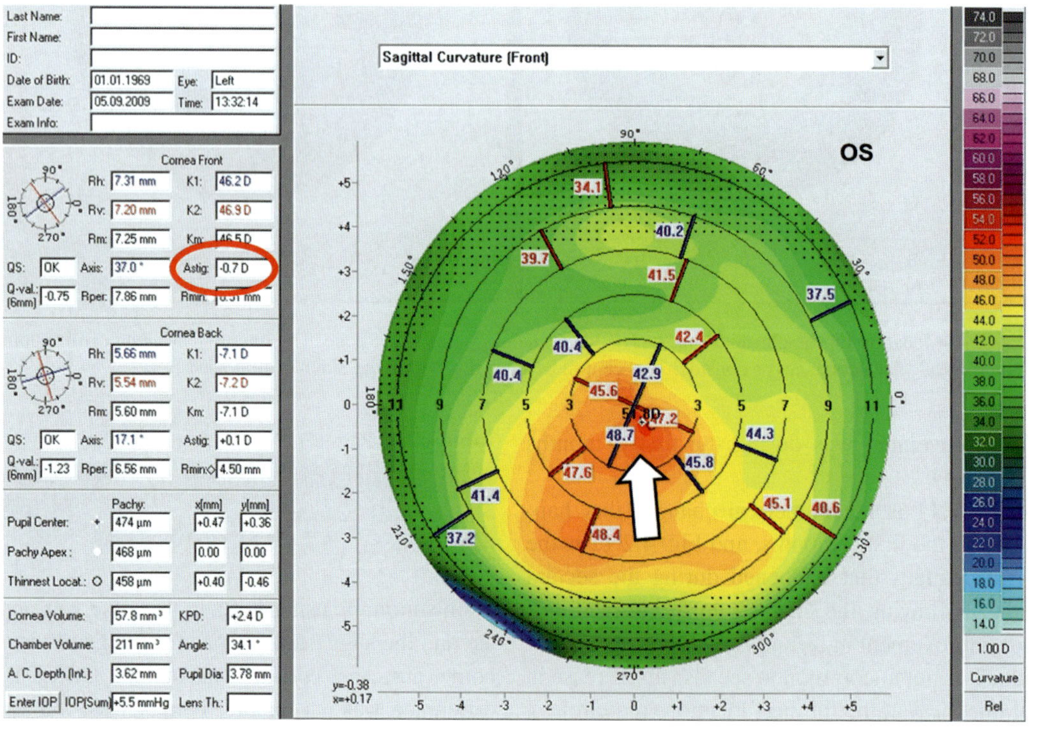

Fig. 4.2.6 Anterior curvature map 3 months after ICR implantation. The central cornea is more regular, K-max improved (*white arrow*), and corneal astigmatism is insignificant (*red circle*)

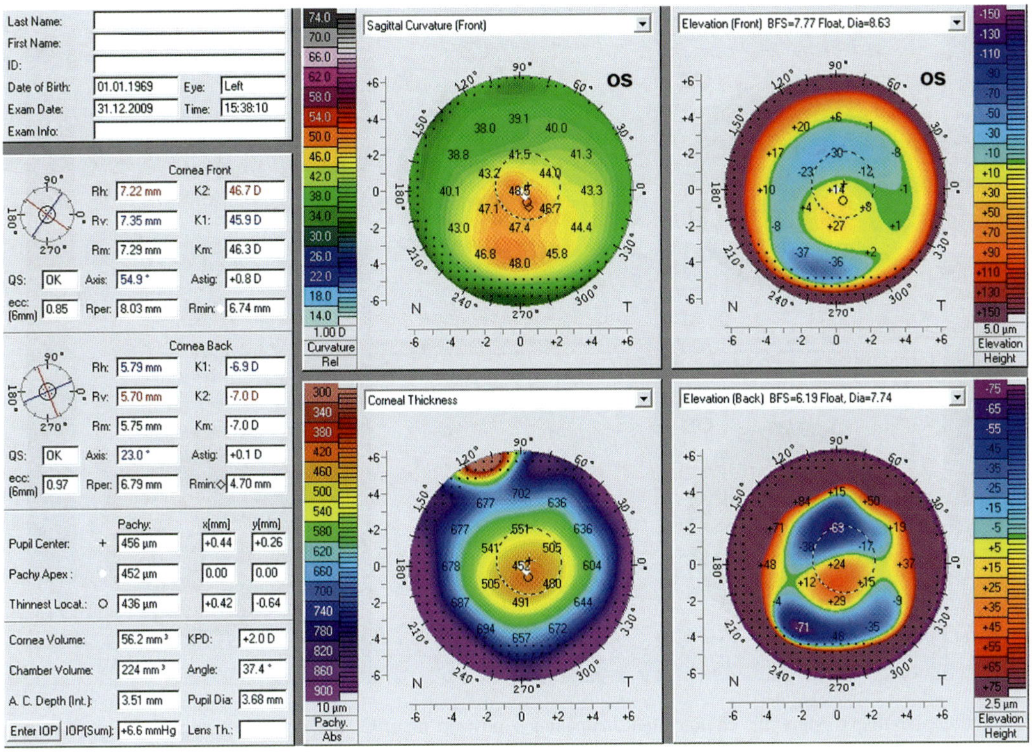

Fig. 4.2.7 Corneal topography 6 months after ICR implantation. In comparison with Fig. 4.2.5, the case was relatively stable during the second 3 months after implantation

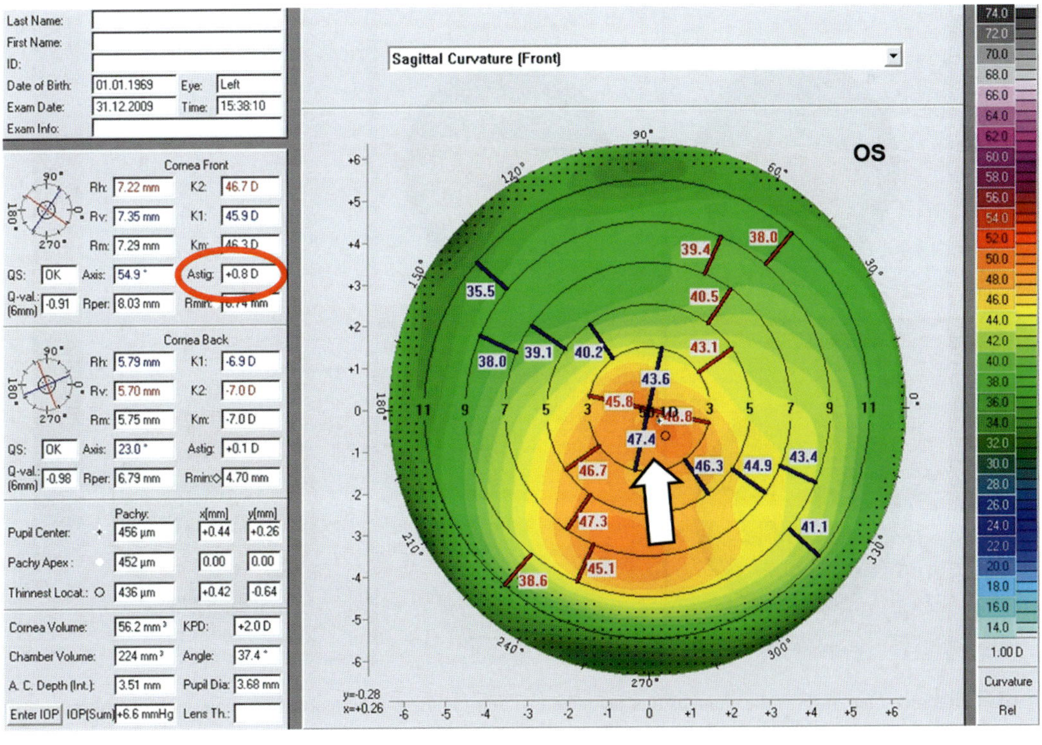

Fig. 4.2.8 Anterior curvature map 6 months after ICR implantation. In comparison with Fig. 4.2.6, there are few changes. Look at the K-max (*white arrow*) and corneal astigmatism (*red circle*)

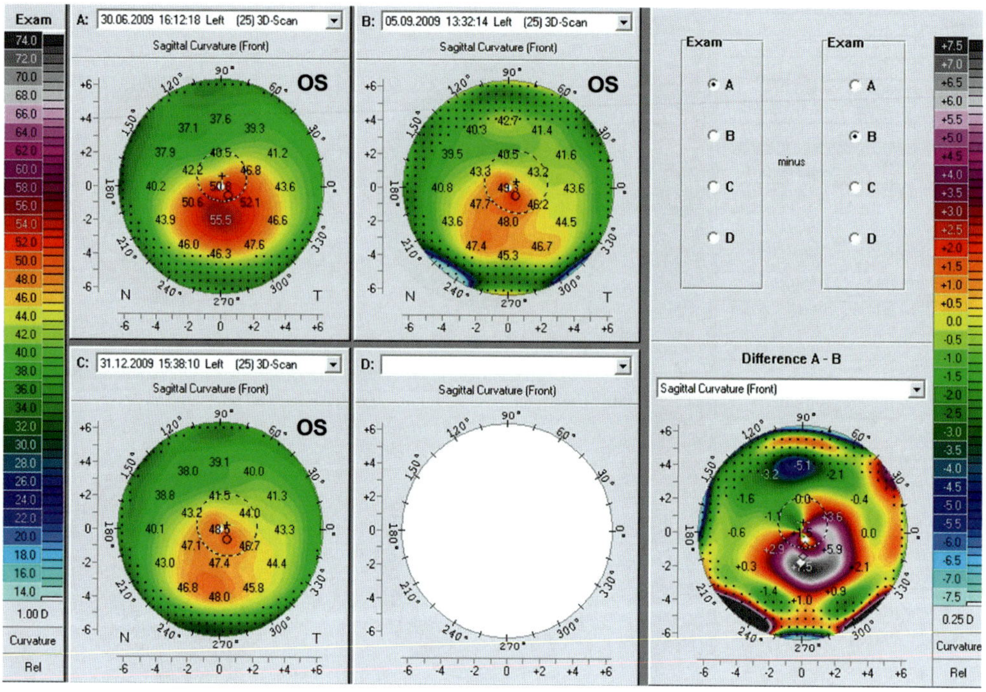

Fig. 4.2.9 Difference map to show the changes that happened during the first 3 months after the operation, the effect of the rings on the anterior corneal surface is visible. A (upper left map) is the pre-op map; B (upper right map) is the 3-months post-op map; C (the lower left map) is the 6-months post-op map; and the column on the right is the difference map representing the changes during the first 3 months post operatively

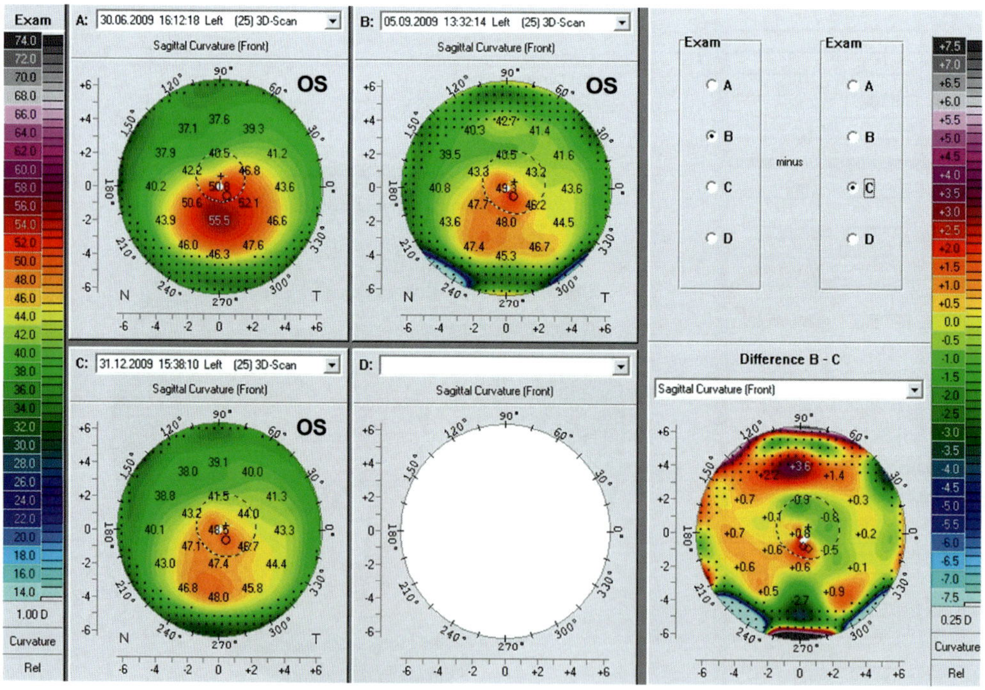

Fig. 4.2.10 Difference map to show the changes that happened during the second 3 months postoperatively. There was still some improvement. A (upper left map) is the pre-op map; B (upper right map) is the 3-months post-op map; C (the lower left map) is the 6-months post-op map; and the column on the right is the difference map representing the changes during the second 3 months post operatively

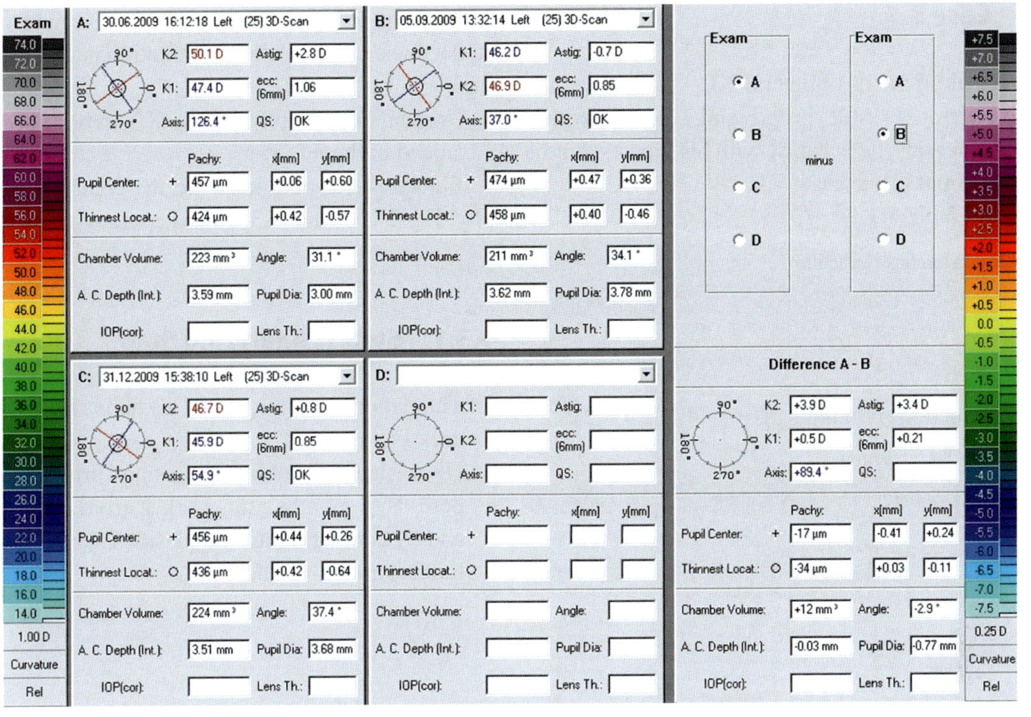

Fig. 4.2.11 Numerical changes that happened during the first 3 months. A (upper left) is the pre-op; B (upper right) is the 3-months post-op; C (lower left) is the 6-months post-op; and the column on the right is the numerical changes during the first 3 months post operatively

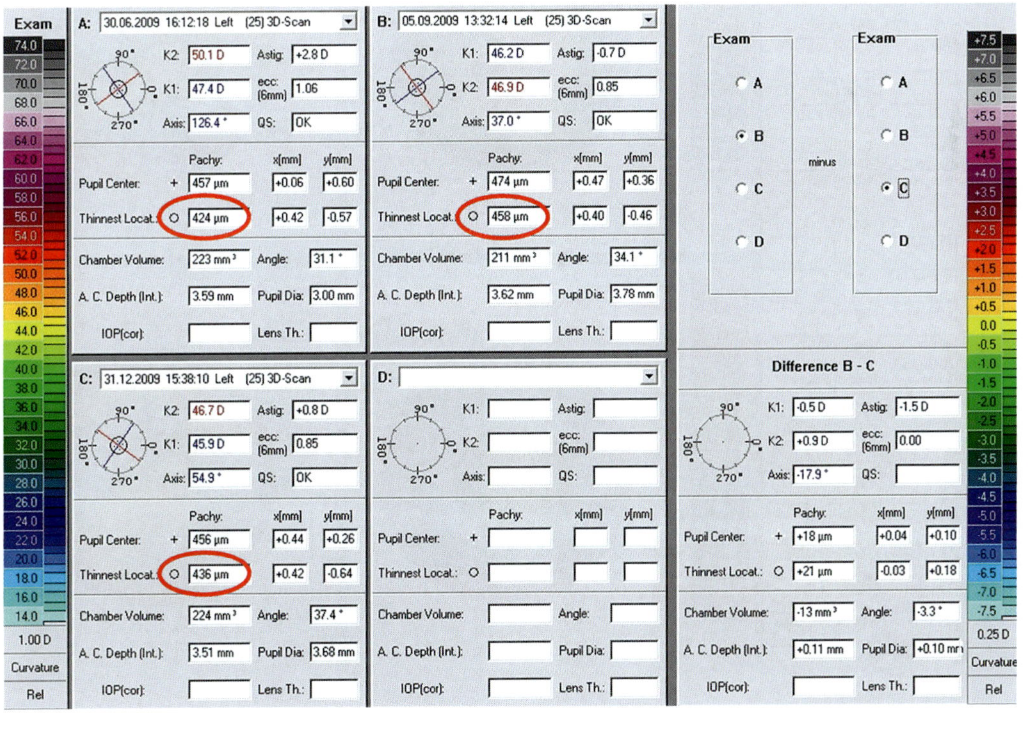

Fig. 4.2.12 Numerical changes that happened during the second 3 months. *Red circles* indicate changes in corneal thickness at the thinnest location. A (upper left) is the pre-op; B (upper right) is the 3-months post-op; C (lower left) is the 6-months post-op; and the column on the right is the numerical changes during the second 3 months post operatively

4.3 Case 3

A 20-year-old male has bilateral KC. As he says, the refractive error is still progressing slowly within 6 months intervals, he is happy with his glasses, but he is worried about his disease.
His MR is (Table 4.3.1):

Table 4.3.1 Manifest refraction

Eye	Sphere	Cylinder	Axis	UCVA	BSVCA
OD	0	−2.5	45	0.6	1.0
OS	−1.5	−3.5	130	0.3	1.0

His old correction (6 months ago) is (Table 4.3.2):

Table 4.3.2 Old refraction

Eye	Sphere	Cylinder	Axis
OD	0	−1.25	45
OS	−0.75	−2.5	120

Slitlamp examination shows clear cornea with no stress lines. Other ocular examination is within normal limits.

Corneal Topography reveals KC in both eyes more advanced in the left eye.

Figures 4.3.1 and 4.3.2 are the right eye topography; Figs. 4.3.3 and 4.3.4 are the left eye topography.

4.3.1 Step 1: Analyzing Step

1. The patient is 20 years old, so he is still in the progressing age.
2. His refractive error is progressing during reasonable periods (6 months); this is clear from his complaint and by comparing his old glasses (Table 4.3.2) with his recent MR (Table 4.3.1).

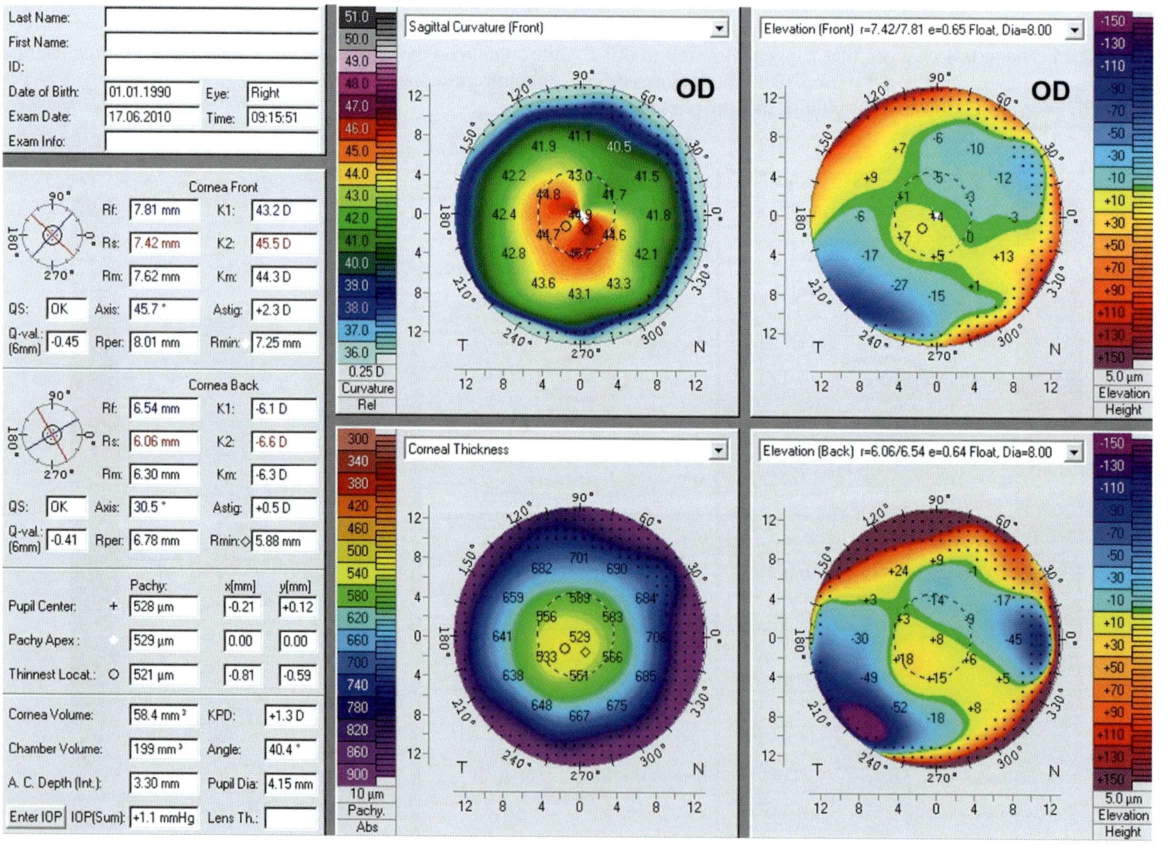

Fig. 4.3.1 Corneal topography of the right eye: mild KC

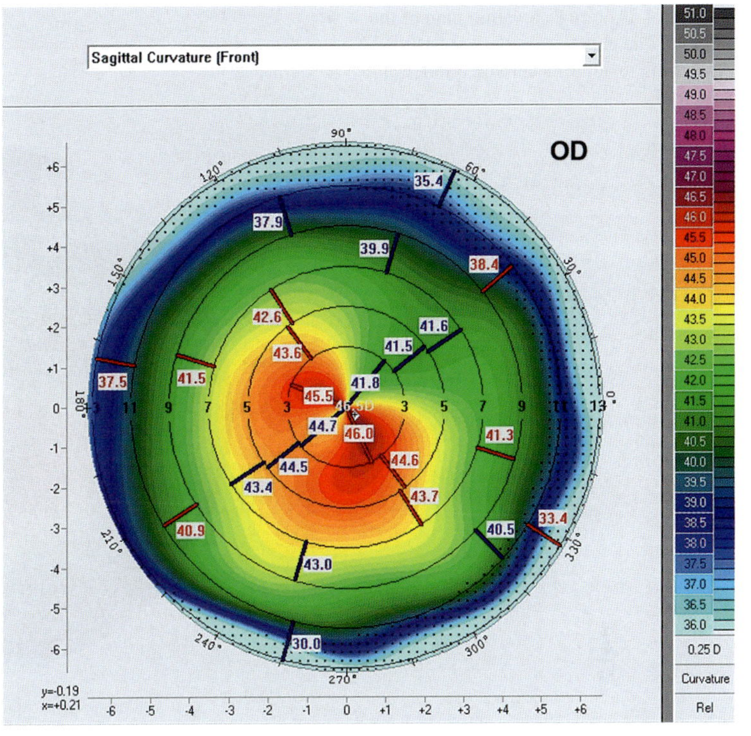

Fig. 4.3.2 Anterior curvature map of the right eye. The curvature pattern is SB/SRAX. According to author's classification, it is pattern 4

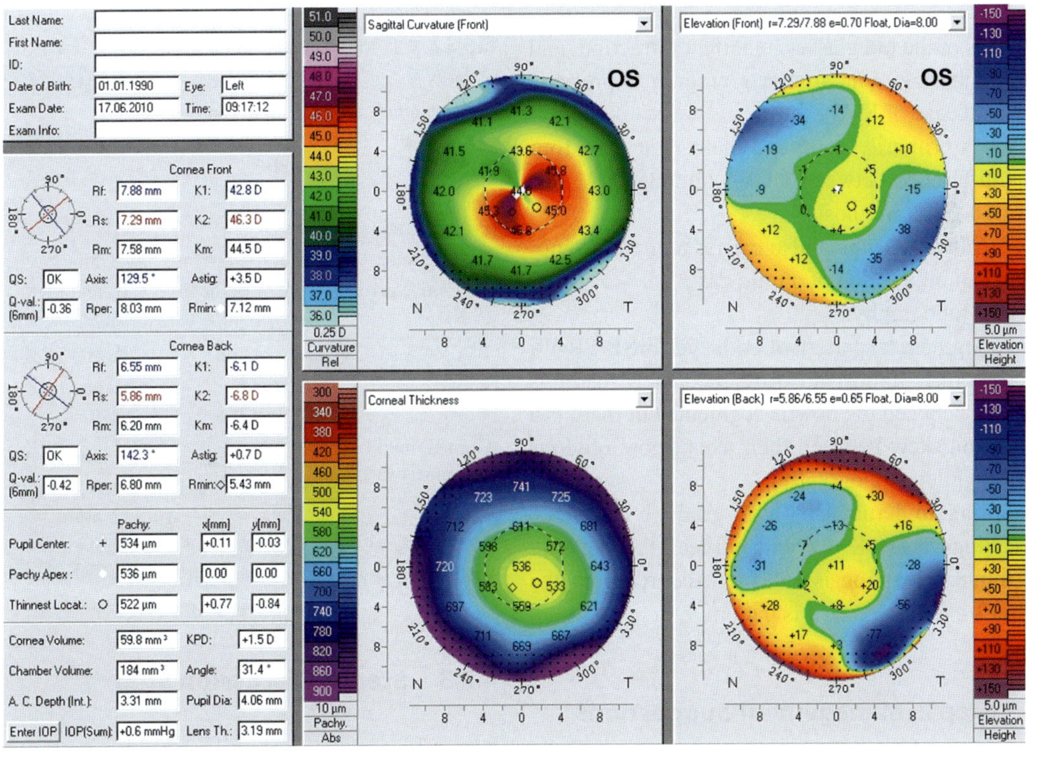

Fig. 4.3.3 Corneal topography of the left eye: mild KC

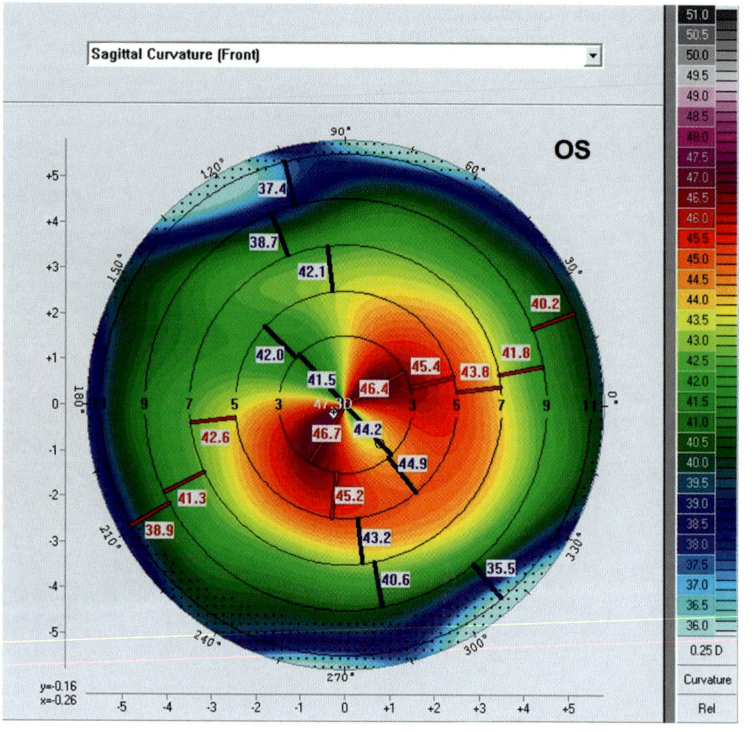

Fig. 4.3.4 Anterior curvature map of the left eye. The curvature pattern is SB/SRAX. According to author's classification, it is pattern 4

3. The axes of the old glasses, manifest refraction, and topography are quite similar giving an impression of a mild case of KC.
4. UCVA is primarily good and there is at least four lines difference between UCVA and BSCVA, this carries a good prognosis.
5. BSCVA is 10/10 which also carries a good prognosis and an impression of a mild case.
6. Corneal topography:
   The topographical pattern of both eyes is SB/SRAX since there is almost no difference in K-readings and size between the bowtie segments but there is a significant skew between their axes (more obvious in the right eye topography).
7. According to Krumeich, it is grade I KC since K-readings are<48 dpt and corneal thickness at the thinnest location is>500 μ. According to the author's classification, it is pattern 4.

4.3.2 Step 2: Management Suggestions

Table 4.3.3 summarizes patient data and the corresponding individual suggestion(s) for treatment, and presents a final summary of the best management.

Table 4.3.3 Management suggestions

Factors	Patient data	Suggested treatment
Transparency and stress lines	Transparent with no stress lines	
Age	20	
Progression	Yes	CxL
CL tolerance	Not tried before	One choice
Refractive error (S.E)	−1.25 dpt R.E −3.25 dpt L.E	CxL and PRK
BSCVA Vs UCVA	Very good	CxL and PRK or ICRs
K-max	46 dpt R.E 47 dpt L.E	CxL and PRK or ICRs
Corneal thickness at thinnest location	521 μ R.E 522 μ L.E	CxL and PRK or ICRs
Sex	Male	
Management summary	CXL to stop the progression and to prepare the cornea for PRK	

4.3.3 Step 3: Discussion Step

It is a typical case of mild KC in a young patient. Since the case is progressive, it is recommended to cross-link the cornea. The conditions for CxL are ideal in this case; corneal thickness at the thinnest location is more than enough even if TG PRK is within the plan, especially that the refractive error is small (<−4 dpt S.E) and can be corrected within the allowed 40–50 μ. Nevertheless, the BSCVA is optimal which means that there are small amount of aberrations and, therefore, the results will be promising.

On the other hand, ICRs are also another option, especially if only one segment is used because the cornea is not very irregular and both astigmatism and K-readings are not too high (<48 dpt).

Personally, I prefer CxL with or without TG PRK since the case is still mild and there is no need to expose the cornea to more invasive procedures.

4.4 Case 4

A 26-year-old female has a refractive error. As she says, her refractive error began when she was 15-year-old. The refractive error thereafter progressed slowly and became stable about 3 years ago. She is pregnant now and she feels that her vision is blurred again. She is worried especially that she has been told by the optometrist 1 month ago that she had KC.

Her MR is (Table 4.4.1):

Table 4.4.1 Manifest refraction

Eye	Sphere	Cylinder	Axis	UCVA	BSVCA±PH
OD	+1.0	−3.0	180	0.4	0.9
OS	+1.5	−2.0	160	0.4	0.9

Her old correction (2 years ago) is (Table 4.4.2):

Table 4.4.2 Old refraction

Eye	Sphere	Cylinder	Axis
OD	+1.0	−2.75	180
OS	+1.5	−2.25	160

Slitlamp examination shows clear cornea with no stress lines. Other ocular examination is within normal limits.

Corneal topography reveals posterior KC in both eyes.

For educational purposes, the right eye will be taken as an example.

Figure 4.4.1 is the right eye topography.

4.4.1 Step 1: Analyzing Step

1. The patient is 26-year-old, so her age is in the border line regarding the progression of KC. But her refractive error – as she claimed and the old glasses showed – is stable.
2. She is pregnant, so she may be prone to re-progression of the disease during pregnancy.
3. Her BSCVA is very good, and therefore, treatment results will be promising.

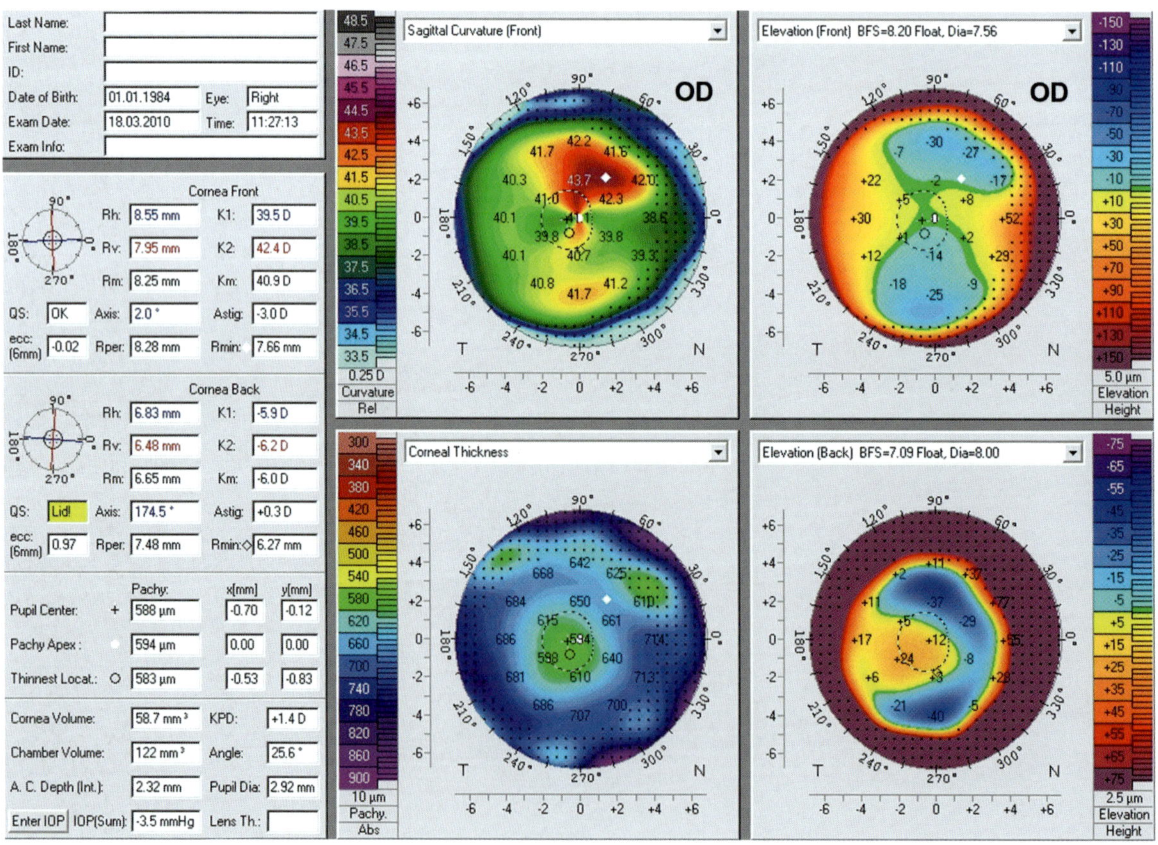

Fig. 4.4.1 Corneal topography of the right eye: mild posterior KC

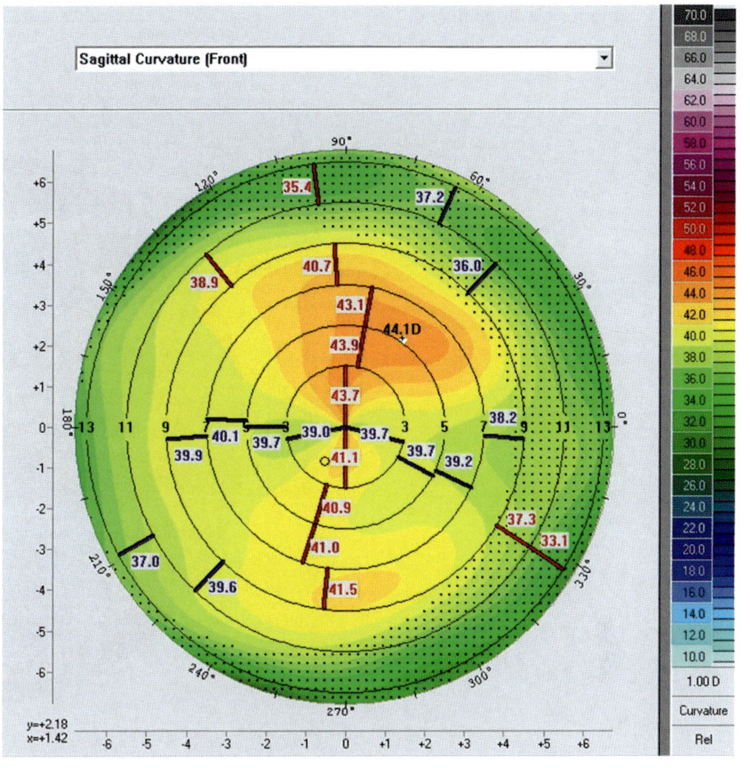

Fig. 4.4.2 Anterior curvature map. The curvature pattern is AB/SS. According to author's classification, it pattern 3

4. Corneal topography of the right eye will be taken as an example:
   (a) The curvature map (Fig. 4.4.2): The axes of the central part of the bowtie are not skewed. The K-readings in the upper segment are higher than those in the inferior segment by more than 2.5 dpt. Therefore, the pattern is asymmetric bowtie / superior steep (AB/SS).
   (b) The elevation maps: Fig. 4.4.3 is the anterior elevation map with the BFS reference body, Fig. 4.4.4 is the anterior elevation map with the BFTE reference body, Fig. 4.4.5 is the posterior elevation map with the BFS reference body, and Fig. 4.4.6 is the posterior elevation map with the BFTE reference body. The anterior elevation map with both reference bodies shows normal shape and values, while the posterior elevation map with both reference bodies shows abnormal shape and values. Therefore, the diagnosis is posterior KC.
5. According to Krumeich classification, it is grade 1 KC since K-readings are < 48 dpt and corneal thickness at the thinnest location is > 500 µ. According to the author's classification, it is pattern 3.

4.4.2 Step 2: Management Suggestions

Table 4.4.3 summarizes patient data and the corresponding individual suggestion(s) for treatment, and presents a final summary of the best management.

Table 4.4.3 Management suggestions

Factors	Patient data	Suggested treatment
Transparency and stress lines	Transparent with no stress lines	
Age	26	
Progression	No	
CL tolerance	Not tried before	One choice
Refractive error (S.E)	−0.5 dpt R.E +0.5 dpt L.E	CxL and PRK
BSCVA Vs UCVA	Very good	CxL and PRK or ICRs
K-max	44.1 dpt R.E	CxL and PRK or ICRs
Corneal thickness @ thinnest location	583 µ R.E	CxL and PRK or ICRs
Sex	Female and pregnant	close monitoring
Management summary	Close monitoring of corneal topography. Maybe CxL after delivery.	

Fig. 4.4.3 Anterior elevation map in the BFS float mode. Normal shape and values

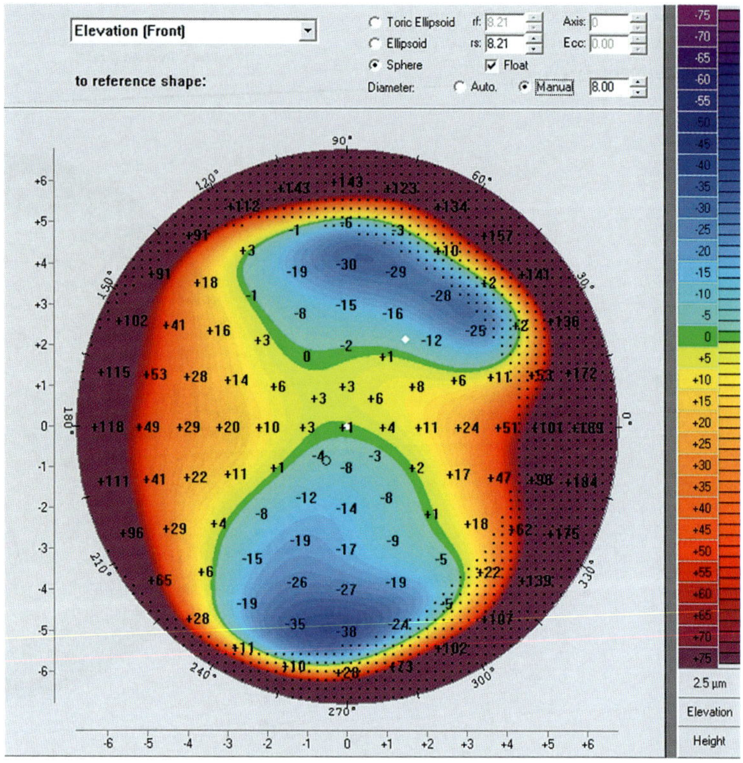

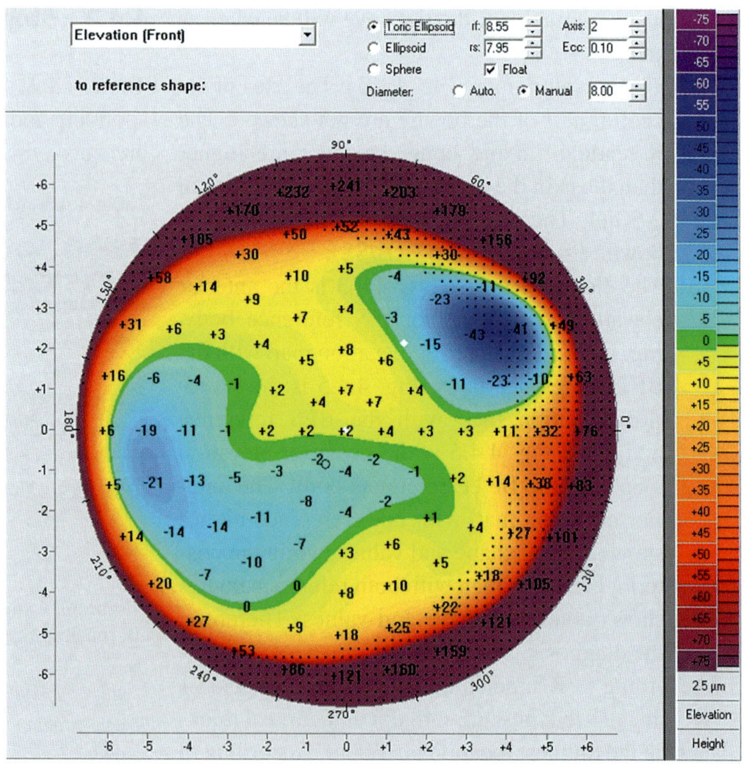

Fig. 4.4.4 Anterior elevation map in the BFTE float mode. Normal shape and values

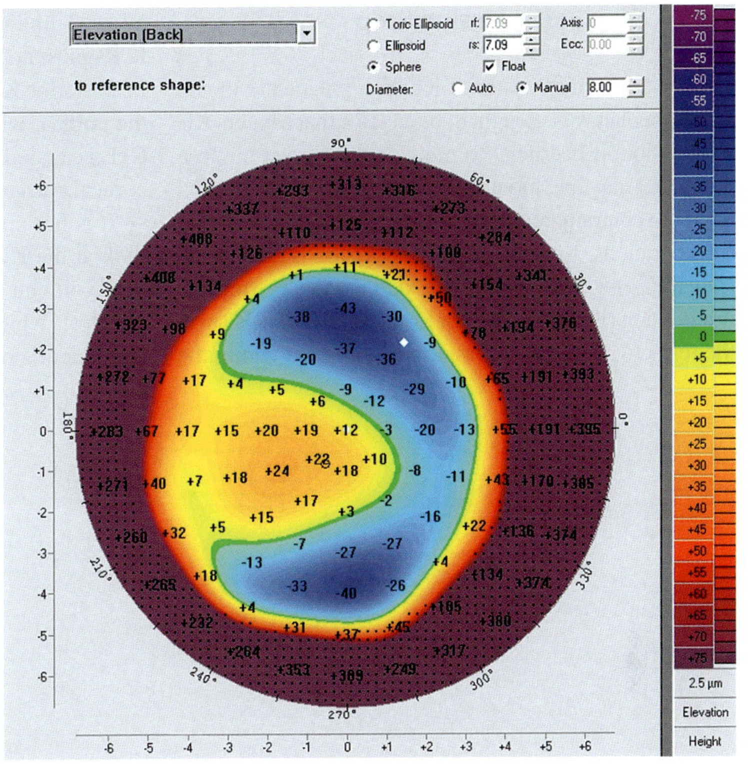

Fig. 4.4.5 Posterior elevation map in the BFS float mode. Abnormal shape and values

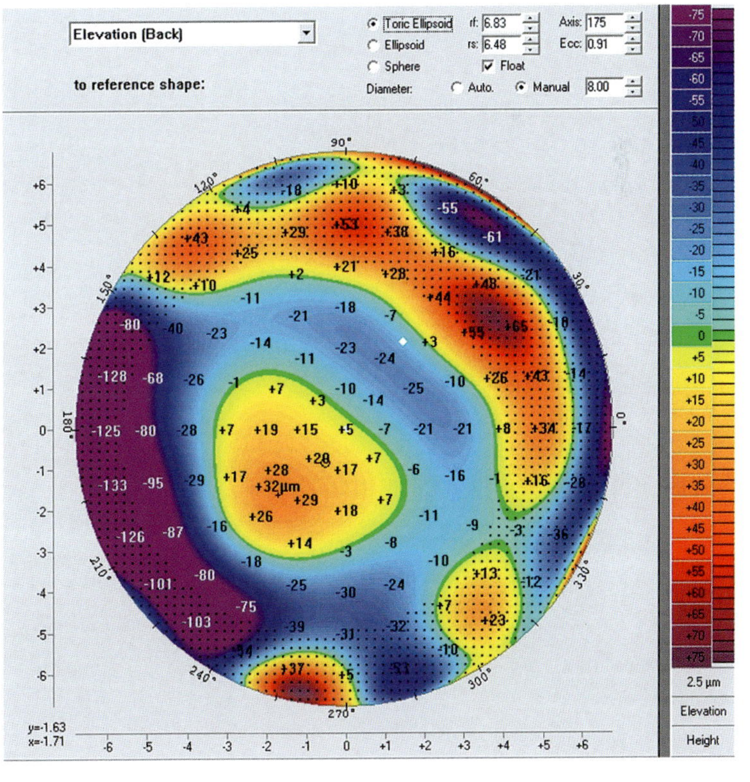

Fig. 4.4.6 Posterior elevation map in the BFTE float mode. Abnormal shape and values

4.4.3 Step 3: Discussion Step

This case is a mild posterior KC in a pregnant woman. Since pregnancy is thought to be a factor that triggers KC progression, it is crucial to monitor the cornea in close intervals (may be monthly) especially that ICRs and CXL are contraindicated during pregnancy due to social considerations. After delivery, if a decision is taken to do something for this case, it is CxL in order to stop the progression (if it happened) or to perform TG PRK since the refractive error and corneal thickness are within the allowed limits. The most important thing here is that ICRs must not be used at all because it is a posterior KC. In posterior KC, the problem is in the posterior part of the cornea, which is out of field of action of the ICRs. CxL is a good choice because it strengthens the anterior corneal barrier against the posterior out-bulging.

It is not uncommon to see hyperopia in KC. If you look at the K-readings in the central 3 mm of the cornea, you can find that there are some low k-readings (39 dpt), which explains the hyperopic component of the patient's refractive error (Table 4.4.1).

4.5 Case 5

A 33-year-old patient complaining of blurred vision in both eyes, more severe in his right eye. He was previously diagnosed to have KC in both eyes, more advanced in the right eye. He is contact lens intolerant, his glasses are not efficient, and he has been advised to have corneal graft. His MR is (Table 4.5.1):

Table 4.5.1 Manifest refraction

Eye	Sphere	Cylinder	Axis	UCVA	BSVCA ± PH	BCVA over RGP contact lenses
OD	−1.0	−6.0	40	CF 2 m	0.3	0.5
OS	+1.5	−4.5	115	0.2	0.6	0.7

His old correction is (Table 4.5.2):

Table 4.5.2 Old correction

Eye	Sphere	Cylinder	Axis
OD	−1.0	−5.5	40
OS	0	−4.5	110

Slitlamp examination shows stress lines (Vogt's striae) in the right cornea with no scars, the left cornea is clear. Other ocular examination is within normal limits.

Figures 4.5.1–4.5.6 are right eye maps, and Figs. 4.5.7–4.5.12 are left eye maps.

4.5.1 Step 1: Analyzing Step

1. Patient's age is 33 years, KC is supposed to be stable in this age.
2. The UCVA and BSCVA are severely compromised in the right eye and relatively better in the left eye.
3. There is a gain of two lines in BCVA over RGP contact lenses in both eyes, but still not completely corrected, which means an amblyopic component may be present.
4. The right cornea has stress lines (Vogt's striae) indicating an advanced KC.
5. Corneal topography.
   (a) Right eye:
      - Figure 4.5.1 is the main four maps.
      - Figures 4.5.2 and 4.5.3 represent the anterior curvature map before and after color scale modification to clarify the cone shape. K-readings are very high (K-max = 71.4: arrow).

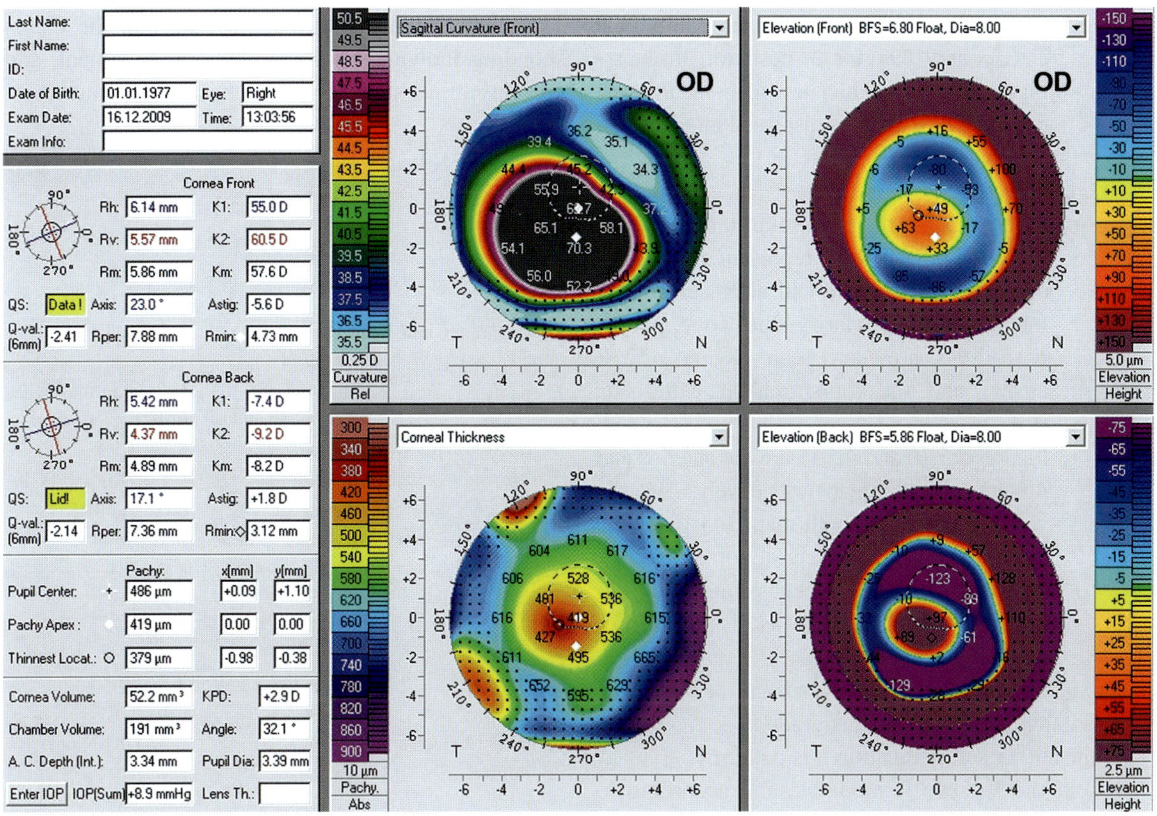

Fig. 4.5.1 Corneal topography of the right eye: advanced KC

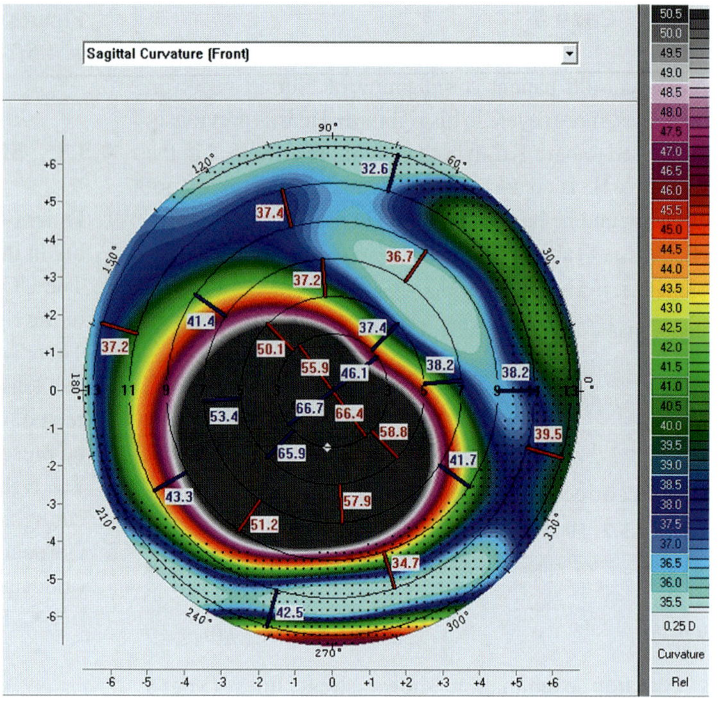

Fig. 4.5.2 Anterior curvature map. The shape of the cone cannot be identified in this color scale

- Figures 4.5.4 and 4.5.5 are the anterior and posterior elevation maps respectively. Elevation values are very high on both maps (88 μ for the anterior and 169 μ for the posterior: arrows).
- Figure 4.5.6 is the thickness map, the thinnest point is 379 μ and it is displaced inferior-temporally (arrows).

(b) Left eye:

- Figure 4.5.7 is the main four maps.
- Figures 4.5.8 and 4.5.9 represent the anterior curvature map before and after color scale modification to clarify the cone shape. K-readings are very high (K-max = 52.4: arrow) and the topographical pattern is PLK.
- Figures 4.5.10 and 4.5.11 are the anterior and posterior elevation maps respectively. Elevation values are high on both maps (44 μ for the anterior and 81 μ for the posterior: arrows).
- Figure 4.5.12 is the thickness map, the thinnest point is 473 μ and it is displaced inferior-temporally (arrows).

6. KC in the right eye is advanced and according to Krumeich classification it is grade 3–4. According to the author's classification it is pattern 1.
7. KC in the left eye is moderate and according to Krumeich classification, it is grade 2. According to the author's classification, it is pattern 5.

4.5.2 Step 2: Management Suggestions

Table 4.5.3 summarizes patient data and the corresponding individual suggestion(s) for treatment, and presents a final summary of the best management.

Table 4.5.3 Management suggestions

Factors	Patient data	Suggested treatment
Progression	Most likely stable	
CL tolerance	No	
Age	33	
Sex	Male	
Transparency and stress lines	R.E: stress lines with no scars	R.E: DALK
	LE: transparent with no stress lines	L.E: CxL and PRK or ICRs
Refractive error (S.E)	R.E: –4.0 dpt	R.E: ICRs
	L.E: –0.75 dpt	L.E: CXL and PRK
BSCVA Vs UCVA	R.E: Poor UCVA with almost 2 lines difference between UCVA and BSCVA.	CxL and PRK? ICRs?
	L.E: Poor UCVA with 4 lines difference.	
K-max	R.E: 71.4 dpt	R.E: DALK
	L.E: 52.4 dpt	L.E: ICRs
Corneal thickness at thinnest location	R.E: 379 μ	R.E: DALK or ICRs
	L.E: 473 μ	L.E: ICRs or CxL and PRK
Management summary:	DALK for the right eye. ICRs or CXL and PRK for the left eye.	

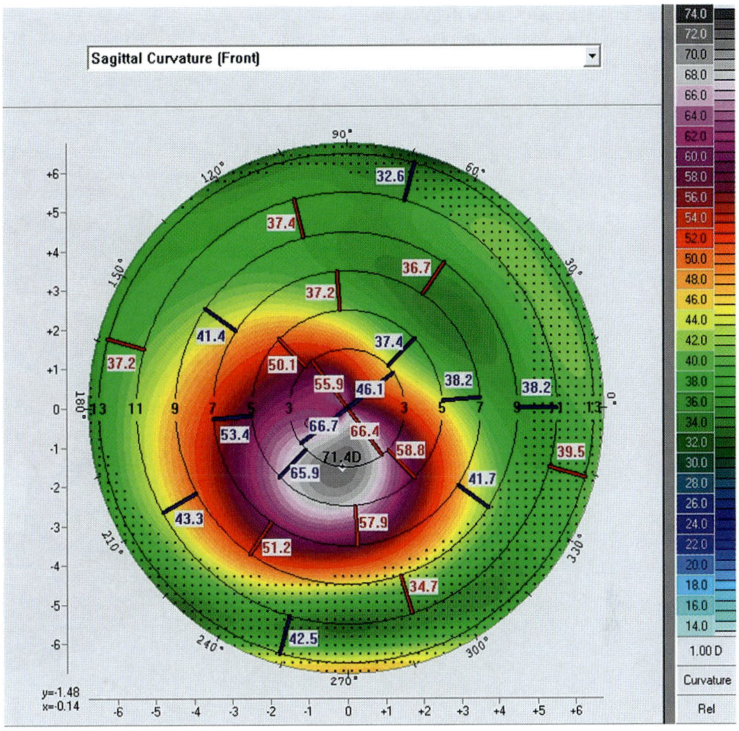

Fig. 4.5.3 Anterior curvature map of the right eye after color modification. The curvature pattern is AB/IS. According to author's classification, it is pattern 1

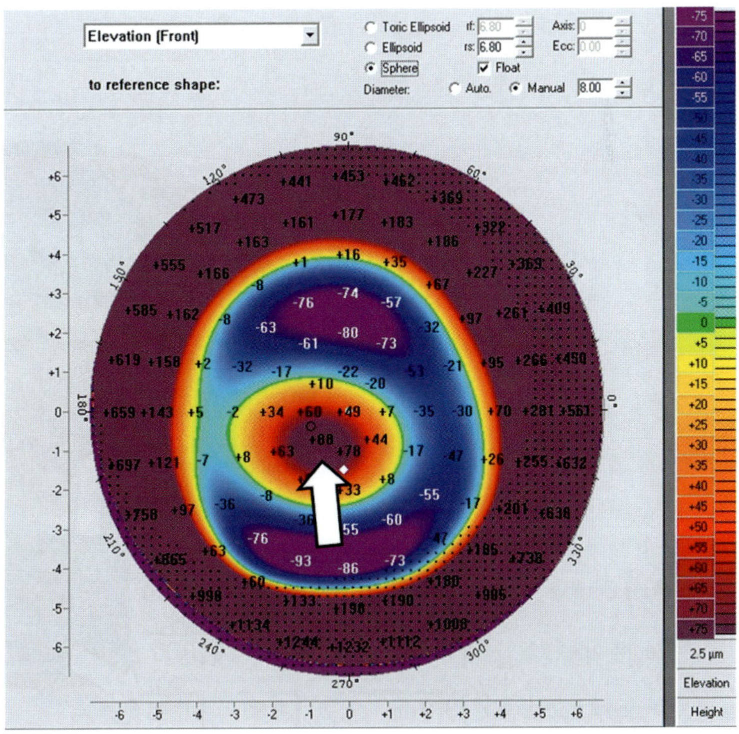

Fig. 4.5.4 Anterior elevation map of the right eye in the BFS float mode. There is a severe cone. The cone location is central

Fig. 4.5.5 Posterior elevation map of the right eye in the BFS float mode. There is a severe cone. The cone location is central

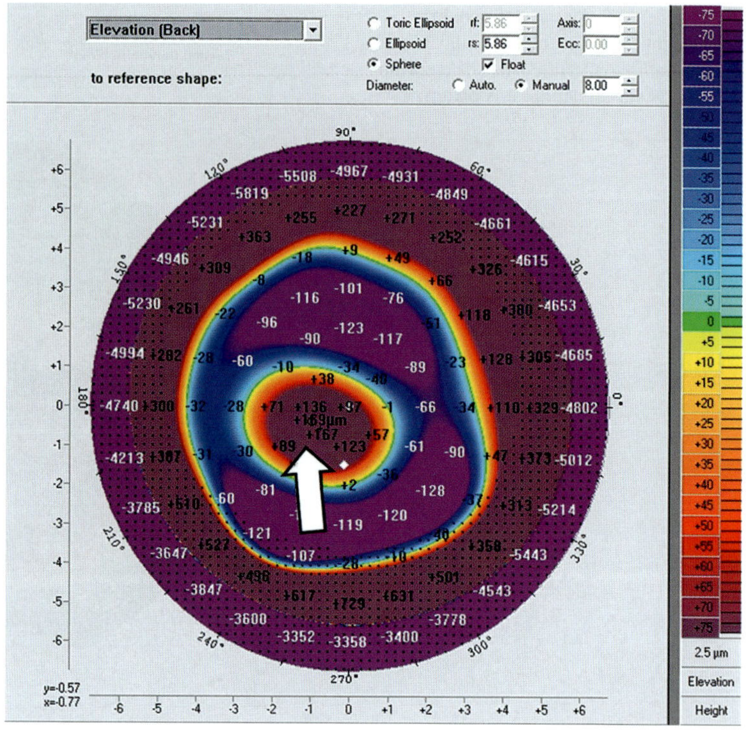

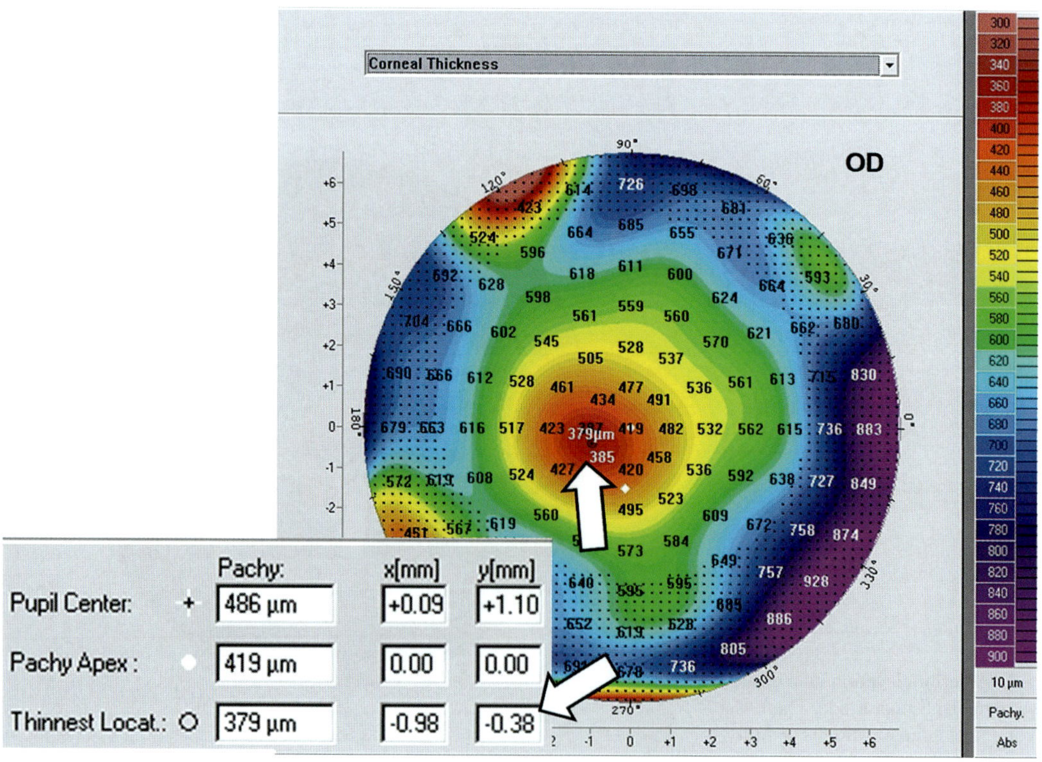

Fig. 4.5.6 Corneal thickness map of the right eye. The thinnest location is displaced inferotemporally (*white arrows*)

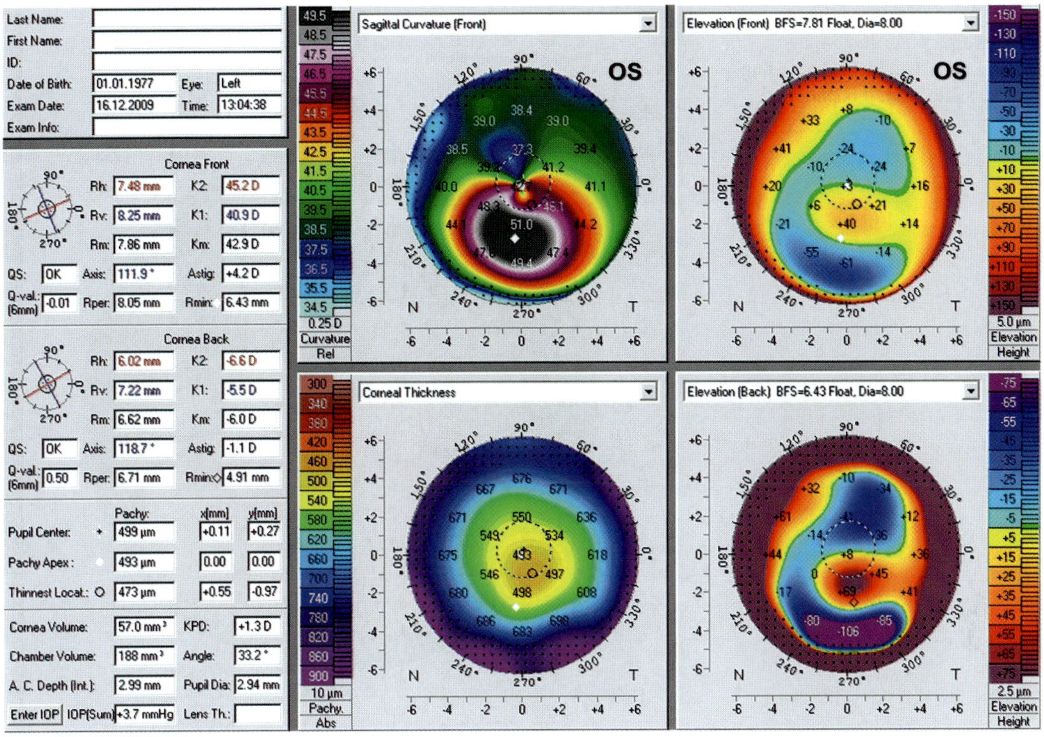

Fig. 4.5.7 Corneal topography of the left eye: mild PLK

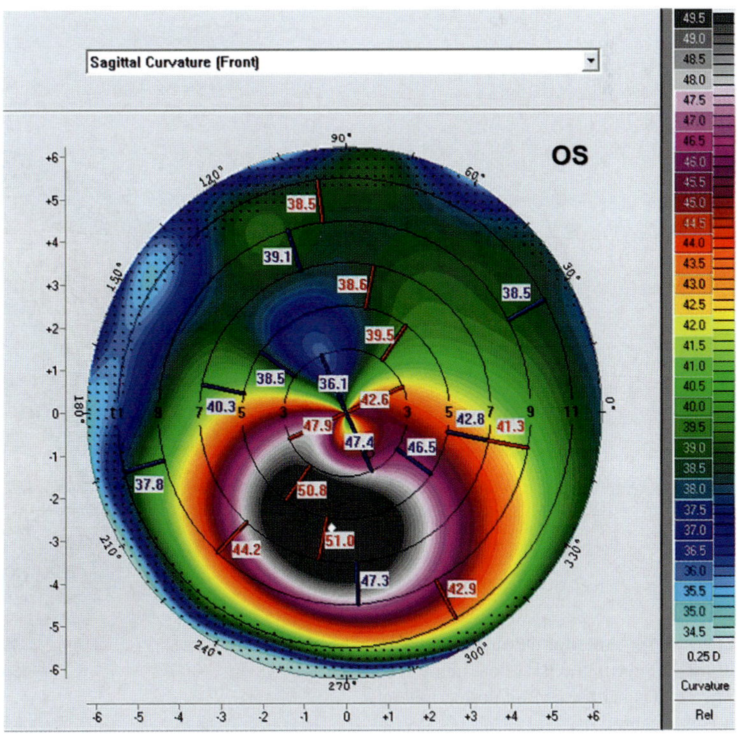

Fig. 4.5.8 Anterior curvature map of the left eye before color modification

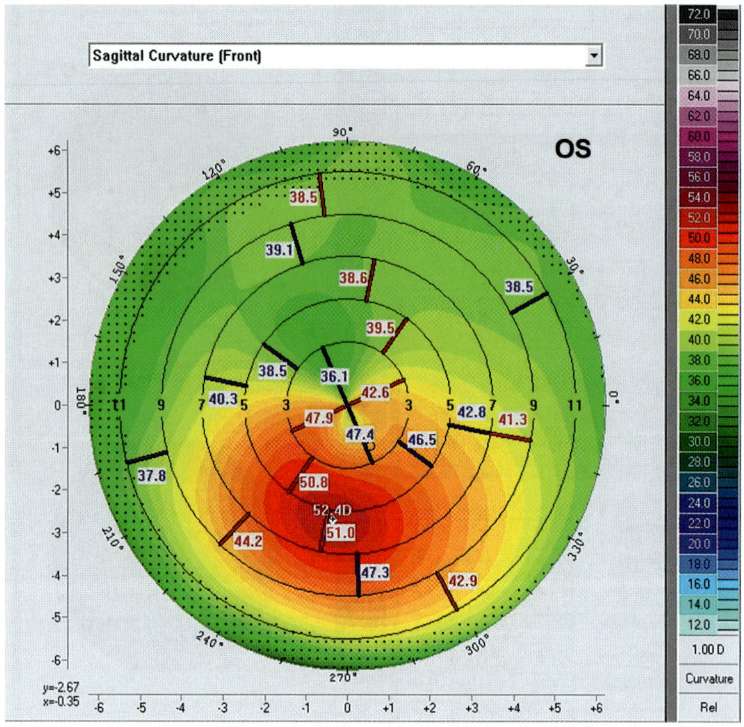

Fig. 4.5.9 Anterior curvature map of the left eye after color modification. The curvature pattern is PLK. According to author's classification, it is pattern 5

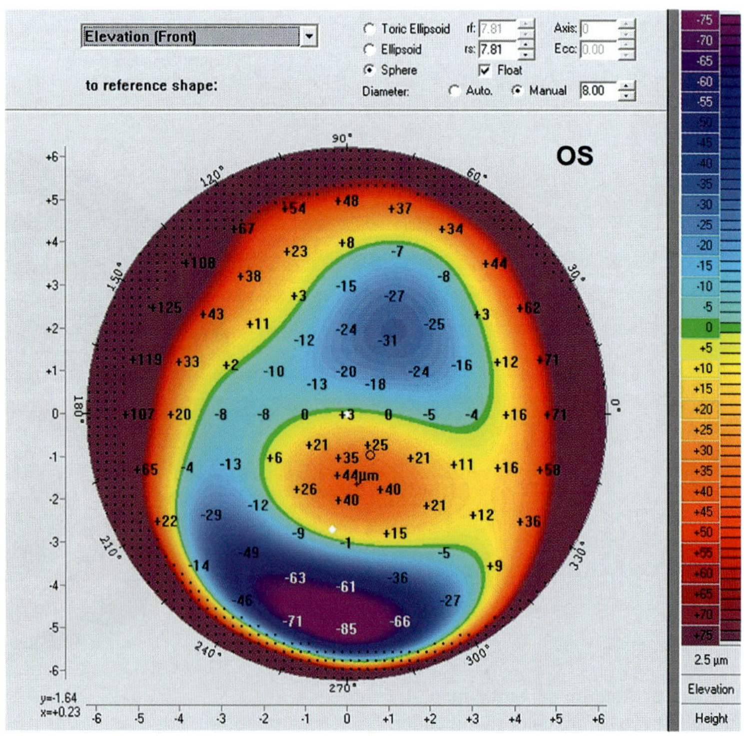

Fig. 4.5.10 Anterior elevation map of the left eye in the BFS float mode. The cone is neither central nor peripheral, it is paracentral

Fig. 4.5.11 Posterior elevation map of the left eye in the BFS float mode. The cone is neither central nor peripheral, it is paracentral

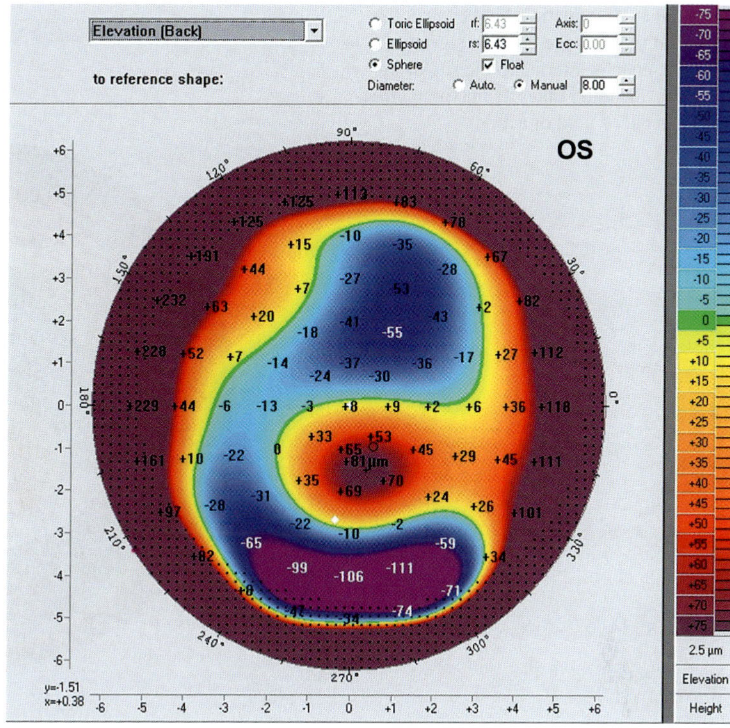

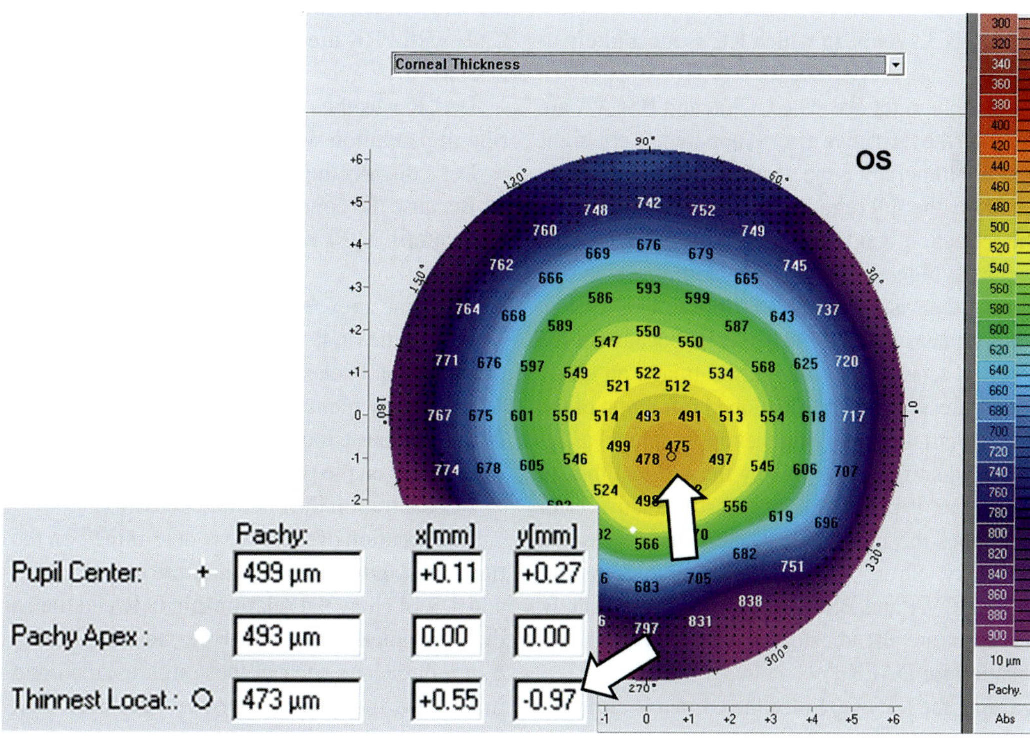

Fig. 4.5.12 Corneal thickness map of the left eye. The thinnest point is inferotemporally displaced (*white arrows*)

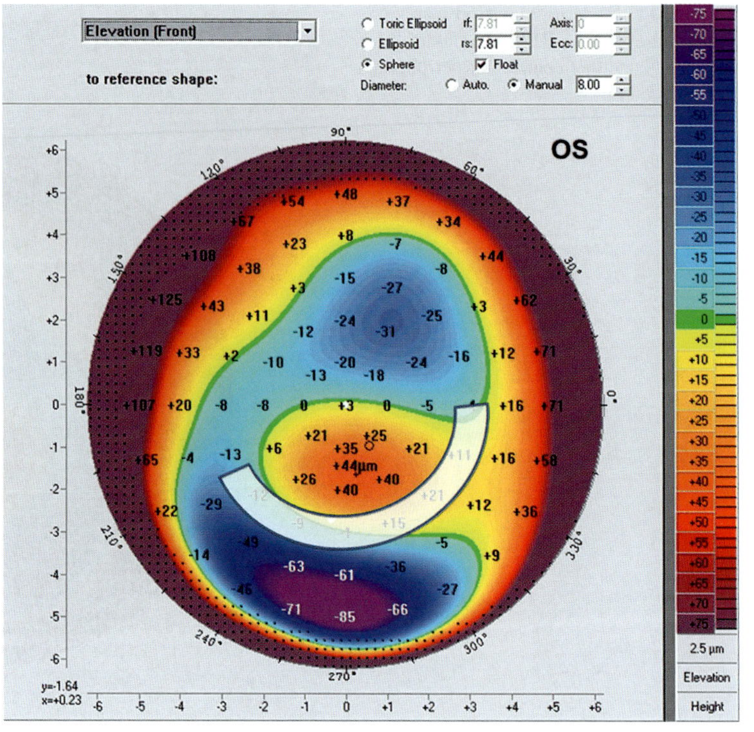

Fig. 4.5.13 The relationship between the implanted ring and the anterior elevation map. The cone is internal to the site of the ring; thus, the latter takes its maximal effect since it is out of field of action

4.5.3 Step 3: Discussion Step

Patient's age is 33 years, in which KC is most likely to be stable.

Regarding the right eye: The UCVA and BSCVA are poor although the refractive error is apparently not high! This is a very important issue; the manifest refraction is not necessarily the full refraction of the patient, it represents the refraction that gives the best visual acuity but still the eye has bigger refractive error adding which will not improve the visual acuity any more. This patient indeed has immeasurable refractive error because of the much skewed scissors and the blurred image on skiascopy due to stress lines. The mentioned refraction of the patient was on trial by applying the topographical astigmatism and identifying the axis by the fan and the slit tests. Therefore, it is only the manifest refractive error that determines the management, but in some cases it may be tricky. Stress lines, immeasurable refractive error, poor UCVA and BSCVA, very high K-readings, and thin cornea are all indicators of advanced KC, hence the indication for DALK.

Regarding the left eye: Since the cornea is clear, the refractive error is measurable, BSCVA is acceptable although the UCVA is poor, the K-readings are moderate and corneal thickness is>450 μ, both ICRs and CXL with PRK are suitable and less invasive than the DALK.

DALK was the choice for the right eye and corneal ring implantation was the choice for the left eye.

Let's discuss the option of ICRs for the left eye.

Because the cone is paracentral and the topographical pattern is PLK, there are two concepts in this regard:

1. The cone apex: When the cone apex lies on the passage of the ring, the ring might form a barrier against the action because it is within the field of action as previously mentioned.
2. The thinnest location: When the thinnest location happens on the passage of the ring, it carries the risk of penetration during tunnel creation.

The location of the cone is determined on the elevation maps and not on the curvature map. Figures 4.5.13 and 4.5.14 show the relationship between the cone and the implanted ring. The ring was implanted at the 6 mm circle. As seen in these figures, the cone is still internal to the implanted ring; therefore, there is no interference between the cone apex and the ring.

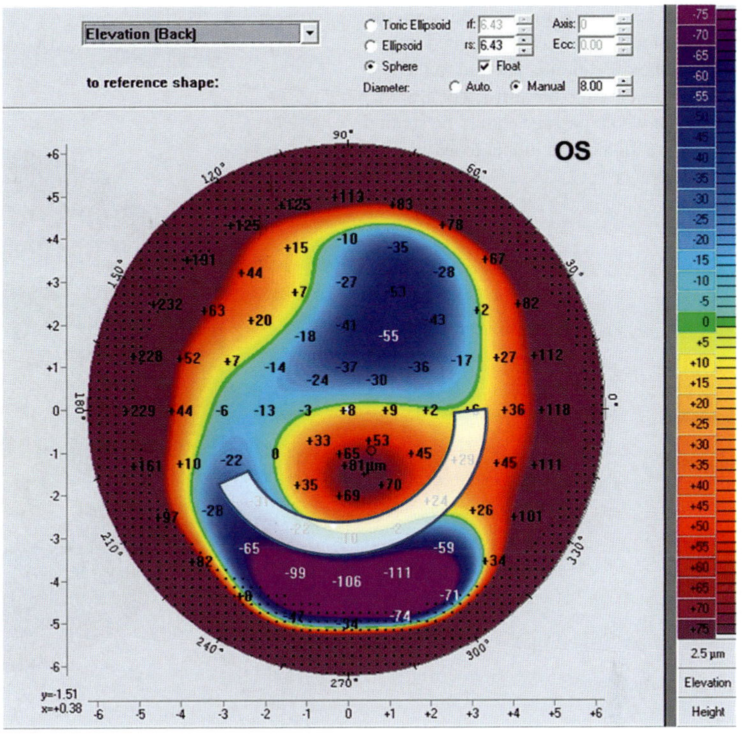

Fig. 4.5.14 The relationship between the implanted ring and the posterior elevation map. What is mentioned in Fig. 4.5.13 can be said here

Figure 4.5.15 shows the relationship between the thinnest location and the implanted ring. As seen in this figure, the thinnest location is internal to the passage of the ring. In spite of this fact, there is no guarantee of prevention of perforation during creation of the tunnel especially if this is to be done by femtosecond. Therefore, it is strongly recommended to study all the proposed passage and take 80% of the thinnest part in this passage as a level to create the tunnel.

Figure 4.5.16 shows the anterior sagittal curvature map nearly 6 months after the operation. Figure 4.5.17 is the difference map between the preoperative and postoperative curvature maps. Note the significant improvement in the shape, K-readings, maximal K-reading (white arrows), and the amount of astigmatism (red arrows).

Six months after the left eye operation, the patient's MR was (Table 4.5.4):

Table 4.5.4 Postoperative MR

Eye	Sphere	Cylinder	Axis	UCVA	BSVCA ± PH
OS	0	−1.5	125	0.7	0.9

The improvement in both corneal topography and clinical refraction can be referred to the following reasons:

1. The patient is still young.
2. The cornea is clear with no stress lines.
3. The refractive error is not high (<−5 dpt).
4. The k-readings are not high (K-max < 55 dpt).
5. Corneal thickness is still good (thinnest location > 400 µ).
6. The topographical pattern is type 5 in the author's classification (PLK with straight central axes).

Fig. 4.5.15 The relationship between the thinnest location and the implanted ring. The thinnest location is internal to the passage of the ring, but this is not always safe. The whole passage should be studied before creation of the tunnel to avoid penetration

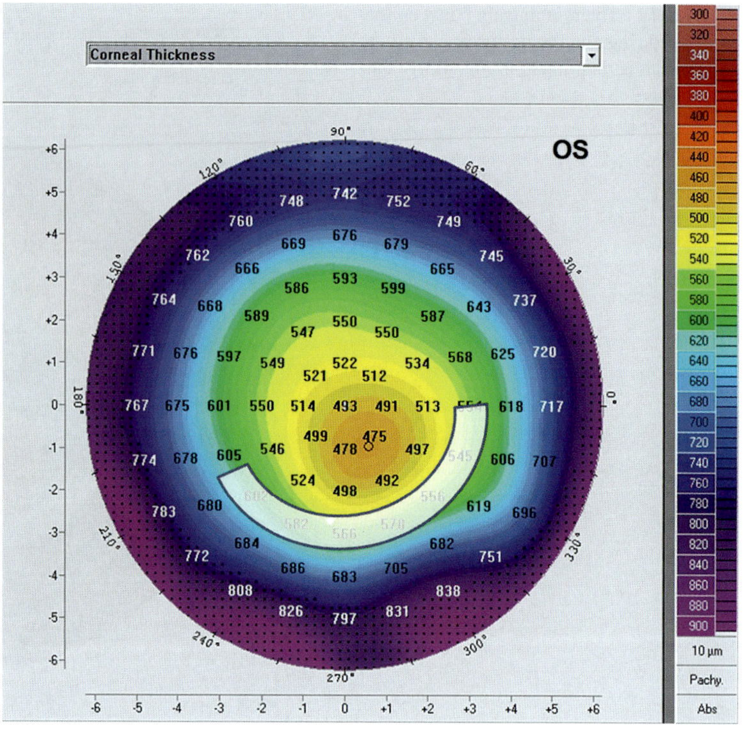

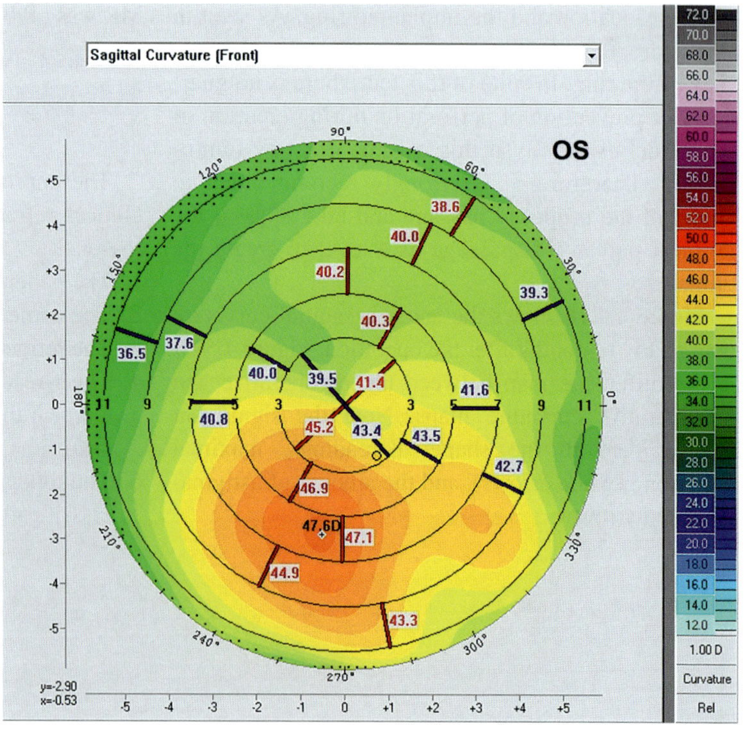

Fig. 4.5.16 The anterior curvature map about 6 months after ICR implantation. The shape of the central cornea is more regular

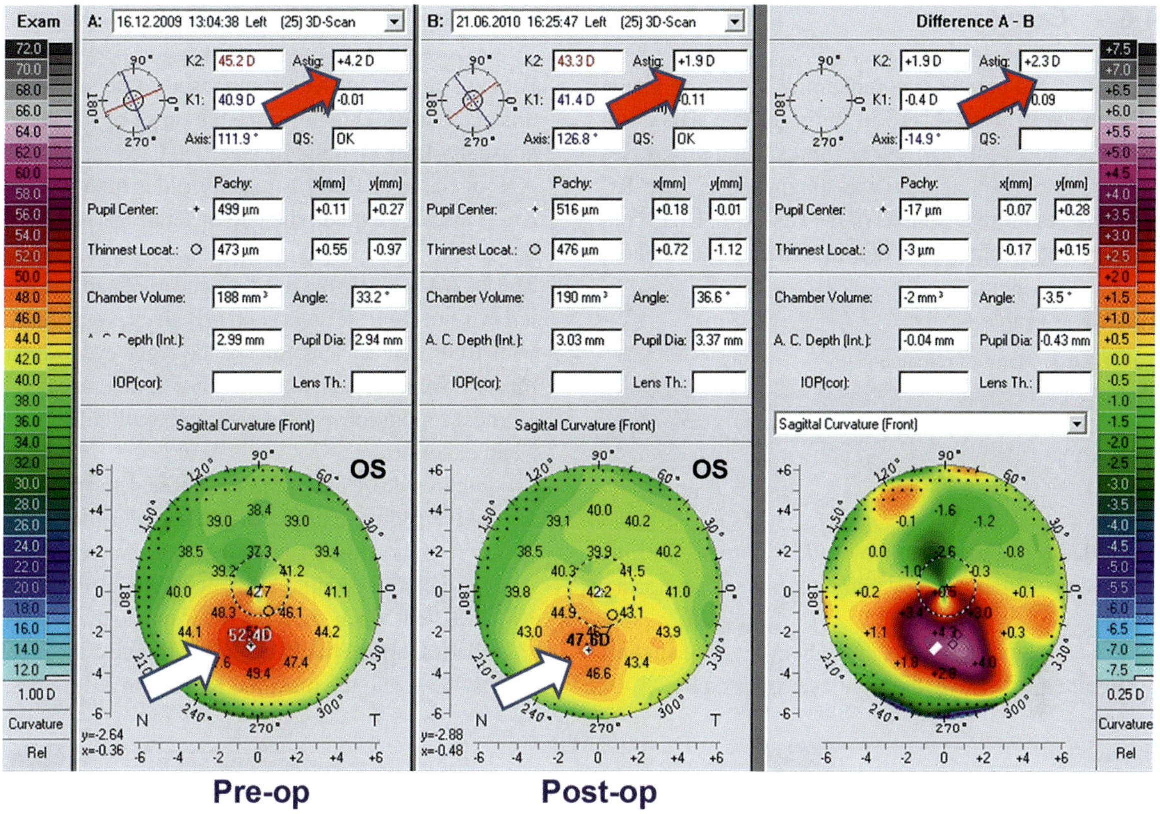

Fig. 4.5.17 The difference map. There is a significant improvement in the shape, K-readings, K-max (*white arrows*), and the amount of corneal astigmatism (*red arrows*)

4.6 Case 6

A 34-year-old patient is complaining of blurred vision in both eyes, more severe in his right eye. His complaint began 5 years ago and he thinks that it progresses slowly. Two years ago, he was diagnosed to have KC in both eyes more advanced in the right eye. He is contact lens intolerant and he does not like glasses and did not even try them.

His MR is (Table 4.6.1):

Table 4.6.1 Manifest refraction

Eye	Sphere	Cylinder	Axis	UCVA	BSVCA ± PH	BCVA over GPCL
OD	+1.5	−3.0	75	0.1	0.4	0.9
OS	+1.5	−2.5	100	0.6	0.9	1.0

Slitlamp examination shows clear corneas with no stress lines. Other ocular examination is within normal limits.

For educational purpose, the right eye will be studied. Figure 4.6.1 shows the right eye topography.

4.6.1 Step 1: Analyzing Step

1. Patient's age is 34. KC is supposed to be stable in this age but PMD is not since the onset of the latter is usually later than the former.
2. Age of onset of PMD is usually older than that of KC. This may explain the late onset of the patient's complaint.
3. The UCVA is low in the right eye and acceptable in the left eye, but the BSCVA is good in both eyes especially with RGP contact lens trial in the right eye, which means no amblyopia and gives sense to treatment.
4. Corneal topography of the right eye will be studied as an example:
   (a) Figures 4.6.1 and 4.6.2 are corneal topography of the right eye before and after color modification to show the shape of the cone. According to the anterior sagittal map, it is either PMD or PLK, but when studying other maps, the case is PLK. Corneal thickness at the thinnest location is 443 μ and the maximal K-reading is 52.2 dpt.

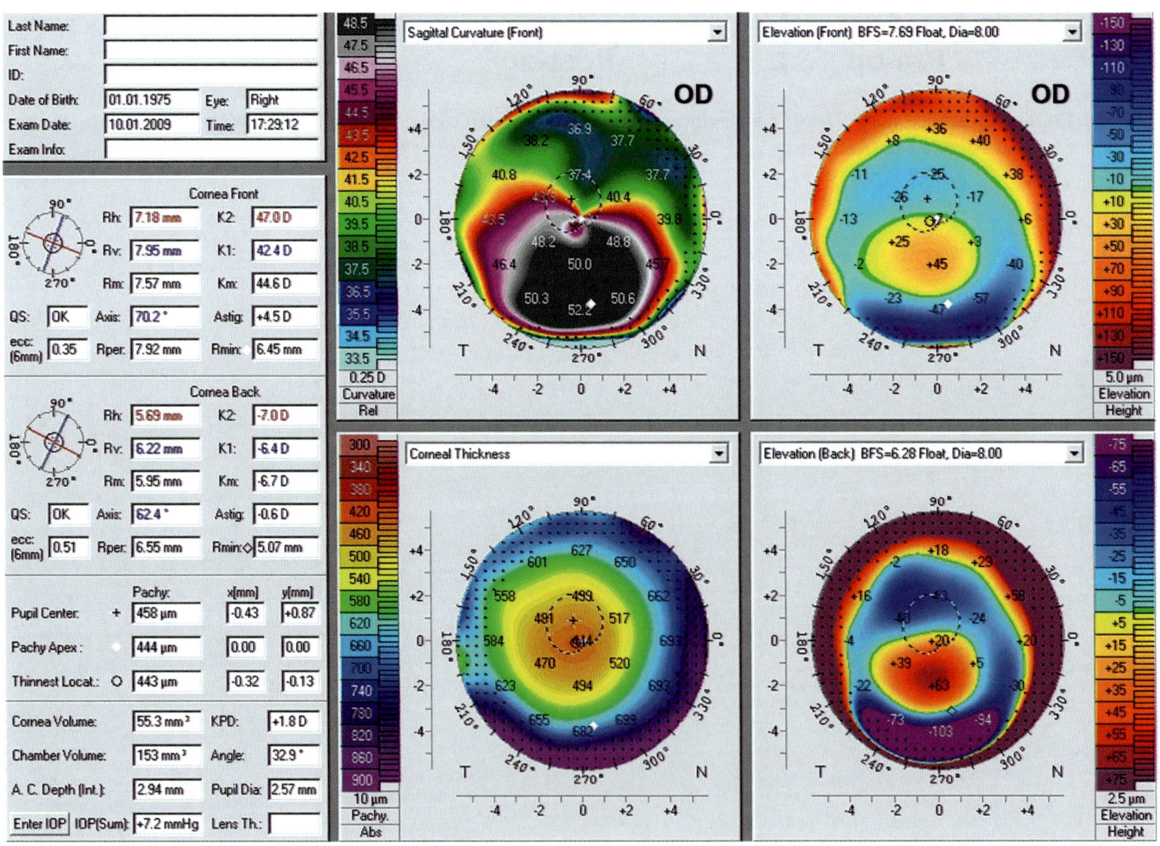

Fig. 4.6.1 Corneal topography of the right eye: moderate PLK

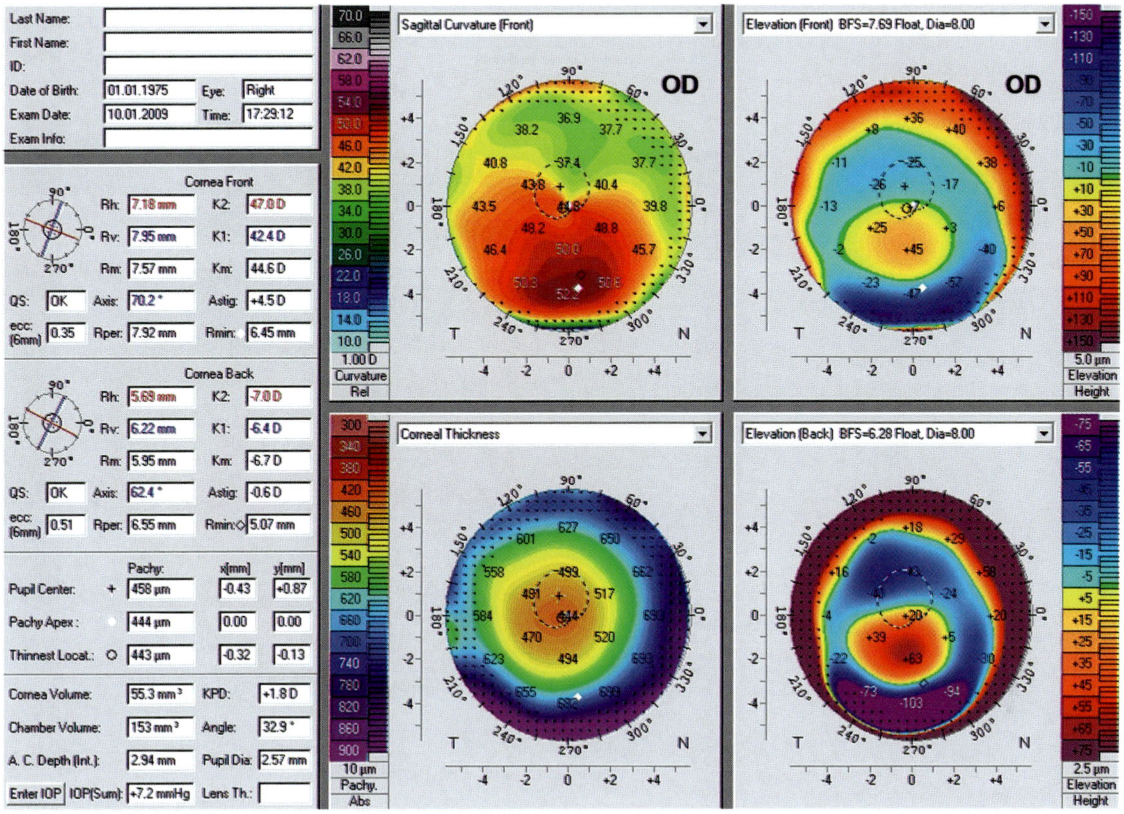

Fig. 4.6.2 Corneal topography of the right eye after color modification, the shape of the cone is better identified. The location of the cone is central

(b) Figure 4.6.3 is the anterior curvature map. There is a significant skew in the central part and according to the author's classification, it is pattern 6.

5. According to Krumeich classification, it is grade 2.

4.6.2 Step 2: Management Suggestions

Table 4.6.2 summarizes patient data and the corresponding individual suggestion(s) for treatment, and presents a final summary of the best management.

Table 4.6.2 Management suggestions

Factors	Patient data	Suggested treatment
Progression	?	Observation
CL tolerance	No	
Age	34	
Sex	Male	
Transparency and stress lines	Clear	CxL and PRK or ICRs
Refractive error (S.E)	0.0	CxL and PRK or ICRs
BSCVA Vs UCVA	Acceptable	CxL and PRK or ICRs
K-max	52.2 dpt	CxL and PRK or ICRs
Corneal thickness at thinnest location	443 µ	ICRs
		CxL for progression not for PRK
Management summary:	ICRs	

4.6.3 Step 3: Discussion Step

Since the BSCVA is 0.4 in the right eye and 0.9 in the left eye and the patient has not tried the spectacles yet, it is strongly recommended to try spectacles first. If the patient is not happy with the spectacles, his explanation of unsatisfactory should be discussed with him. If the cause was just that he does not like spectacles, he should know that there is no optimal treatment that guarantees getting rid of them. If the cause was aberrations, he should know that ICR implantation which is the only suitable interventional procedure in this case can reduce (but not eliminate) aberrations and the rings themselves may induce halos that will disappear most often after 6 months.

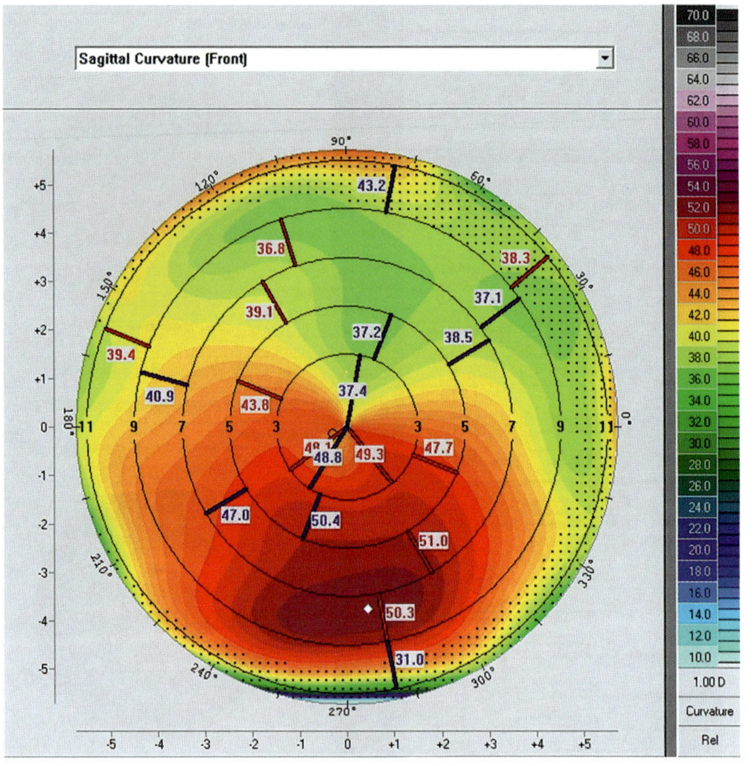

Fig. 4.6.3 Anterior curvature map of the right eye. The curvature pattern is PLK. According to author's classification, it is pattern 6

CxL is indicated in this case if the disease is still progressing, but it is not indicated for TG PRK since corneal thickness is not sufficient for both procedures.

However, ICR implantation was performed in the right eye. Figures 4.6.4 and 4.6.5 are corneal topography 1 year after the operation. Figure 4.6.6 is a comparison between the preoperative and postoperative topography. In this comparison, the following can be seen:

1. The center of the cornea became more homogenous.
2. There is a decrease in K-readings (arrow) from 42.4 dpt to 41.2 dpt for K_1 and from 47 dpt to 43.8 dpt for K_2.
3. There is a decrease of almost 2 dpt in *topographical* astigmatism.

The postoperative MR is (Table 4.6.3):

Table 4.6.3 Postoperative manifest refraction

Eye	Sphere	Cylinder	Axis	UCVA	BSVCA ± PH	BCVA with toric CL
OD	+3.0	−3.0	85	0.4	0.4	0.9

Clinically, the right eye gained 3 lines in UCVA; it became 0.4, but surprisingly it is uncorrectable. The patient was unsatisfied and he began complaining of halos especially when driving at night. When comparing the pre- and postoperative refraction, the *clinical* astigmatism is still the same with an increase in hyperopia! This is logical because the K-readings decreased shifting the refractive error toward hyperopia. On the other hand, a soft toric contact lens was suggested and applied; the BVCA with this lens was 0.9. That is because the corneal surface became more regular after implantation allowing for soft lens application.

Looking at the site at which the ring was inserted (Fig. 4.6.7) reveals that the ring was close to the cone and part of the cone is on the passage of the ring. This may give an explanation of the small effect of the ring on either *topographical* or *clinical* astigmatism. Implanting a ring at 6- or 7-mm zone might have been better in such a case.

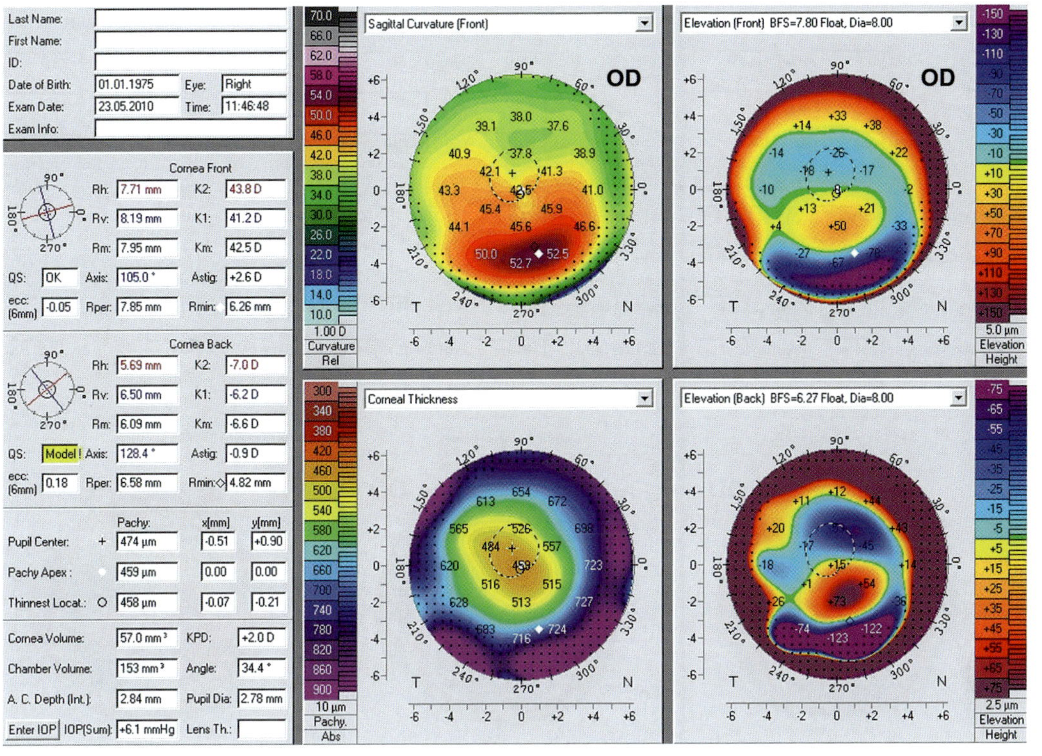

Fig. 4.6.4 Corneal topography of the right eye 1 year after ICR implantation

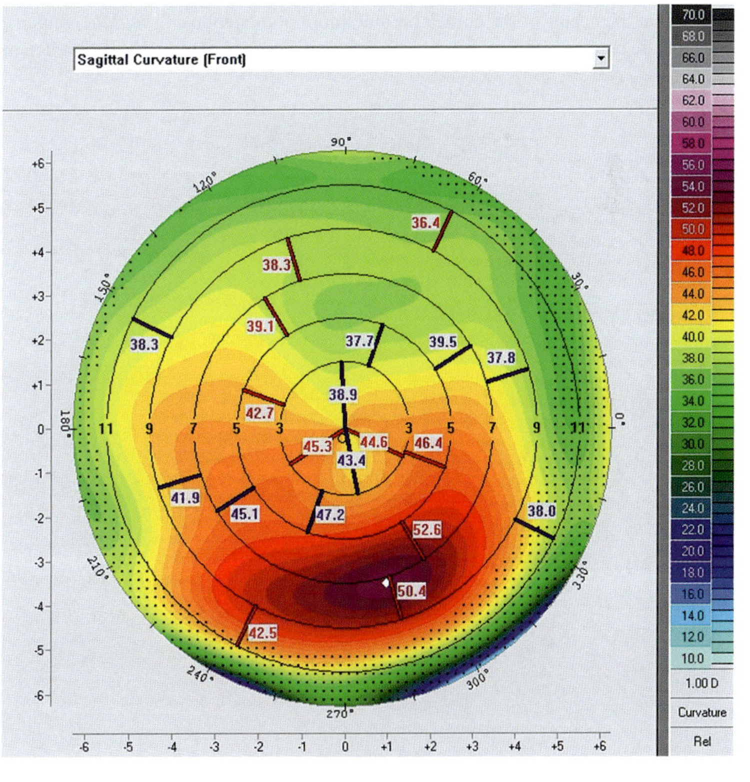

Fig. 4.6.5 Anterior curvature map of the right eye 1 year after ICR implantation. The central cornea is more regular

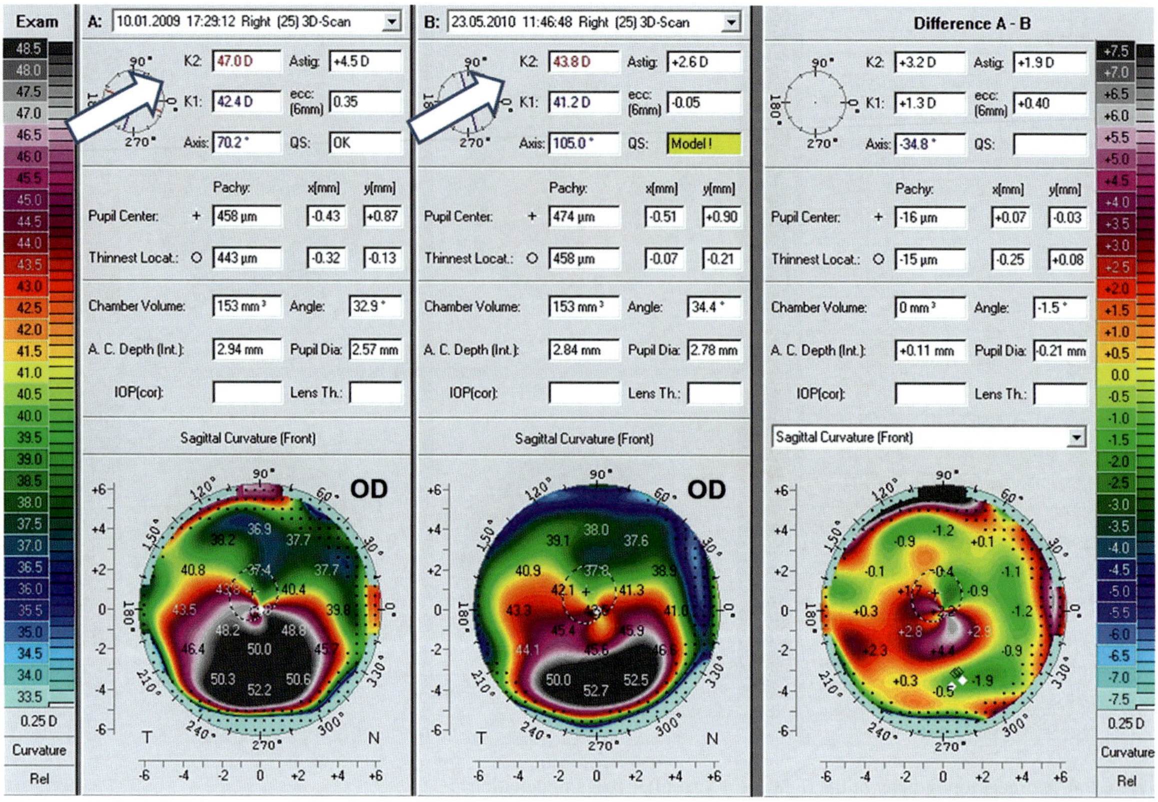

Fig. 4.6.6 Topographical changes after ICRs implantation. Notice that the center of the cornea became more homogenous, and both K-readings and topographical astigmatism decreased (*white arrows*). A (*the left column*) is the pre-op map; B (*the middle column*) is the post-op map; and C (*the right column*) is the difference map representing the achieved results

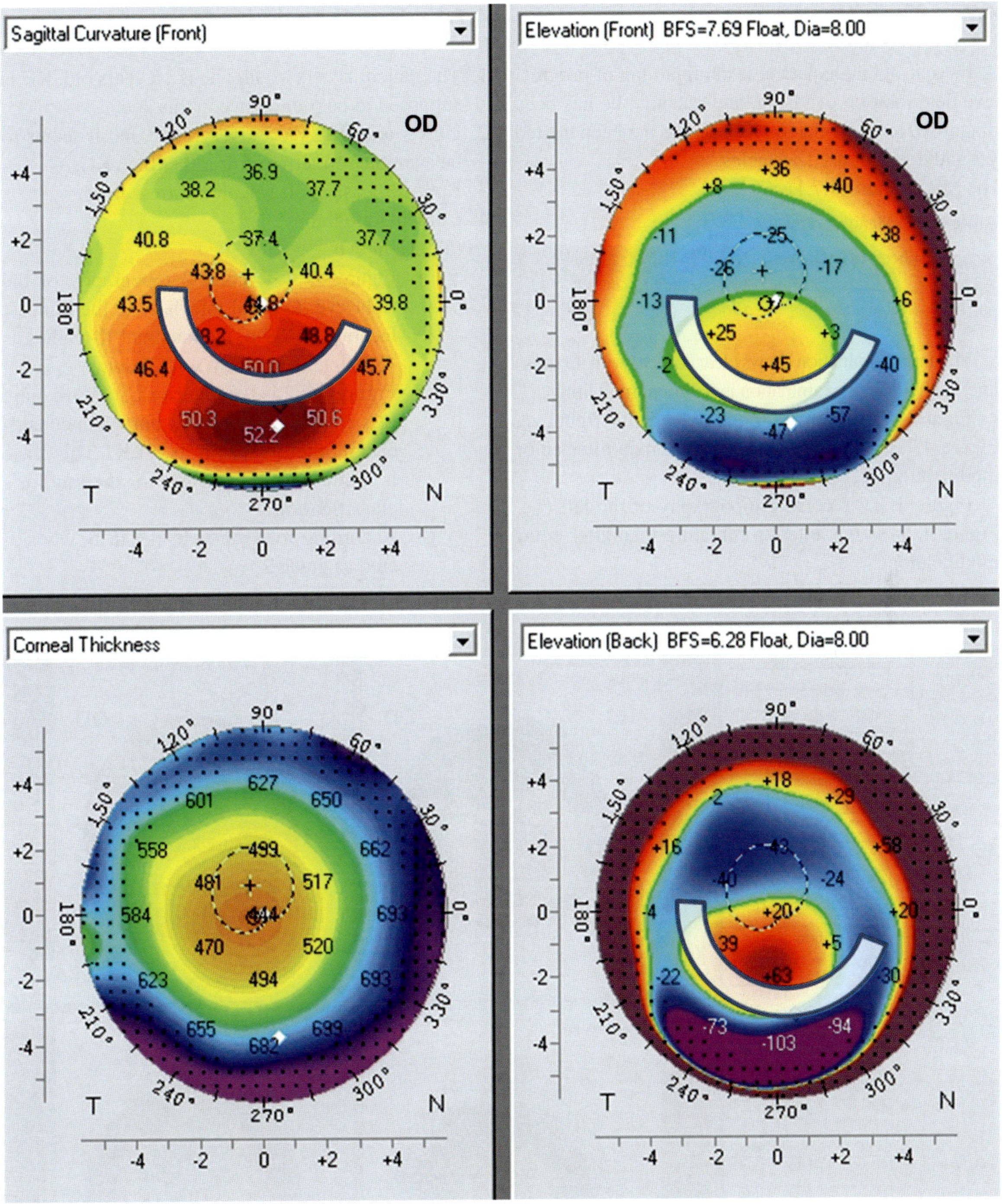

Fig. 4.6.7 The site of insertion of the segment. It passes through the cone as shown on the elevation maps. This may explain the small effect that the patient had either clinically or topographically. Additionally, this case is of pattern 6 according to author's classification where patterns 5, 6, and 7 have less favorable results than others

4.7 Case 7

A 16-year-old male patient is complaining of progressive deterioration of vision, and recently, he has been diagnosed to have bilateral KC. He has not been treated yet and does not use spectacles.

His MR is (Table 4.7.1):

Table 4.7.1 Manifest refraction

Eye	Sphere	Cylinder	Axis	UCVA	BSVCA
OD	0	−1.75	60	0.7	1.0
OS	−0.5	−0.5	120	0.7	1.0

Slitlamp examination shows clear corneas with no stress lines. Other ocular examination is within normal limits.

Figure 4.7.1 is corneal topography of the right eye. Figure 4.7.2 is the anterior curvature map after color modification.

Figure 4.7.3 is corneal topography of the left eye. Figure 4.7.4 is the anterior curvature map after color modification.

4.7.1 Step 1: Analyzing Step

1. The patient is very young; he is 16 years old. KC is supposed to be progressive in this age.
2. UCVA and BSCVA are very good and it seems to be a simple refractive error rather than KC.
3. Both corneas are clear with no stress lines.
4. Corneal topography.
   (a) Right eye:
      - Figure 4.7.1 is corneal topography of the right eye. Corneal thickness at the thinnest location is 489 μ, the maximal K-reading is 48.7 dpt, and the Km is 45.7 dpt.
      - Figure 4.7.2 is the anterior curvature map. It is either PMD or PLK, but when considering other maps, it is PLK. This case is pattern 5 according to the author's classification.
      - According to Krumeich, it can be considered as grade 2.

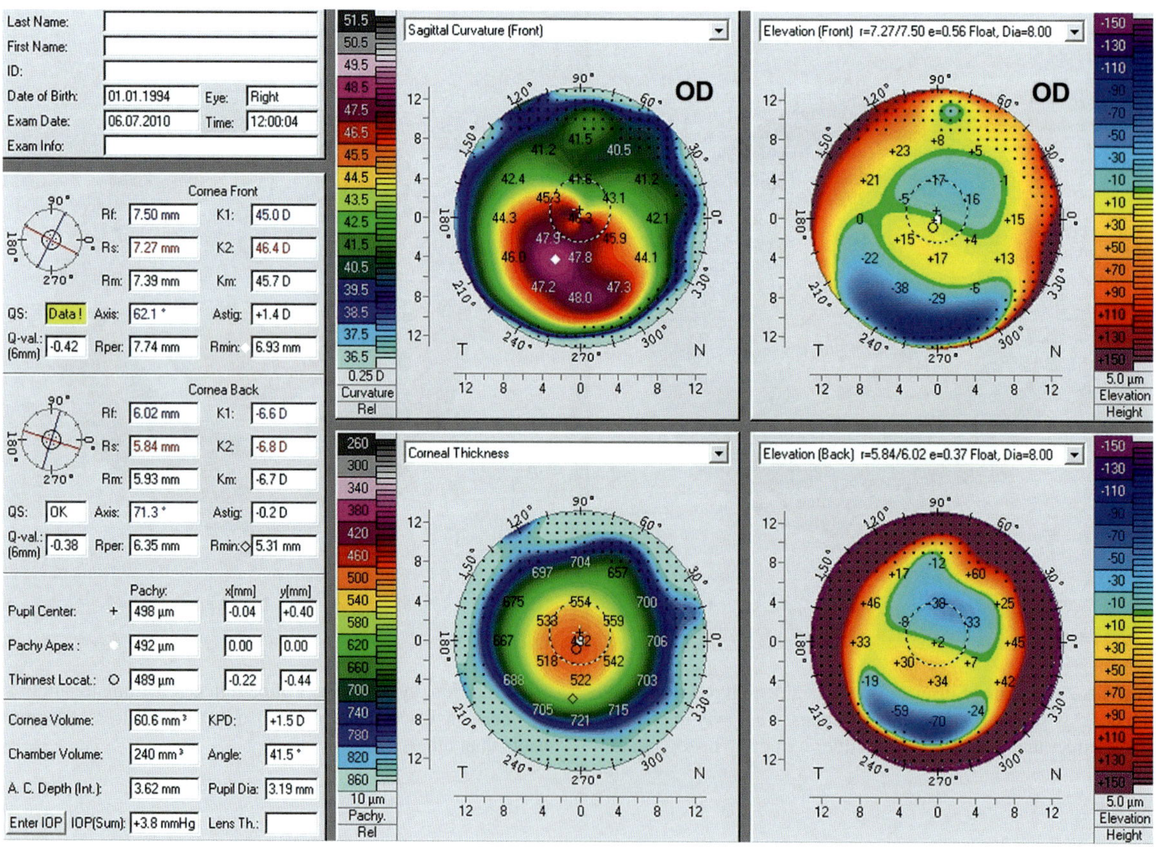

Fig. 4.7.1 Corneal topography of the right eye: mild PLK

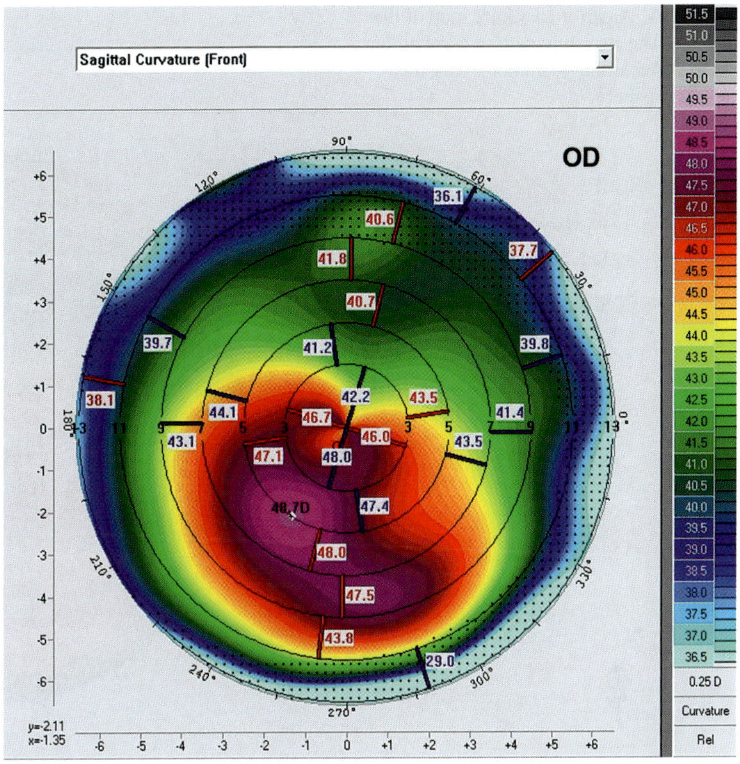

Fig. 4.7.2 Anterior elevation map of the right eye. The curvature pattern is PLK. According to author's classification, it is pattern 5

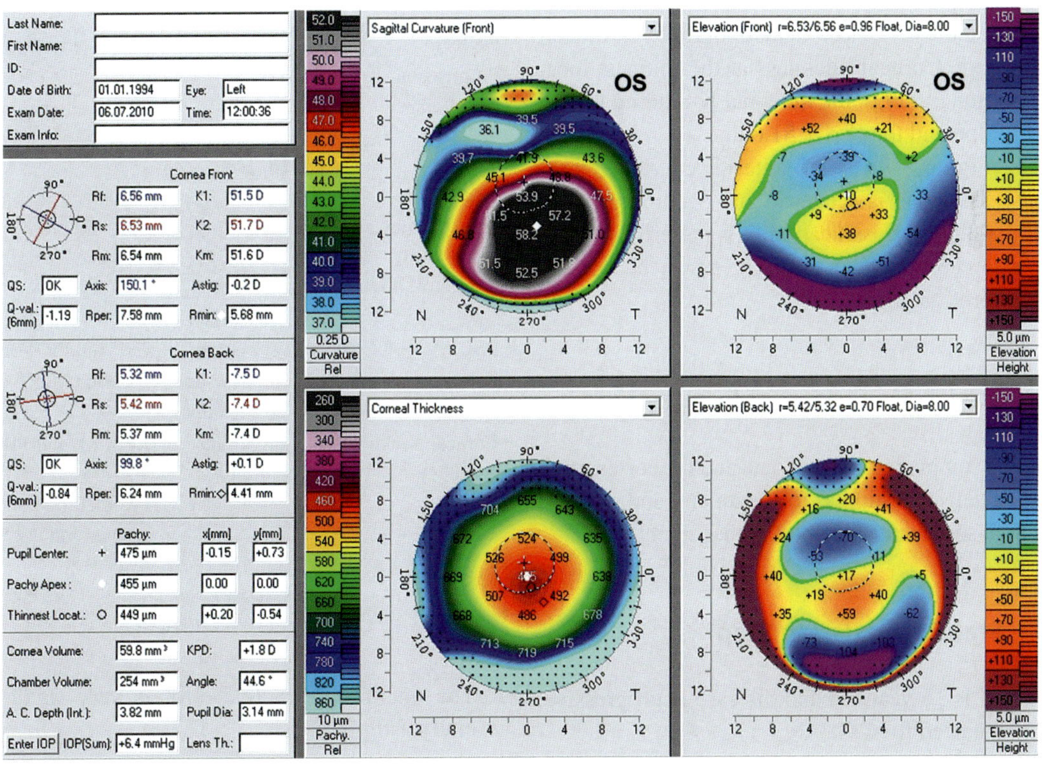

Fig. 4.7.3 Corneal topography of the left eye

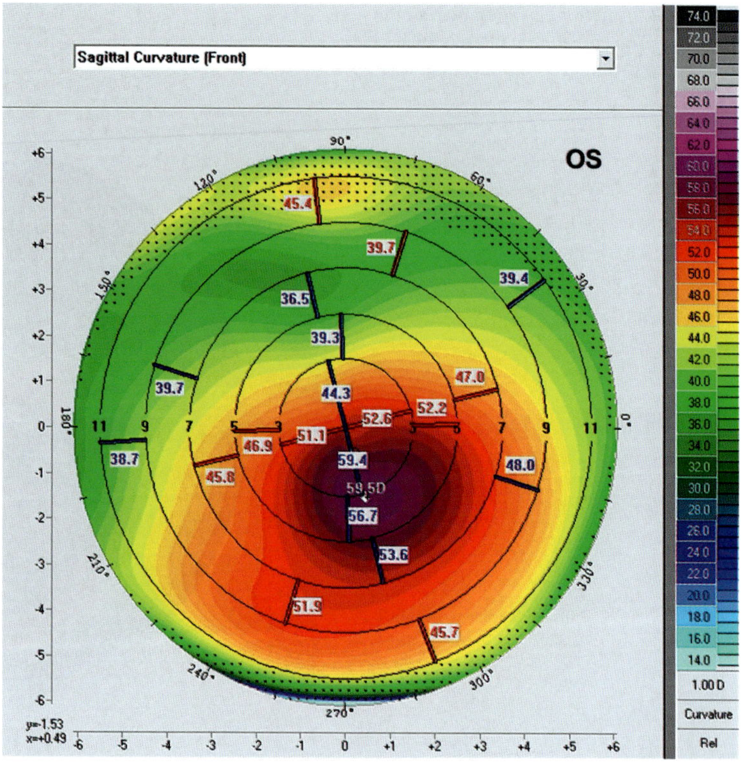

Fig. 4.7.4 Anterior curvature map of the left eye. The curvature pattern is round hot spot IS. According to author's classification, it is pattern 7

(b) Left eye:
- Figure 4.7.3 is corneal topography of the left eye. Corneal thickness at the thinnest location is 449 μ, the maximal K-reading is 59.5 dpt, and the Km is 51.6 dpt.
- Figure 4.7.4 is the anterior curvature map. The cone is eccentric and according to the author's classification, it is pattern 7.
- According to Krumeich, it can be considered as grade 2.

4.7.2 Step 2: Management Suggestions

Table 4.7.2 summarizes patient data and the corresponding individual suggestion(s) for treatment, and presents with a final summary of the best management.

Table 4.7.2 Management suggestions

Factors	Patient data	Suggested treatment
Progression	Yes	CxL
CL tolerance	?	Can be tried after CxL
Age	16	
Sex	Male	
Transparency and stress lines	Clear	CxL and PRK or ICRs
Refractive error (S.E)	RE: −1.0 LE: −0.75 LE	CxL and PRK
BSCVA Vs UCVA	very good	CxL and PRK or ICRs
K-max	RE: 48.7 dpt LE:59.5 dpt	CxL and PRK or ICRs
Corneal thickness @ atthinnest location	RE: 489 μ LE: 449 μ	RE: CxL and PRK or ICRs LE: CxL for progression not for PRK
Management summary:	CxL ± PRK	

4.7.3 Step 3: Discussion Step

The patient is 16-year-old and his case is progressive, yielding the need for CxL.

ICRs are not suitable for this case due to the following reasons:

1. The manifest refractive error is very small especially astigmatism.
2. The topographical astigmatism is not reasonable enough to indicate implanting ICRs. It is noticed

that the left eye is more advanced than the right eye although the topographical astigmatism is smaller in the left eye. That is because the cone in the left eye is more eccentric than that in the right eye.

3. Implanting rings usually pushes the cone toward the center of the cornea leading – in such a case – to increase in both spherical and astigmatic components of the refractive error!

PRK and CxL may be suitable to regularize the central 5 mm of the cornea and therefore improve the quality of vision. This is possible because of the suitable thickness, but it is to remember that 40 μ of maximal ablation depth is an important issue and the priority is for the irregular astigmatism.

What are suitable also are glasses after CxL. That is probably the most logic choice since the refractive error is so small and both UCVA and BSCVA are very good. The patient has not tried the spectacles yet, so it is appropriate to persuade him to have CxL and continue with glasses.

4.8 Case 8

A 22-year-old male is complaining of a refractive error which is stable since 3 years ago. He has been diagnosed to have KC and he is suffering from his glasses because of aberrations.

His MR is (Table 4.8.1) is:

Table 4.8.1 Manifest refraction

Eye	Sphere	Cylinder	Axis	UCVA	BSVCA
OD	−2.75	−1.25	45	0.1	0.6
OS	−2.5	−1.75	100	0.3	0.6

His old correction is (Table 4.8.2):

Table 4.8.2 Old correction

Eye	Sphere	Cylinder	Axis
OD	−2.5	−0.75	40
OS	−2.5	−2.0	120

Slitlamp examination shows clear corneas with no stress lines. Other ocular examination is within normal limits.

For educational purpose, only the right eye will be studied.

Figure 4.8.1 is corneal topography, and Fig. 4.8.2 is the anterior curvature map of the right eye.

4.8.1 Step 1: Analyzing Step

1. The patient is young; he is 22 years old, but according to his complaint and to his old refraction, his refractive error seems to be stable.
2. The BSCVA is acceptable.
3. Both corneas are clear with no stress lines.
4. Corneal topography of the right eye:
   - Figure 4.8.1 is corneal topography of the right eye. Corneal thickness at the thinnest location is 441 μ, the maximal K-reading is 50.2 dpt, and the Km is 46.3 dpt.

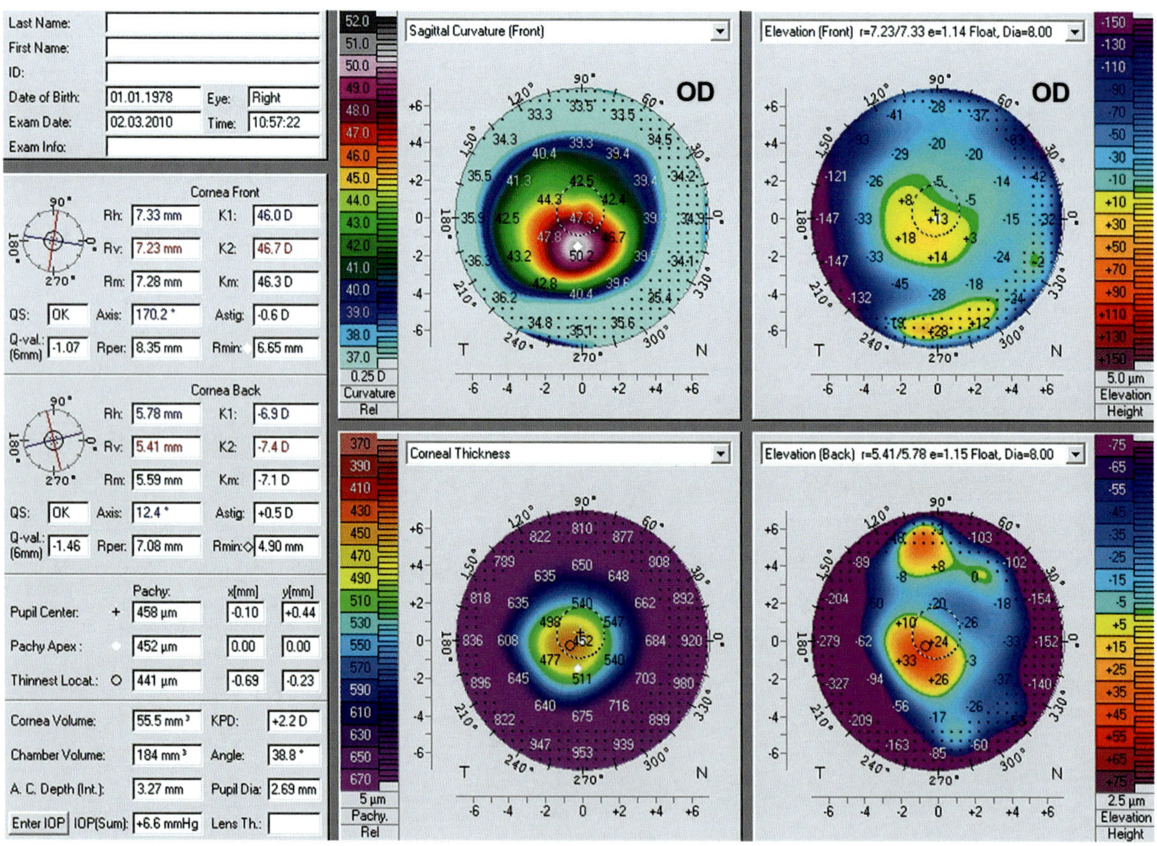

Fig. 4.8.1 Corneal topography of the right eye: mild to moderate KC

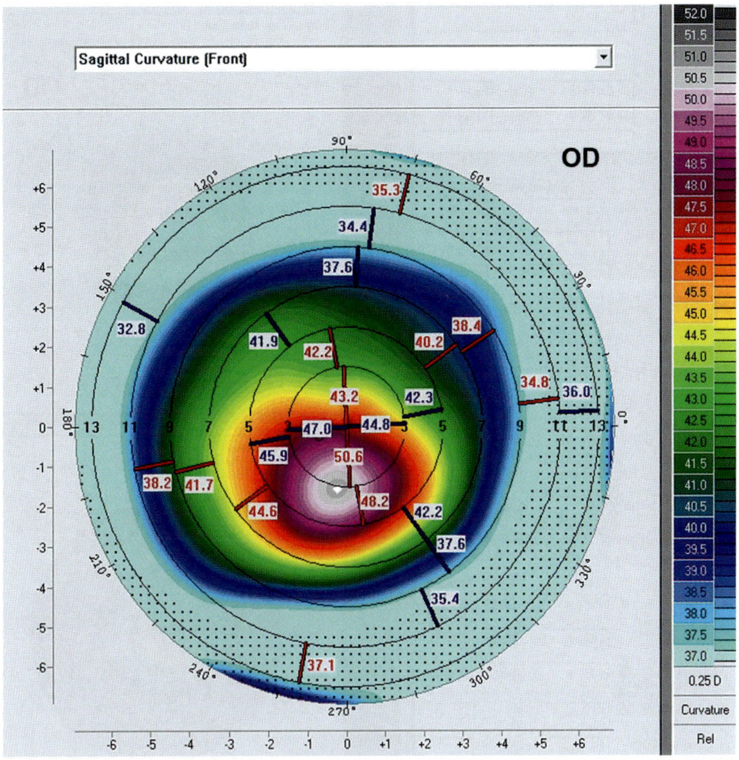

Fig. 4.8.2 Anterior curvature map of the right eye. The curvature pattern is round hot spot IS. According to author's classification, it is pattern 7

- Figure 4.8.2 is the anterior curvature map. The cone is eccentric, and according to the author's classification, the pattern is 7.

5. According to Krumeich, it can be considered as grade 1–2.

4.8.2 Step 2: Management Suggestions

Table 4.8.3 summarizes patient data and the corresponding individual suggestion(s) for treatment, and presents with a final summary of the best management.

Table 4.8.3 Management suggestions

Factors	Patient data	Suggested treatment
Progression	No	
CL tolerance	?	Can be tried
Age	22	
Sex	Male	
Transparency and stress lines	Clear	CxL and PRK or ICRs
Refractive error (S.E)	RE: −3.0	CxL and PRK or ICRs
BSCVA Vs UCVA	Acceptable	CxL and PRK or ICRs
K-max	RE: 50.2 dpt	CxL and PRK or ICRs
Corneal thickness at thinnest location	RE: 441 μ	CxL and PRK? or ICRs
Management summary:	CXL and PRK? or ICRs	

4.8.3 Step 3: Discussion Step

Supposing that the case is stable, there are several options for management:

1. Contact lenses: This option should be always kept in mind.
2. CxL and TG PRK: Attention should be paid to the available thickness and to the allowed amount of ablation, here is 40 μ, which may be enough to regularize the central 5 mm of the anterior corneal surface especially that its astigmatism is very small.
3. ICR implantation is also an option.

ICR implantation was performed to the right eye. Four months after the operation, the patient was unsatisfied and the results were unsatisfactory!

His postoperative MR is (Table 4.8.4):

Table 4.8.4 Postoperative manifest refraction

Eye	Sphere	Cylinder	Axis	UCVA	BSVCA
OD	−4.0	−1.25	35	0.1	0.4

It is clear that both spherical and astigmatic components increased. UCVA remained the same and the patient lost 2 lines of his BSCVA!

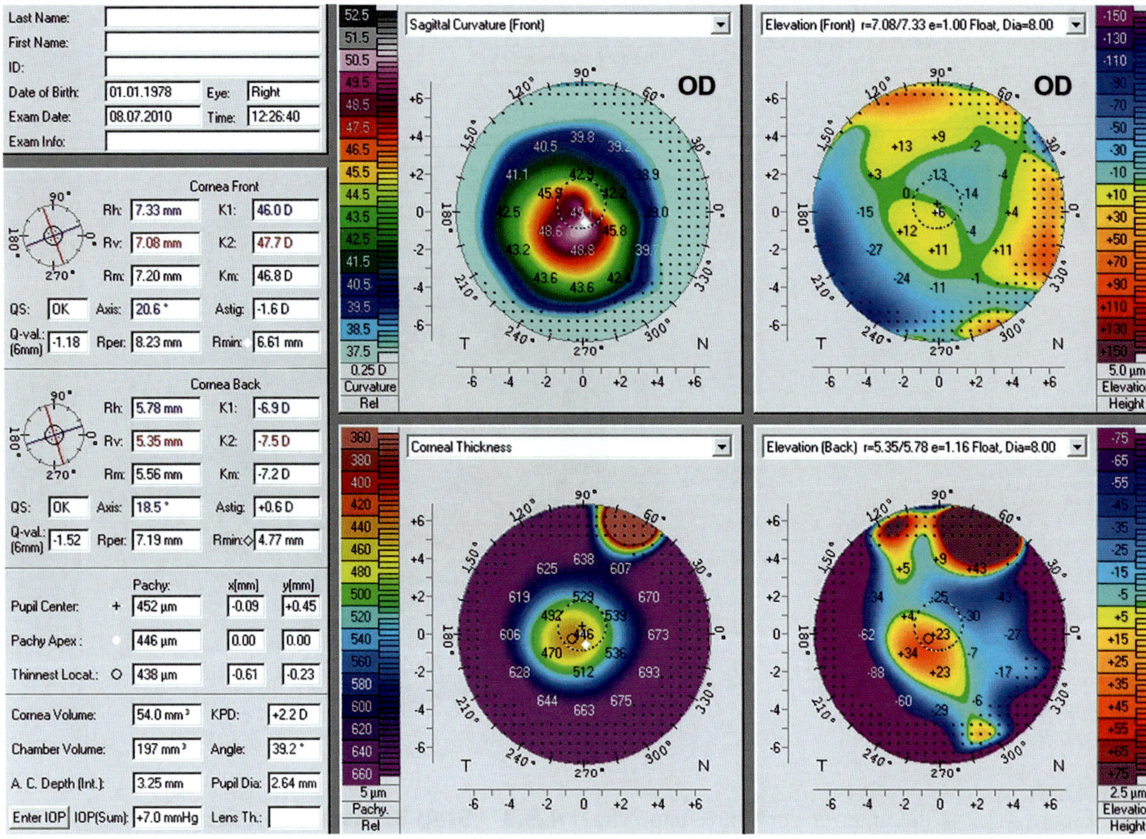

Fig. 4.8.3 Corneal topography after ICR implantation. Changes on the elevation maps are very few if any

To understand the cause behind this clinical problem, the change that happened on corneal topography should be studied carefully. Figure 4.8.3 is postoperative corneal topography. Figure 4.8.4 is postoperative curvature map. Going back to Fig. 4.8.2, it is an eccentric cone and the pattern is 7 (author's classification), in which the steep axis cannot be identified, the topographical axis is 90º, whereas the clinical axis is 135º! Fig. 4.8.5 is a comparison between the preoperative and postoperative topography, there is an induced astigmatism (red circles), and the cone was pushed toward the center of the cornea resulting in more irregular astigmatism and iatrogenic spherical component as shown in the postoperative manifest refraction (see Table 4.8.4).

Finally, this case is presented to show that the results in this pattern are unpredictable and the ICR choice was not correct. May be CxL with TG PRK was a better alternative.

Fig. 4.8.5 Topographical changes after ICRs implantation. There is an induced astigmatism (*red circles*), and the cone was pushed toward the center of the cornea resulting in more irregular astigmatism and iatrogenic spherical component. A (the left column) is the post-op map; B (the middle column) is the pre-op map; and C (the left column) is the difference map representing the achieved results

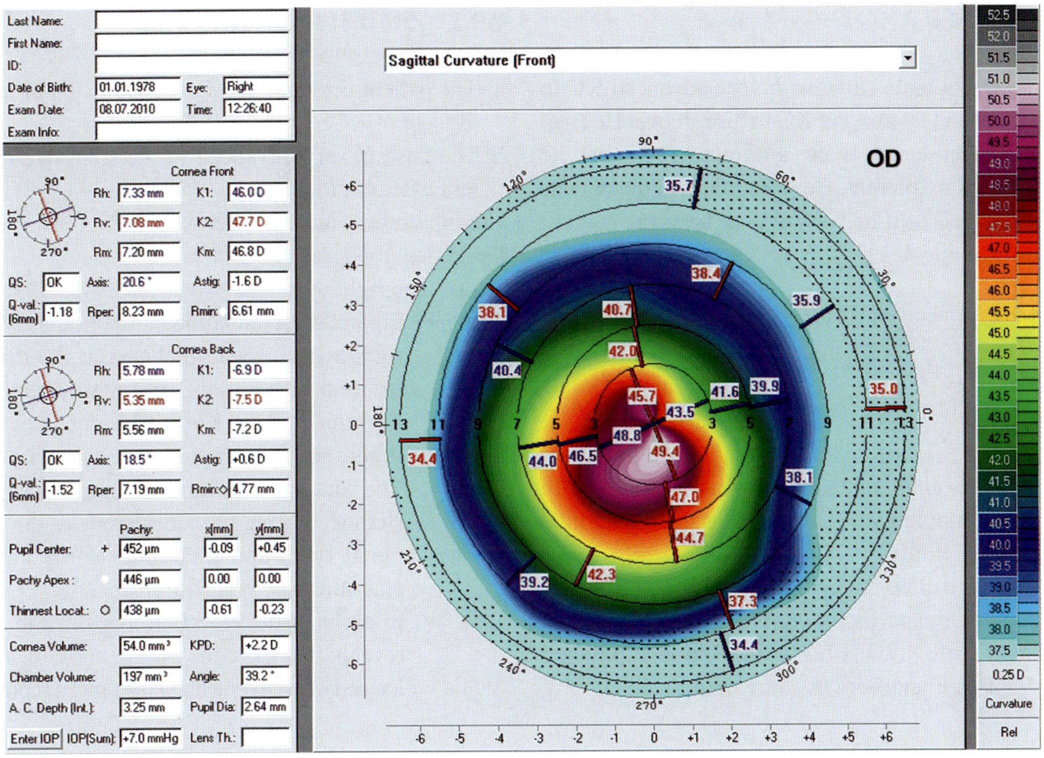

Fig. 4.8.4 Anterior curvature map after ICR implantation. The cone was pushed by the rings and became central increasing central corneal irregularity and topographical astigmatism

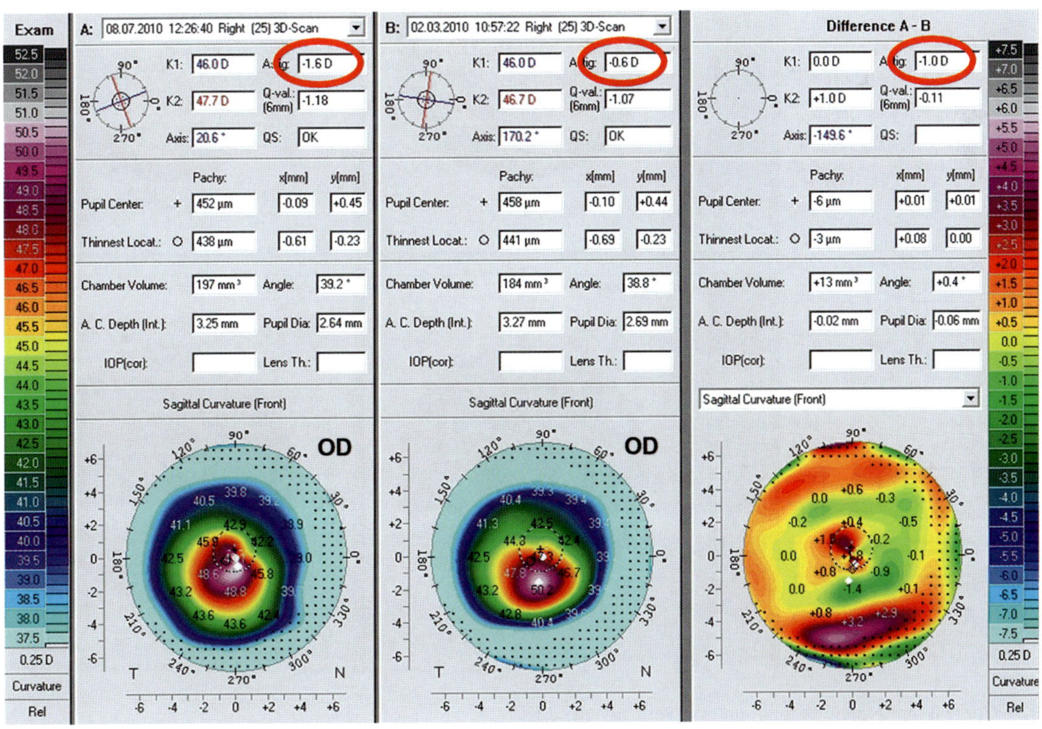

4.9 Case 9

An 18-year-old male came with very advanced KC in his right eye and less severe KC in his left eye. He used to use contact lenses with different types, but he became no more tolerant. He is a student in the university and he feels as if he was blind as he says.

His MR is (Table 4.9.1):

Table 4.9.1 Manifest refraction

Eye	Sphere	Cylinder	Axis	UCVA	BSVCA
OD	Un-recordable			CF 3 m	??
OS	−8	−4.5	100	0.05	0.4

Slitlamp examination shows clear corneas with stress lines in both eyes. Other ocular examination is within normal limits.

Both eyes will be studied: Figure 4.9.1 is R.E corneal topography and Fig. 4.9.2 is R.E anterior curvature map. Figure 4.9.3 is L.E corneal topography and Fig. 4.9.4 is L.E anterior curvature map.

4.9.1 Step 1: Analyzing Step

1. The patient is young; his age is within the progressing age of KC.
2. The case is very advanced in the right eye and to less extent in the left eye.
3. Both corneas are clear but with stress lines.
4. Corneal topography.
   (a) The right eye:
   - Figure 4.9.1 is corneal topography of the right eye. Corneal thickness at the thinnest location is 289 μ, the maximal K-reading is 74.9 dpt, and the Km is 61.9 dpt.
   - Figure 4.9.2 is the anterior curvature map. The pattern of the curvature map is relatively strange, it can be considered as the junctional type, and according to the author's classification, it is pattern 1.
   - Looking at the elevation maps in Fig. 4.9.1 reveals that the cone on the anterior map is located inferiorly; at the same time, it represents

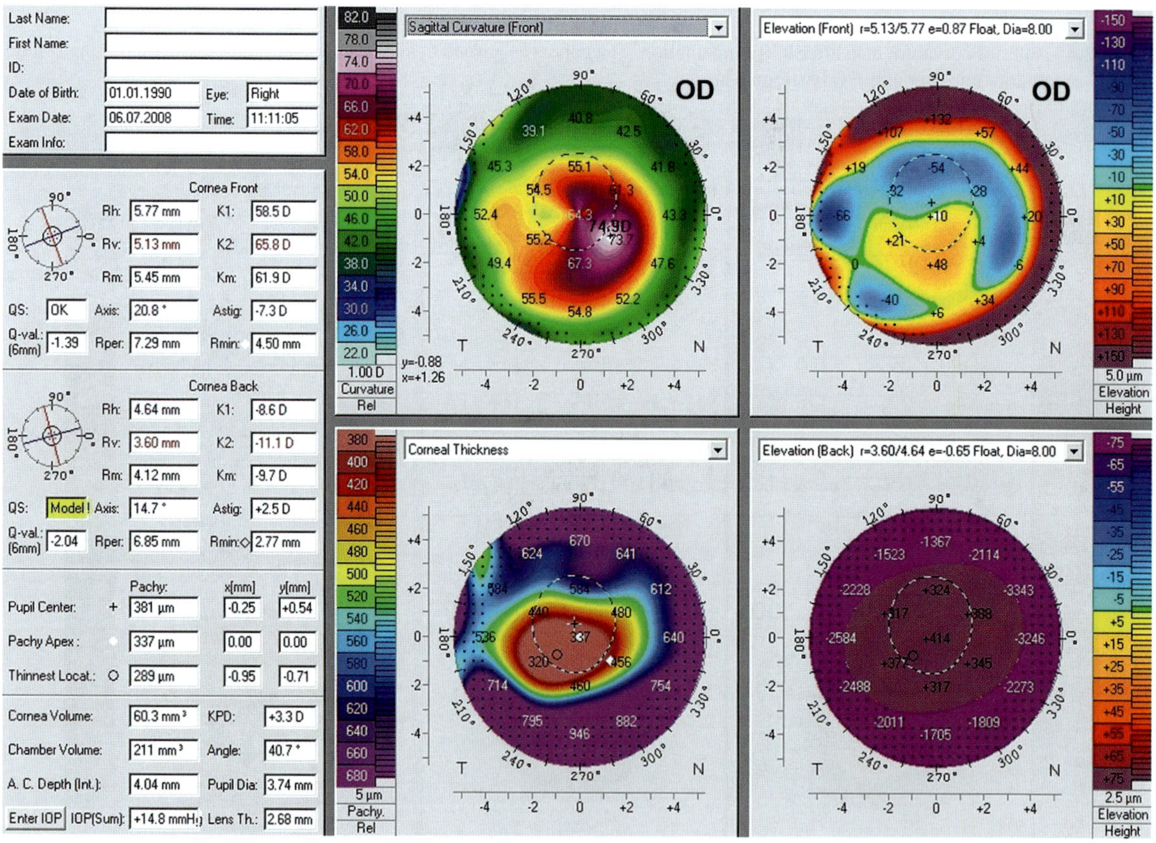

Fig. 4.9.1 Corneal topography of the right eye: very advanced KC

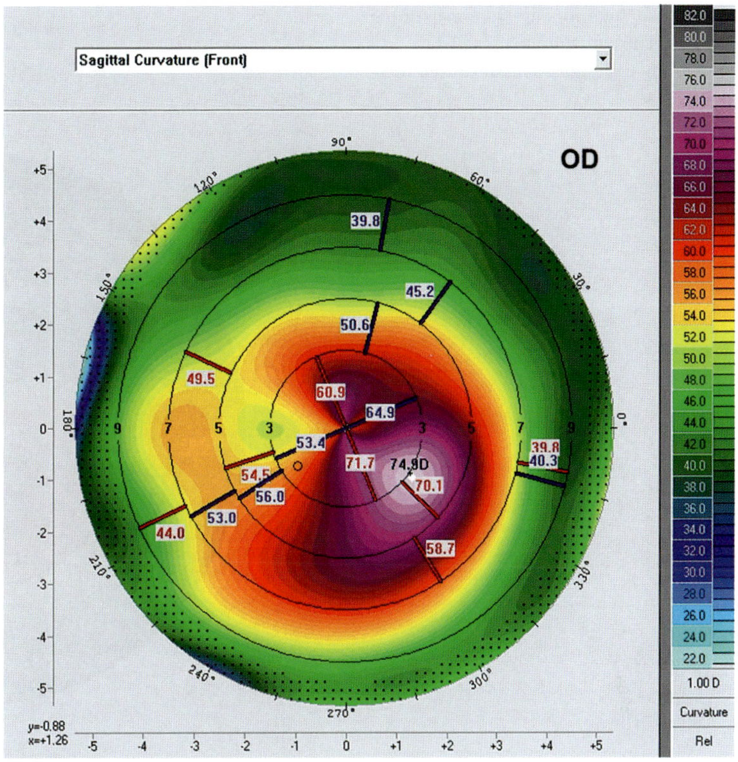

Fig. 4.9.2 Anterior curvature map of the right eye. The curvature pattern is AB/IS and can be considered as the junctional pattern. According to author's classification, it is pattern 1

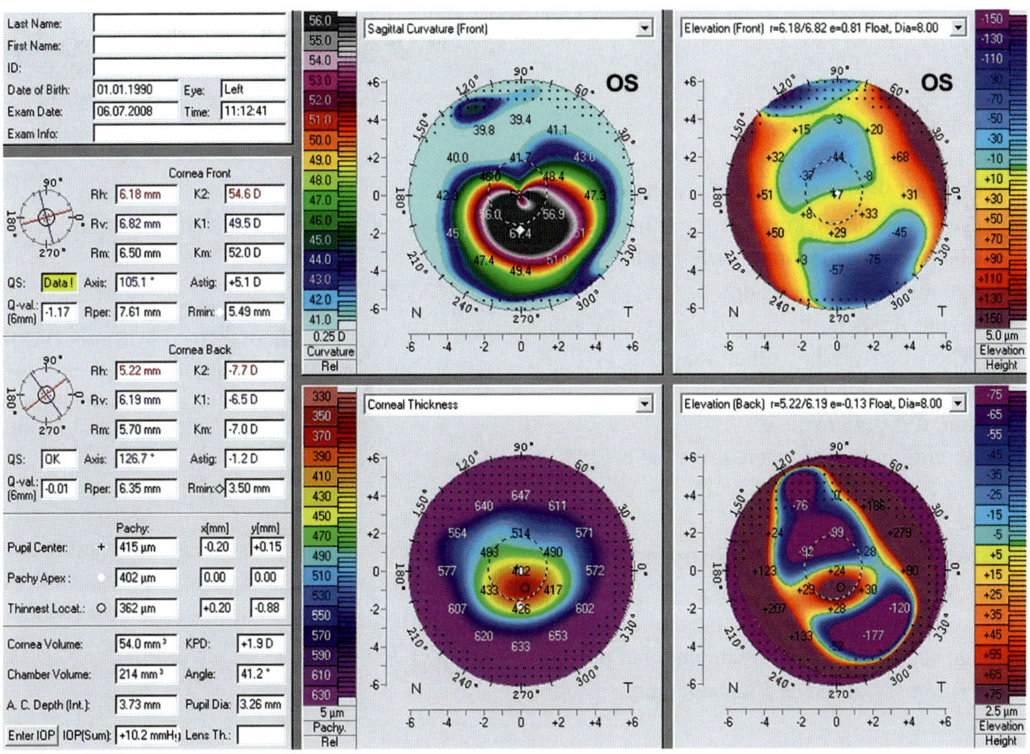

Fig. 4.9.3 Corneal topography of the left eye: advanced PLK

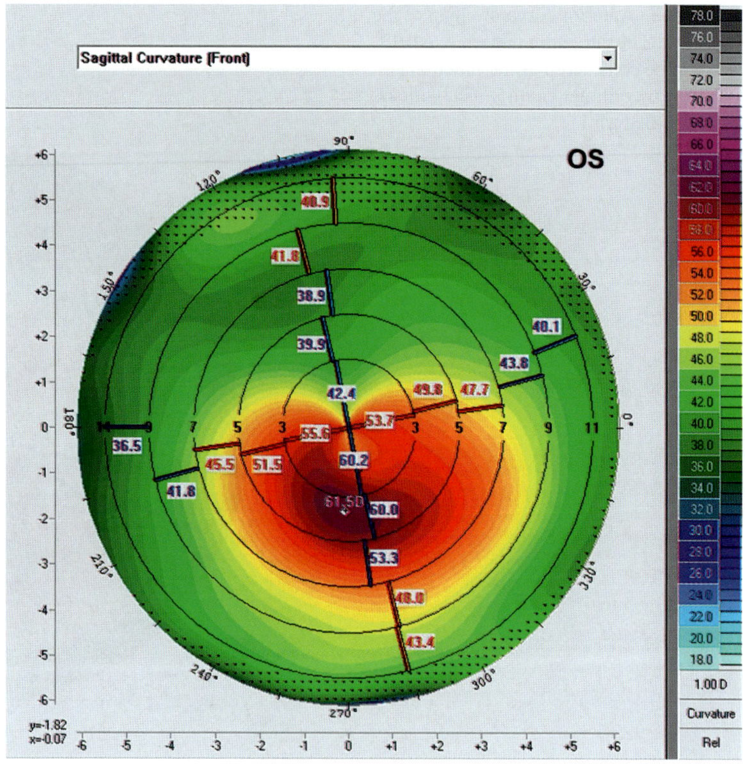

Fig. 4.9.4 Anterior curvature map of the left eye. The curvature map is PLK. According to author's classification, it is pattern 5

a very big posterior out-bulging on the posterior elevation map.
  - According to Krumeich, this case can be considered as grade 4.

(b) The left eye:
  - Figure 4.9.3 is corneal topography of the left eye. Corneal thickness at the thinnest location is 362 μ, the maximal K-reading is 61.4 dpt, and the Km is 52 dpt.
  - Figure 4.9.4 is the anterior curvature map. When considering other maps, it is PLK, and according to the author new classification, it is pattern 5.
  - According to Krumeich, this case is grade 3.

4.9.2 Step 2: Management Suggestion

Table 4.9.2 summarizes patient data and the corresponding individual suggestion(s) for treatment, and presents with a final summary of the best management.

Table 4.9.2 Management suggestions

Factors	Patient data	Suggested treatment
Progression	?	Observation
CL tolerance	Intolerant	Other modalities
Age	18	CxL
Sex	Male	
Transparency and stress lines	Clear but with stress lines	DALK
Refractive error (S.E)	R.E: Un-recordable	DALK
	L.E: −10.25	IORLs or DALK
BSCVA Vs UCVA	R.E: very poor	DALK
	L.E: very good	CxL and PRK or ICRs or IORLs
K-max	R.E: 74.9	R.E: DALK
	L.E: 61.4	L.E: ICRs or IORLs
Corneal thickness at thinnest location	R.E: 289 μ	R.E: DALK
	L.E: 362 μ	L.E: ICRs or IORLs or DALK
Management summary:	R.E: DALK	
	L.E: ICRs or IORLs or DALK	

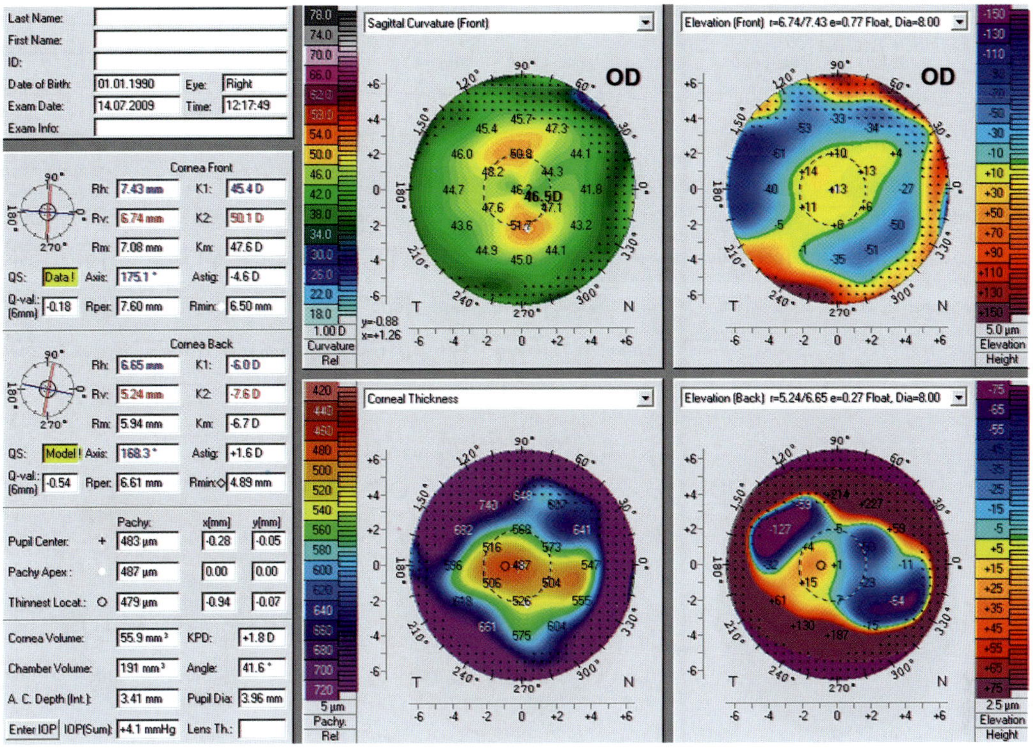

Fig. 4.9.5 Corneal topography of the right eye 6 months after DALK

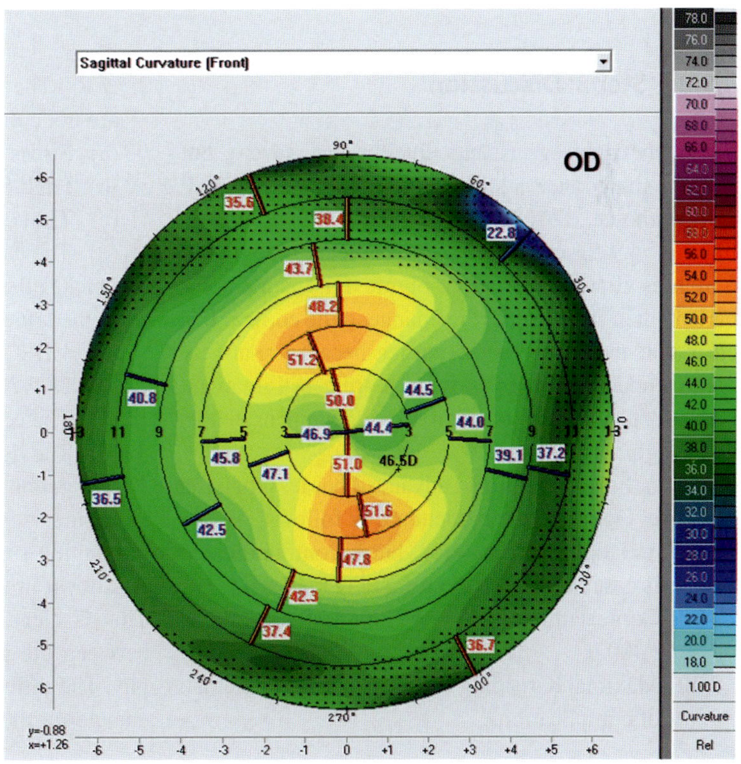

Fig. 4.9.6 Anterior curvature map of the right eye 6 months after DALK. There is with-the-rule astigmatism. The cornea is very regular. If removal of sutures is done under control of topography, the cornea will be regular and homogenous

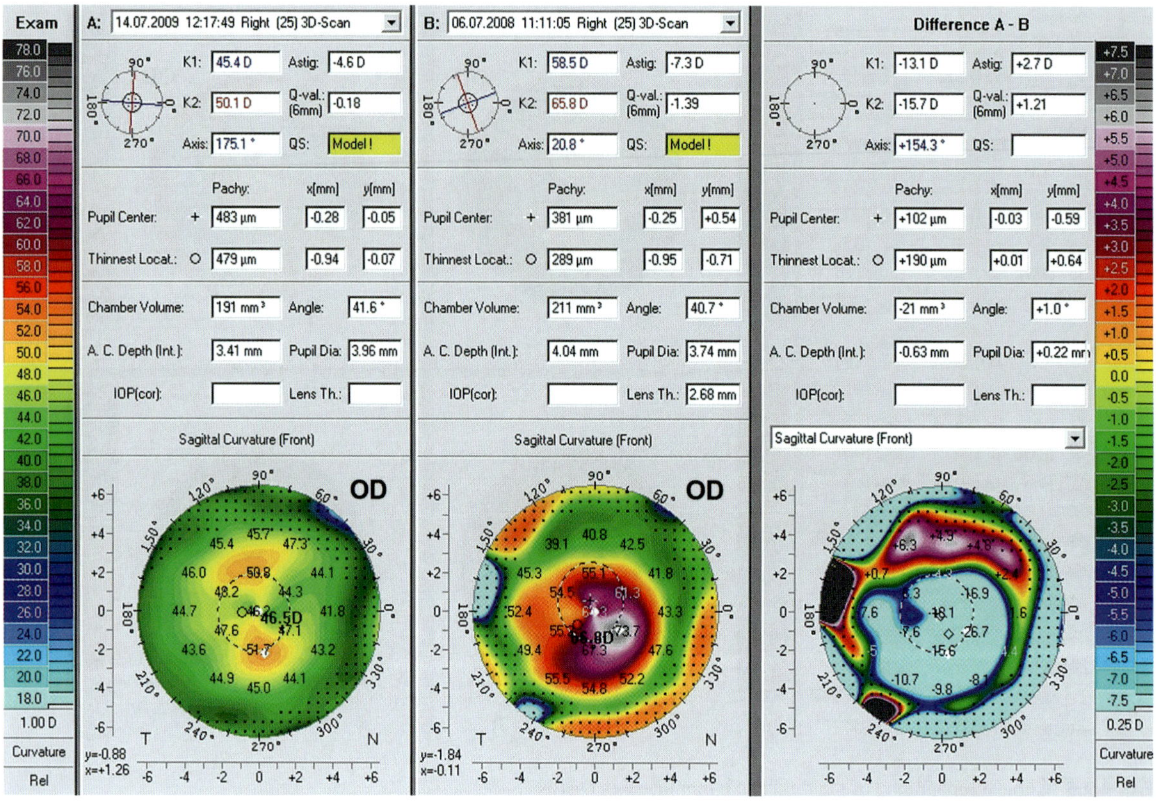

Fig. 4.9.7 Topographical changes after DALK. The map on the left is postoperative, the map in the middle is preoperative, and the map on the right is the difference map showing the change achieved by DALK

4.9.3 Step3: Discussion

KC in the right eye is undoubtedly very severe, but because the cornea is still clear, DALK and not PKP is the choice. DALK was done to the right eye. Figures 4.9.5 and 4.9.6 are corneal topography 6 months after the operation. Figure 4.9.7 is the comparison map showing the big change in the cornea. It is clear that the shape of the cornea became relatively homogenous and there is with-the-rule astigmatism. Controlled releasing of sutures will compensate for this astigmatism.

KC in the left eye is also advanced but less than the right eye. Options for treatment are as follows:

1. CxL to stop the progression, but is contraindicated in this case because of the following reasons:
   (a) Corneal thickness at the thinnest location is <400 µ.
   (b) Maximal K-reading is > 58 dpt carrying the risk of complications.
2. ICRs: The conditions for using the ICRs in this case are not completely suitable because of:
   (a) Stress lines.
   (b) High K-readings.
   (c) Thin cornea.
   (d) The case is still progressing.
3. On the other hand, ICR implantation was performed in the left eye for the following reasons:
   (a) 1.BSCVA and the difference between the UCVA and BSCVA is favorable.
   (b) The cornea is still clear.
   (c) The right eye needs an emergent DALK and the patient refused a future DALK for his left eye.

Figures 4.9.8 and 4.9.9 are corneal topography after implanting one inferior segment at the 5 mm circle. As shown in these figures, there is an overcorrection! This is clear in Fig. 4.9.10 which is a comparison between the preoperative and postoperative topography. The difference map on the right shows a very big change on the vertical axis, which is just opposite to

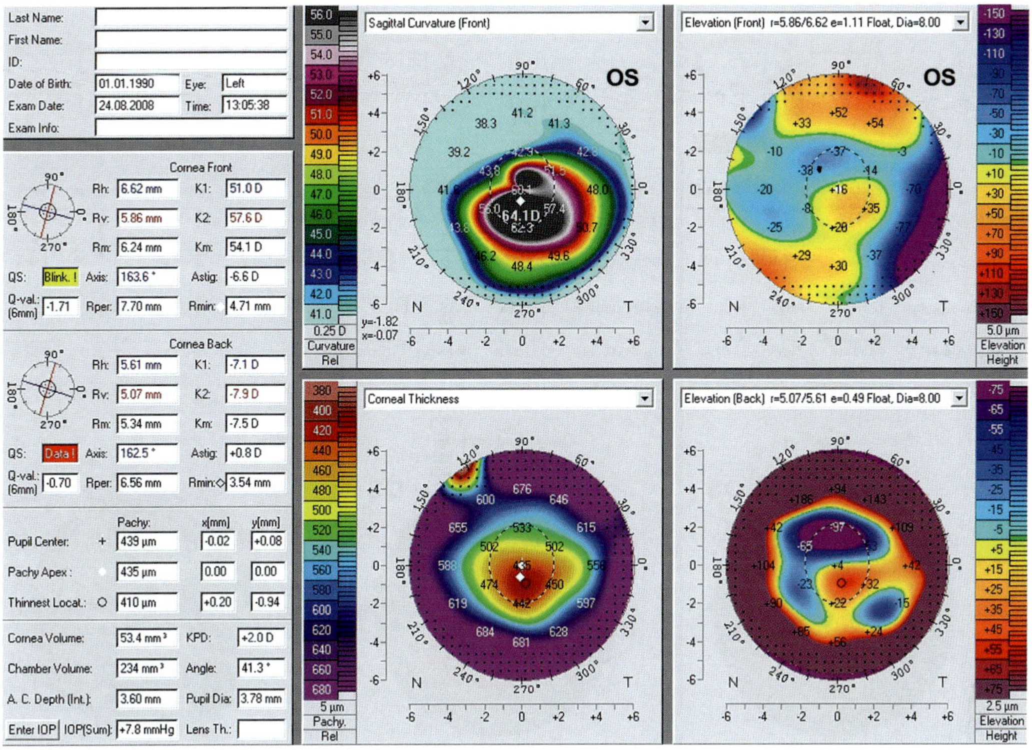

Fig. 4.9.8 Corneal topography of the left eye after implanting one inferior segment on the 5 mm zone

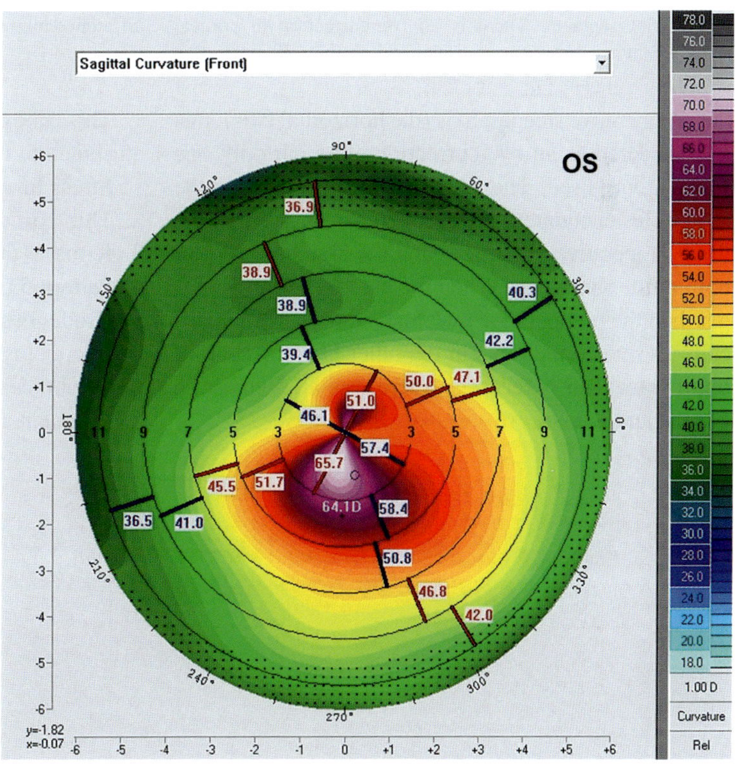

Fig. 4.9.9 Anterior curvature map of the left eye after implanting one inferior segment on the 5 mm zone. When compared with the preoperative curvature map in Fig. 4.9.4, it is clear that the cone became central and a with-the-rule astigmatism was induced

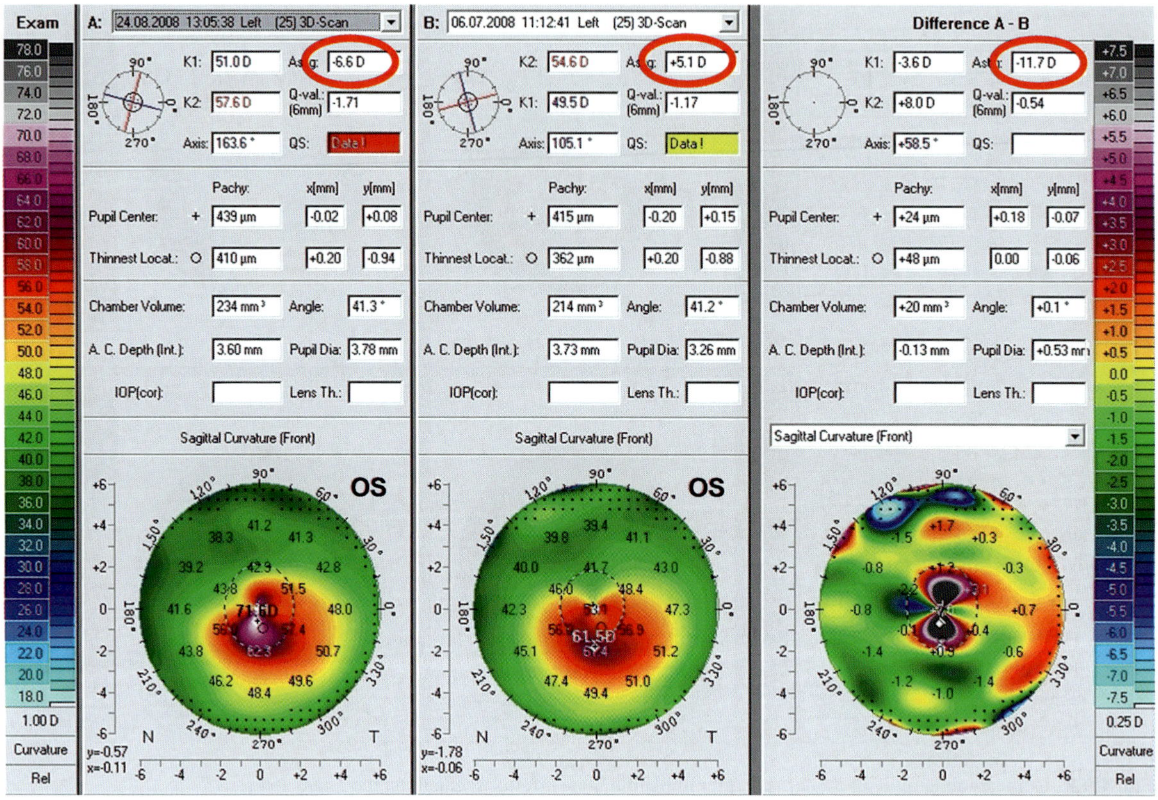

Fig. 4.9.10 Topographical changes after ICR implantation. The difference map shows the changes achieved by implanting the inferior segment. There is an overcorrection in corneal astigmatism as shown in *red circles* and on the difference map on the right. A (the left column) is the post-op map; B (the middle column) is the pre-op map; and C (the right column) is the difference map representing the achieved results

the preoperative steepest axis (the horizontal axis); this is considered as an overcorrection although only one segment was used! The astigmatism shown within the red circles encounters the preoperative in the middle, the postoperative in the left, and the algebraic sum of both in the right map. When the algebraic sum is bigger than the preoperative astigmatism, it is mathematically an overcorrection. On the other hand, instead of improvement in K-readings, there was an increase in K_1, K_2, and K-max.

This unexpected and undesirable result can be attributed to the following factors:

1. Stress lines
2. Thin cornea
3. K-max > 60 dpt
4. Pattern 5 (author's classification)
5. Grade 3 (Krumeich classification)

In conclusion, ICR implantation was not an appropriate choice. The patient underwent an explanation of the segment and a DALK was finally performed.

Index

M.M. Sinjab, *Quick Guide to the Management of Keratoconus*,
DOI 10.1007/978-3-642-21840-8, © Springer-Verlag Berlin Heidelberg 2012

Printing and Binding: Stürtz GmbH, Würzburg